Principles of CHILDHOOD

LANGUAGE

DISABILITIES

Principles of | # CHILDHOOD

LANGUAGE

DISABILITIES

EDITED BY

JOHN V. IRWIN / Memphis State University

MICHAEL MARGE/United States Office of Education

APPLETON – CENTURY – CROFTS

Education Division

MEREDITH CORPORATION

New York

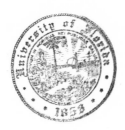

Copyright © 1972 by
MEREDITH CORPORATION

All rights reserved

72 73 74 75 76/10 9 8 7 6 5 4 3 2 1

Library of Congress Card Number: 77-180170
PRINTED IN THE UNITED STATES OF AMERICA

390-47768-0

*For those who have dedicated their lives
to serve those who suffer.*

Contributors

Richard A. Chase, M.D.
Associate Professor, Department of Psychiatry and Behavioral Sciences
Johns Hopkins University School of Medicine
Baltimore, Maryland

John S. Hicks, Ph.D.
Chairman, Department of Special Education and Rehabilitation
Hofstra University
Hempstead, New York

John V. Irwin, Ph.D.
Pope M. Farrington Professor
Department of Audiology and Speech Pathology
Memphis State University
Memphis, Tennessee

Corinne Kass, Ph.D.
Associate Professor, Special Education Department
Coordinator, Learning Disabilities Program
University of Arizona
Tuscon, Arizona

Delores Kluppel, Ph.D.
Associate Professor
Department of Communicative Disorders
University of Wisconsin
Madison, Wisconsin

Michael Marge, Ed.D.
Deputy Associate Commissioner for International Education
United States Office of Education
Department of Health, Education, and Welfare
Washington, D. C.

Jacklyn Minnick Moore, M.A.
Director of Speech Pathology and Audiology
Arlington State Hospital and School
Arlington, Tennessee

Donald F. Moores, Ph.D.
Director, Research Development and Demonstration Center in Education of Handicapped
    Children
University of Minnesota
St. Paul, Minnesota

Michael H. O'Malley, Ph.D.
Assistant Professor of Linguistics
University of Michigan
Ann Arbor, Michigan

Donald L. Rampp, Ph.D.
Associate Professor of Speech Pathology
Coordinator of Research
Department of Audiology and Speech Pathology
Memphis State University
Memphis, Tennessee

Sylvia O. Richardson, M.D.
Associate Clinical Professor of Pediatrics
Assistant Director University Affiliated Program for Children with Learning Disabilities
University of Cincinnati College of Medicine
Cincinnati, Ohio

Richard Schiefelbusch, Ph.D.
Director, Bureau of Child Research
University of Kansas
Lawrence, Kansas

Roger Shuy, Ph.D.
Director of Scoiolinguistics Programs
Georgetown University
Washington, D.C.

David Swinney, M.A. *
Research Associate
Center for Applied Linguistics
Washington, D.C.

*On leave at University of Texas, Austin

Orlando Taylor, Ph.D.
Professor, Department of Communication Sciences
Federal City College
Washington, D.C.

Ronald Tikofsky, Ph.D.
Chairman, Department of Psychology
Florida International University
Miami, Florida

Empress Zedler, Ph.D.
Professor and Chairman of Department of Special Education
Director, Speech, Hearing and Language Clinic
Southwest Texas State University
San Marcos, Texas

Preface

Language disabilities in children, whether regarded as an area of basic research or as a problem in health and educational management, have been characterized more by divisiveness than by synthesis. The purpose of this book is to bring together the most current findings from basic research and from management relevant to these disabilities.

Agreement is increasing that many of the problems confronting our society are in part related to language difficulties. Increasing professional acceptance of this point of view may lead to revision in the environmental and sociological concepts of current management philosophy. Such acceptance may also lead to an ever-closer cooperation between those behavioral and natural scientists who are involved in this particular problem. The problem of childhood language disabilities constitutes a very vital area for such synthesis.

Among the reasons why a straightforward and successful attack on the problem of language disabilities has not been made is the lack of sound criteria in defining the condition, establishing firm techniques of evaluation, and laying out accepted patterns of management and treatment. This combination of problems accounts, at least in part, for the wide variation in prevalence estimates, for the confusion and disagreement as to the nature of the condition, and for the virtual chaos in contemporary management and education. An additional complication is that the condition clearly is the concern of many disciplines. Understanding and solution can only be achieved by an interdisciplinary approach.

Major professional areas are aware that they have a stake in the evaluation and treatment of childhood language disabilities. In the field of education, preschool, elementary and secondary teachers, special education teachers, language arts specialists, mathematics teachers, and administrators are faced in their programs with the management responsibility for many children with language disabilities. In the field of medicine, the pediatrician, pediatric neurologist, child psychiatrist, human geneticist, and ophthalmologist are increasingly aware and concerned. And finally, professionals in relevant areas such as speech pathology and audiology, psychology, linguistics, and child development are demonstrating a new sense of responsibility.

Needed today is a synthesis of the data which are presently known concerning childhood language disabilities. This multidisciplinary text, in its orientation, will serve three purposes:

1. It will serve as a guide for the professional who, in a wide variety of public and private environments, must deal today with the needs of these children.

2. It will serve as a text book or as a basic resource book for educational and medical training centers.

3. It will serve as a basis for assessing the present state of the art and for stimulating imperatively needed future research.

To accomplish these purposes, the authors have provided the most current information about the a) new linguistic and psycholinguistic approaches to understanding language and its acquisition by the child, b) the characteristics of childhood language disabilities viewed by major etiological categories, c) relevant diagnostic and evaluative techniques, both medical and nonmedical, d) and management procedures. An interdisciplinary team of distinguished authors represents pediatrics, pediatric neurology, speech pathology and audiology, psychology, child development, psycholinguistics, sociolinguistics, and special education.

An essential theme of this book is that language disabilities must be viewed within the context of expected behavioral outcomes and not just as etiological categories. A second major theme is that the value of diagnosis should be assessed in terms of its contribution to the development of an effective program of management. Therefore, from an essentially behavioristic approach to the analysis and modification of language, this book takes a fresh look at the significant issues in childhood language disabilities as well as provides practical recommendations for the diagnosis and management of this disorder.

The authors wish to stress that this book is about children who are suffering and future children who will suffer from language problems. Though the information contained in the pages which follow have been written for those who assume professional responsibility for these children, our contribution can only be realistically judged if it assists in the reduction, elimination, and prevention of the suffering which this disability imposes. Therefore, the significant question becomes not "What will this book do for professionals?" but "What will this book do for children with language disabilities?"

JOHN V. IRWIN
MICHAEL MARGE

Contents

xiii

Part 1: Linguistic approaches

1: The structure of language

Michael H. O' Malley and Ronald Tikofsky

Man is distinguished by his acquisition and utilization of complex codes for the purpose of communication. Only man can talk, and the codes he evolves for talking are embodied in more than 2,000 different spoken languages. Yet while the number of different languages is great, all share many properties. Linguists have been studying language structures for at least 3,000 years. The discovery of those characteristics and underlying features which link the languages of the world to one another has been a major focus of study. For all the effort that linguists and others have put forth in their studies of languages, relatively little is known concerning the way languages are put together, and even less is known about how we come to "understand," "generate," or "acquire" the language we speak. There are many different and often incompatible linguistic theories which are invoked to explain the facts of language and there are many facts about language which are not taken into account by any theory. However, it is abundantly clear that, whether or not the theories provide adequate explanations of language, man in his daily use of language as his primary communication tool goes on talking. Unfortunately, those who are concerned with problems of communication can ill afford such a blasé attitude toward the study of language structure.

Failure to acquire language, or a disruption of the language acquisition process, is one of the most devastating and isolating events which can occur to a human being. Results of such disruptions can and do have far-reaching educational and societal implications. There is ample evidence to show that there are great numbers of children who for one reason or another have not achieved a level of language acquisition which permits them to enter fully into the life of the community. That there are such children has led to a search for techniques of assessment and treatment by which the impairment of communicative function can be alleviated. If this goal is to be achieved, those concerned with disabilities of language should have some understanding of the structure of language in order to be better able to assess and treat the child with a language impairment.

3

This chapter is designed to present the reader with a basic introduction to the structure of language. The aim is to present the facts of language, as they now seem to be established, in a clear and concise manner. No prior background in linguistics on the part of the reader has been assumed. Some of what appears below will be familiar to the reader, but may be at variance with some of his traditional views of language. No effort will be made to deal with problems of normal or delayed language acquisition. Rather, the goal is to provide a base from which to examine such problems.

As prologue let us review briefly what it is that the linguist has as a goal when attempting to discover the structure of language. His goals and methods are frequently quite different from those of the psychologist, speech pathologist, or educator. The arguments that so often arise out of statements made about language by the various disciplines concerned with language and language users result from a failure to appreciate differences in points of view. The next section attempts to provide a brief account of some of the different approaches to language structure.

The relationship between a linguistic description of a language and a psychological or neurological model of a language user is very controversial. The goal of linguistics is the development of a theory of language, not a theory of language users. The description of the language user is left to psychology and psycholinguistics.

Linguistics attempts to describe the structure of a language; the elements can be used to communicate information. In short, a linguistic description contains the information which is necessary to understand and create utterances in a language. Almost by definition, a language user must know how to create and understand utterances in order to engage in successful verbal communication. Therefore, in some sense, a linguistic description is a description of what it is that a person who knows a language knows. This abstract knowledge of a language is called linguistic *competence.* Of course, the language user cannot necessarily describe his knowledge explicitly; if he could, the linguist would be out of a job.

The speaker's linguistic knowledge must, of course, be represented in his brain. Furthermore, similarities in the structure of apparently diverse languages and similarities in the acquisition of these languages suggest that many aspects of linguistic structure are biologically determined (Lenneberg, 1967). On the other hand, it is quite unlikely that the elements in a description of linguistic competence will bear any resemblance to neurological or psychological processes. Linguistic rules attempt to describe what a speaker knows—his competence; they do not describe the processes he uses to produce or understand language. There is an analogue between the rules which describe linguistic competence and the rules of arithmetic or chess. The rules for these activities describe valid calculations and legitimate chess games, but they do not say anything about the mental activity involved in calculation or chess playing.

Language users make mistakes, they forget what they were talking about, they hesitate, they change their minds. A description of what a language user actually says, a description of his *performance*, will be related to, but by no means be identical to, a description of his knowledge, his competence. The distinction between competence and performance can be important in therapy. Does a particular case of language pathology represent a deficit in competence or performance?

COMPONENTS OF A LINGUISTIC DESCRIPTION

A linguistic description or grammar is generally organized into three components: syntax, semantics, and phonology. Before discussing these components in detail, brief definitions of the terms are in order.

Syntax is the study of the order in which the elements of a language can occur and the relationships among these elements in an utterance. Syntactic rules associate a syntactic structure with each sentence which indicates how the information in that sentence is organized.

Semantics is concerned with the meaning of utterances and how utterances are related to other utterances and to the world. Semantic rules operate on syntactic structures to describe the way in which an utterance is used and understood.

Phonology is concerned with the relationship between linguistic elements and their physical realization. Phonological rules thus relate a sequence of linguistic units to a sequence of articulatory, acoustic, or neural events.

The preceding definitions did not specify particular linguistic elements. In general, the smallest unit of syntax is the morpheme and the largest is the sentence. Traditionally, that part of syntax dealing with the formation of words is called *morphology*. Other linguistic units, such as phonemes and distinctive features, will be described later.

In the preceding paragraphs the word "rule" was used rather frequently. The concept of "rule" as used in a discussion of language structure requires clarification. Every language possesses a structure, and this structure is described in terms of a complex system of rules. What is of great importance for those who are making their first formal contact with linguistics to keep in mind is that the rules being discussed *are not prescriptive*, as are ethical rules or traffic laws. Neither are they inviolable, as are the laws of physics. Rather, rules as used in this chapter are constitutive. That is, as the rules of chess serve to constitute or define the game, so the rules of English define what it means to know English.

Languages are productive, which is to say that given a vocabulary it is possible to construct an almost infinite variety of word strings. Because of the productivity of languages, rules are required to describe a language. To illustrate this point consider the following example. Suppose that a person with a small vocabulary of 10,000 words began generating English sentences by stringing words together at random. On the average, there would be between 10 and 100 words which could be substituted at any given point and still have the sentences make good sense. About 1,000 words could be substituted to yield English-like nonsense. If only 30 word utterances produced by our speaker were examined, how many such utterances would constitute acceptable and sensible English? It turns out that only between 10^{30} and 10^{60} of such utterances would make sense, 10^{90} might be considered grammatical but nevertheless nonsensical, but the overwhelming majority of the utterances, 10^{120}, would be in complete violation of English structure.

As can be seen from the above example, even if our speaker produced only "good English sentences" it is unlikely that he would speak all the possible good English sentences in a lifetime. In fact, the majority of the possible, perfectly acceptable, short

English sentences have never been and will never be spoken. On the other hand, of all the possible sequences of words, only an infinitesimal fraction of these sequences are potential English sentences. Clearly there must be a finite mechanism or system of rules which specifies the sequences of words which correspond to English structure and those which do not. Rules are also necessary to specify the meaning and pronunciation of each of these potential English sentences. Thus, linguistics could be characterized as the study of the structure of these rules.

A word of caution is necessary. What we have been talking about in the preceding paragraphs have been constitutive or descriptive rules, which are at times confused with or taken to be the same as prescriptive "rules of grammar" that are sometimes learned in school. This is not at all the case. In fact, such a misconception or confusion would for example suggest that the socially prestigious dialect of a language is the "correct" one and that other dialects are degenerate, rule-less forms of the "standard" dialect. What must be remembered, however, is that in each dialect, and in fact for each speaker, there will be some sentences which are acceptable and some which are not. Thus each dialect and each idiolect (personal dialect of an individual speaker) can be described by its own set of rules. And just as no language is structurally more advanced or primitive than any other, so no dialect is better or more communicative than any other.

In teaching grammar in the schools it is tacitly assumed that the student knows the rules for one dialect, since he speaks and is understood by parents, teachers, and peers. What school grammars do is to describe differences between the dialect the child speaks and a standard or written dialect, by concentrating on defective sentences such as

(1)   a. *Me and Bill is going.[1]
            b. *It burns good.
            c. *Looking up from the street, the building seemed very tall.

These sentences demonstrate rather superficial aspects of linguistic structure, while more difficult errors such as the following, tend to be ignored:

(2)   a. *I believe to be sick.
            b. *I tried for Max to leave.
            c. *John seemed leaving.
            d. *Did that Harry left bother you?
            e. *That John hadn't left surprised anyone.

Most speakers of English sense that the sentences in (2) violate English structure. However, prescriptive grammars do not provide rules for rejecting such sentences. More impressive is the fact that with no overt instruction, children who have never been to school can induce a set of rules which will enable them to recognize the defects in this group of sentences.

[1] An asterisk before a word or sentence means that it is not an acceptable form in the dialect under discussion.

As fluent speakers of English, readers of this book already know the structure of at least one English dialect. Perhaps this knowledge can best be made explicit through an examination of the phonology, morphology, syntax, and semantics of the following sentence:

(3)   I challenge your decision to make Harry a senator, since I know he is even more inflexible than most politicians.

If sentence (3) were repeated several times in succession, even by the same speaker, no two repetitions would be physically identical. Each utterance of this sentence would be a continuous movement of the vocal tract with few obvious segments. In linguistic terms, however, each of the repetitions might consist of an identical sequence of phonological units, or *phonemes* as they are usually called. A listener would normally react to these discrete linguistic units rather than to the continuous physical event. This property of discreteness, of chopping up a continuous event and representing it by discrete units, is fundamental to linguistics.

While the phonemes of a language are discrete units, they are also systematically related. For example, the initial phonemes in meat /mit/ and neat /nit/ are identical except for the feature of place of articulation. The dimensions along which the phonemes of a language contrast are called *distinctive features*. It has been suggested that a small number of distinctive features can account for all the phonemic contrasts in every language. A phoneme is thus analyzed as a bundle of distinctive features.

Not every sequence of phonemes can occur in the words of a language. For example, ging /giɔ/ is a possible English word while ngig /ɔig/ is not. If sentence (3) had been

(4)   . . . he is more ging than most politicians.

the listener might assume that *ging* was a new adjective. Had the speaker used *ngig*, the listener would have known that the word was not English. The grammar of the permissible sequences of phonemes is called *phonotactics*.

In addition to the segmental phonemes, the *prosodic* information such as *stress* and *intonation* must be indicated. A word such as politician /palətɪʃən/ has a medium stress on the first syllable and a strong stress on the third. If the main word stress were moved to the second syllable, the first three vowels would all change: /pəlɪtəʃən/. There is a strong interaction between stress placement and vowels in English.

Each word has its own stress pattern. In addition, various words in an utterance receive different degrees of stress according to the grammar of the sentence and the speaker's emphasis. Intonation, which is the pattern of pitch changes during an utterance, also is a function both of the grammar and the speaker's intended message.

One utterance of sentence (3) could be transcribed either as a sequence of phonemes or as a sequence of English words. Phonemes have no meaning. However, words such as *your, decision, senator, inflexible,* and *politician* are obviously made up of meaningful units smaller than words. The smallest or most elementary meaningful units in a language are called *morphemes.*

Morphemes are represented by sequences of phonemes. Sometimes two different morphemes such as the agentive[2] (as in *runner*) and the comparative (as in *hotter*) are represented by the same phoneme sequence. Sometimes a morpheme such as plural has different representations in different environments, as in *dogs, cats, glasses* (/dɔgz, kæt-s, glæs-ɛz/). The study of the representation of sequences of phonemes is called *morphophonemics.*

The complexity of the morphophonemic rules of English is illustrated by the words *decide, decisive,* and *decision.* Adding the adjective-forming morpheme /-ɪv/ to the verb /disaɪd/ changes the final /d/ to /s/: /disaɪsɪv/. Adding the noun-forming morpheme /-iən/ changes the /d/ to /ʒ/ and deletes the /a/ of the verb and the /i/ of the suffix. All these changes are quite regular and can be used productively by fairly young children.

Morphology is the study of how morphemes are put together to make words. Of course, not every sequence of morphemes is a word. Therefore, morphology will include both *morphophonemics* and *morphotactics*, the rules which define the permissible sequences of morphemes. Violations or incorrect use of both morphophonemic and morphotactic rules might be expected to occur as part of the normal course of language development and in language pathology. For example, *foots* for *feet* would be a morphophonemic violation, while *catchdoger* for *dogcatcher* would violate English morphotactics.

To talk of morphotactic rules and violations implies that all morphemes are productive units for the speaker of a language. Most morphemic divisions are apparent to a native speaker. However, a word such as *decide* is made up of two morphemes which were joined in Latin before English even existed. While *de-* is still a slightly productive prefix in that it can be used to form new words (*defrost, de-escalate*), *-cide* is definitely not productive. Psychologically, *decide* is a single unit for most speakers. In the study of language disorders, it is necessary to distinguish between productive morphemes, which enter into morphotactic processes to generate new words, and fixed morpheme sequences, which must be learned as a unit.

One major classification of morphemes is according to whether or not their primary function is to signal grammatical information. Morphemes such as *to, a, is, even, than, PAST, PLURAL,* and *-ing* function almost entirely as grammatical markers; they are called *function* or *system morphemes.* On the other hand, morphemes such as *challenge, decide, senate, flex,* and *politic* seem to have meaning apart from their occurrence in a particular sentence; they are called *content* morphemes.

In general it is easy to add new content morphemes to a language. The content morphemes in a sentence can even be replaced with nonsense syllables without changing the grammatical structure of the sentence. On the other hand, function morphemes belong to small, closed classes such as preposition and article. Function morphemes signal grammatical structure and their meaning is a function of their position within a sentence.

While the content-function distinction is useful, it should not be pushed too far. Prepositions signal syntactic structures in English and generally behave like function words. However, prepositions also have meanings which are independent of their

---

[2] Agentives are morphemes which are attached or affixed to verbs such as *run* to indicate the person or agent performing the action.

syntactic function. On the other side, adverbs such as *here, now,* and *then* are content words which are like function words in that they belong to closed classes.

Morphology is the study of word-forming processes and provides a bridge between phonology and *syntax*. Since not every sequence of words is an English sentence, syntactic rules are necessary to specify which sequences are permissible. As an extreme case, the words in sentence (3) when read in reverse order have no syntactic structure:

(5)   Politicians most than inflexible more even is he know I since, senator a Harry make to decision your challenge I.

On a more subtle level, replacing *is* by *are* results in a sentence which is close to English but which does violate the rules of English syntax.

(6)   I challenge your decision to make Harry a senator, since I know he are even more inflexible than most politicians.

Native speakers know more than just whether or not a particular sequence of words forms an English sentence. In fact, it is their implicit "knowledge" of English syntax that enables them to make such judgments. Thus, although they cannot necessarily make explicit the syntactic rules or names of the syntactic classes and functions of the various words and morphemes in the sentence, native speakers know which groupings of words form phrases, they know the referents of pronouns, they know, in short, a great many syntactic facts about any given sentence. Of course they cannot always articulate their knowledge, even though it is part of their competence. For example, in sentence (3) a speaker would have the following information:

a. *Challenge, make,* and *know* are verbs, and *decision* is a noun which has been derived from a verb.

b. *I*, a pronoun, is the subject of both *challenge* and *know*, and *you* is the subject of *make*.

c. *You* functions as if it were the subject of the verb underlying *decision.*

d. *A senator* is a phrase which can be used in place of most proper nouns.

As shown in the next section, the syntactic rules assign to each sentence of a language a structure which indicates the class membership and grammatical function of the various parts of the sentence. This structure represents the speaker's knowledge in the sense that the syntactic structure is, by definition, necessary for understanding a sentence.

Sometimes a sequence of words can have more than one syntactic structure. In sentence (3) *make Harry a senator* can mean either *make a senator for Harry* or *make Harry be a senator.* In the former interpretation, which is not semantically acceptable, Harry is in apposition to *a senator.* A sequence of words which has several distinct interpretations is said to be *ambiguous.* Syntactic ambiguity is extremely common but usually only one of the interpretations is semantically acceptable.

The converse of ambiguity is the case of *paraphrase* in which two or more sentences have similar meanings. For example, the following sentences are synonymous in ways which can be described by regular transformational processes in English:

(7)   a. John made Harry a Senator.
            b. John made a Senator of Harry.
            c. Harry was made a Senator by John.
            d. It was John who made Harry a Senator.
            e. What John made of Harry was a Senator.

The goal of syntactic analysis is to find rules which can describe ambiguity, paraphrase, grammaticality, and the various relationships within and between sentences.

Syntax is concerned with the internal structure of language; semantics is concerned with the relationship between language and the things it talks about. There are many elaborate theories of syntax, but most syntactic descriptions [e.g., *you* is the subject of *decide* in sentence (3)] depend upon a particular theoretical framework. In contrast, theories of semantics are quite vague, while semantic facts (e.g., *inflexible* and *rigid* are synonymous) are easy to come by.

In spite of the lack of a unifying semantic theory, certain theoretical points can be made. One thing which words do is name or refer to things. In sentence (3) *I, you, he,* and *Harry* refer to particular people. Of course, the people whom these words name will be different for different occasions in which sentence (3) might be uttered. It is important to realize that referring is a property of an utterance—a particular physical act by a particular person—rather than a property of a sentence—an abstract linguistic object.

It is equally important to realize that some words do not refer. Function words such as *to, is,* and *since* clearly do not refer to anything. Words such as *know, make,* and *inflexible* might be said to refer to some abstract concepts of knowledge, making, and inflexibility. Rather than invent new objects for these words to name, it is better to look for their meaning elsewhere.

It might be argued that the primary semantic function of a sentence is to describe or to assert that a particular description is true. This analysis would be reasonable for sentences such as

(8)   The telephone is on the table.

However, sentence (3) would not be said to describe a challenge; rather than describing anything at all, it would be used to question or challenge a decision. In the theory of speech acts (Searle, 1969) the meaning of a sentence is considered to involve the acts which it is used to perform.

An important part of the semantics of an utterance are the *presuppositions* or conditions which are assumed in the making of the utterance. In sentence (3) if the word *most* receives extra stress or prominence, the utterance presupposes that Harry is a politician. However, if the stress is on *politician*, the utterance presupposes that Harry is not a politician.

There are a great many semantic relationships among words and sentences in English which need to be described. However, there is little agreement on the form that such a description must eventually take.

Each of the components of a linguistic description could be the subject matter of an entire volume. In some cases several books have been written on each of these topics. The bibliography which accompanies this chapter will provide selected references for each of the areas discussed. The remainder of the chapter will offer a more detailed discussion of syntax, phonology, and semantics. However, most of the emphasis will be on syntax. There are several reasons for this. Most prominent is the fact that this is the area which is receiving the greatest attention from linguists, psychologists, and psycholinguists, but has only recently become an area of prime interest to the speech pathologist and others concerned with delayed language acquisition. Another reason is that many of the points made with respect to syntax can also be applied to the area of phonology. Semantics will be discussed, but in less detail than phonology or syntax.

SYNTAX

Syntax is concerned with the order in which the elements of a language occur and the relationships among the elements in an utterance. It has become the focal point of modern theories of linguistic structure.

Most current linguistic theories propose that underlying the sentences of a language are rather elaborate syntactic structures. Many people who are not professionally involved in syntactic analysis feel that the structure of language could not be so complex; after all, children learn to talk at a very early age. In order to defend the complexity of current theories, it is necessary to dispose of some simpler and superficially more plausible ones.

Utterances as Responses to Stimuli

One simple and attractive theory of language use might be the following:

Language users have a finite store of responses—words, phrases, simple sentences— from which to create utterances. Each of these responses is associated with extralinguistic stimuli. Utterances are constructed by stringing these responses together, one after another. The sequential order of the responses is determined by the stimuli.

If human speech did consist of learned responses elicited by appropriate situations, there would be little need for syntax. Linguistic structure would be just a catalog of potential responses. However, such a model cannot account for the complexity of actual sentences. If the responses were words and short phrases, the specification of the permissible sequences of words would depend upon possible sequences of stimuli. Stimuli occur relatively independently of each other and so their order does not explain the strong sequential interdependencies found in English sentences (Lashley, 1951). On the other hand, if the responses were entire sentences, it would be impossible to learn the unlimited number of possible English sentences.

Utterances as Substitutions in Patterns

One starting point for a theory of syntax is the observation that a sentence may be extended into an unlimited number of new sentences through the expansion of one of its elementary parts. In spite of this expansion, the relationships in the remainder of the sentence remain unchanged. For example, consider the following sentences:

(9)   a. George distrusted theories.
        b. George distrusted some theories.
        c. George distrusted all poorly tested theories of dysarthric speech.
        d. George distrusted Sam's analysis of Harvey's reaction to all miscalibrated spectrograms.

The noun phrase *theories*, which is the object of the verb *distrusted*, is successively expanded by means of regular English processes. Furthermore, in contexts in which *theories* is used as a noun phrase, it can almost always be replaced by the same set of expansions.

The possibility of expansion illustrated by (9) suggests a theory in which the syntax of a language consists of a set of basic patterns or sequences of substitution points. At each point, either a word or another pattern may be substituted. By starting with the basic patterns and carrying out all possible substitutions, all the potential sentences of the language may be produced.

The set of items which may be substituted at a particular substitution point is called a constituent. For example, the constituent noun phrase (NP) is a set containing such phrases as *Harvey, a spectrogram, a poor spectrogram, a poor spectrogram of Harvey's speech,* and *spectrograms.* The individual phrases which make up the constituent noun phrase may themselves be analyzed as sequences of constituents. A noun phrase, for instance, may consist of a proper noun (N_{pr}) or a determiner (Det) followed by a noun (N). A determiner may be either *a* or *the.* The constituent noun may be either a single noun, an adjective (Adj) followed by a noun, or a noun followed by a prepositional phrase (PP). A prepositional phrase consists of a preposition followed by a noun phrase. Defining a sentence (S) as a noun phrase followed by a verb phrase (VP) and defining verb phrase as a verb (V) followed by a noun phrase completes a grammar for a small fraction of the sentences of English.

This grammar may be written formally as a set of phrase-structure rules (Chomsky, 1963) as follows:

(10)   a. S → NP VP
        b. VP → V NP
        c. NP → N_{pr}
        d. NP → Det N
        e. N → Adj N
        f. N → N PP
        g. N → man, spectrograph, theory . . .
        h. PP → Prep NP
        i. Det → a, the
        j. Adj → green, tall . . .
        k. V → ran, saw
        l. N_{pr} → Harvey, George . . .
        m. Prep → in, on, near . . .

The arrow (→) means rewrite or replace the symbol on the left by the sequence of symbols on the right. The derivation or generation of a sentence starts with the symbol S. Each line in a derivation is derived from the preceding line by applying one of the rules in (10). A derivation may be terminated when all the symbols in the final line belong to the terminal vocabulary. The last line in the derivation is called the terminal string and is said to be generated by the rules of the grammar. The set of terminal strings derived from S by the rules of the grammar is called the language generated by that grammar. The following is an example of the use of the rules in (10) to generate a terminal string:

(11)   *Derivation*   *Rule   Used*

Derivation	Rule Used
NP VP	a
NP V NP	b
NP saw NP	k
NP saw N_{pr}	c
NP saw George	l
Det N saw George	d
Det Adj N saw George	e
Det Adj N PP saw George	f
Det Adj N Prep NP saw George	h
Det Adj Adj N Prep NP saw George	e
Det Adj Adj N Prep Det N saw George	d
The Adj Adj N Prep Det N saw George	i
The tall Adj N Prep Det N saw George	j
The tall green N Prep Det N saw George	j
The tall green man Prep Det N saw George	g
The tall green man on Det N saw George	m
The tall green man on the N saw George	i
The tall green man on the spectrograph saw George	g

This derivation can be represented more clearly by a tree diagram.

(12)

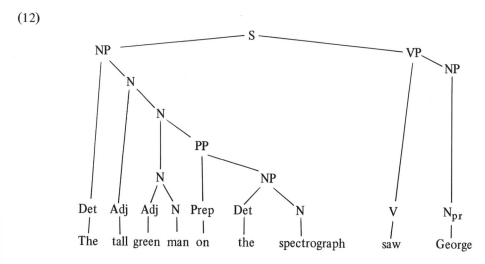

Each of the nodes (NP, VP, and so forth) represents a constituent. The lines leaving the node are called branches and represent rewriting rules. The sequence of words and morphemes at the bottom represents the terminal string or the sentence generated by the derivation. The tree diagram illustrates the way in which the rules generate the sentence.

The tree diagram, which is called the surface structure of the sentence, provides important syntactic information. For instance, it indicates how the elements in the sentence are to be grouped together. The importance of this grouping can be seen in the ambiguous sentence. For example:

(13)   a.

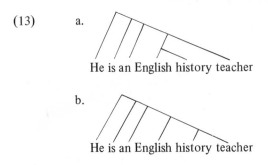

b.

This sentence has two sharply different meanings. The interpretation in which "he" is English is represented by the unlabeled tree (13a), and the interpretation in which "he" teaches English history is represented by (13b). The difference in meaning is a result of the difference in grouping.

Another example of ambiguity is the sentence "Time flies." The ambiguity is shown in the following illustration:

(14)   a.

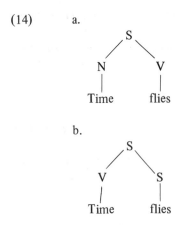

b.

In this case, the groupings for the two interpretations are identical; the difference in meaning can be represented by a difference in the labeling of the nodes in the tree diagram.

The preceding examples show why a surface-structure tree is a good representation for much of the syntactic information of a sentence. The grouping and labeling of its elements provides essential information for using and understanding a sentence. The tree also represents information which is necessary for assigning stress and intonation patterns to the sentence. In fact, the surface-structure tree is such a good representation for syntactic information that only within the last 10 or 15 years have its limitations been recognized.

The following ambiguous sentence illustrates one of the limitations of the surface-structure tree as a representation of syntactic information:

(15)   The lamb is too hot to eat.

This sentence can be about the lamb eating something or about something eating the lamb. Both of these interpretations, however, would probably be assigned identical surface trees. Therefore, the tree diagram would not contain sufficient information to determine the meaning of the sentence. The tree diagram does not indicate whether *lamb* is the subject or object of *eat*.

Once the importance of grammatical relationships such as subject and object is realized, the limitations of surface-structure trees as representations of syntactic information become obvious. For example, both of the following sentences would have the same tree diagram since they differ only in the choice of adjective:

(16)   a. Sarah is anxious to amuse.
          b. Sarah is hard to amuse.

Thus the fact that *Sarah* is the subject of *amuse* in the first sentence and the object of *amuse* in the second sentence would not be represented.

Surface-structure trees also do not adequately represent the structure of sentences with "missing" parts. For example,

(17)   John was found lurking in a culvert and so was Bill.

The information that Bill was lurking in the culvert is not represented in the surface structure of sentence (17).

A third difficulty with surface-structure trees is that they do not indicate the similarity in meaning of sentences such as the following:

(18)   a. Sam gave somebody a bribe.
          b. Sam gave a bribe to somebody.
          c. A bribe was given to somebody by Sam.
          d. Somebody was given a bribe by Sam.
          e. There was a bribe given to somebody by Sam.

nor do they indicate the relationship of these sentences to sentences of the form

(19)   Harry expected there to be a bribe given to someone by Sam.

These and other difficulties (Postal, 1964) suggest that a more complex theory of grammar is required. One such theory, although not the only possible one, is the theory of transformational grammar developed by Chomsky (1957, 1965).

Utterances as Transformed Deep Structures

From the preceding section it should be obvious that a structure more complex than a simple surface-structure tree is required for representing the conceptual structure of most sentences. For instance, sentence (17) would appear to contain four elementary propositions:

(20)   a. Someone found John.
          b. Someone found Bill.
          c. John was lurking in a culvert.
          d. Bill was lurking in a culvert.

The relationship among these propositions might be expressed by structure (21), where the elementary propositions are hung under an S node:

(21)

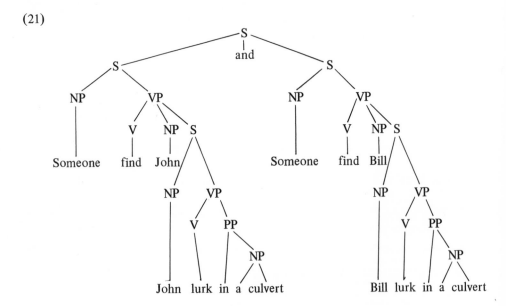

The structure of each elementary proposition can be represented by a modification of the tree diagrams described in the preceding section. Thus the "deep" or conceptual structure of a sentence may be represented by a tree diagram in which sub-trees represent the elementary propositions that make up the sentence.

Structure (21) represents the syntactic information of the sentence more adequately than does the surface-structure tree. Syntactic functions such as the subject and object for each verb are associated with that verb in the elementary proposition. Information which appears only once in the actual sentence may be represented as many times as necessary in the deep structure. In general structure (21) represents the meaning of the sentence far more clearly than does the surface-structure tree. However, the deep-structure tree does not indicate the actual order of the elements in the sentence. Thus it is necessary to devise rules for relating the deep structure of a sentence to its surface structure. The rules proposed by Chomsky (1957) are called transformations and are operations which change one tree into another. The set of transformations is called the transformational component of a grammar.

Some of the operations required in a transformational grammar can be seen in the conversion of the deep structure (21) into a surface structure. The first step would be to embed "John lurked in a culvert" into the structure "Someone found John." The transformation which produces "Someone found John John lurking in a culvert" on the left side of the tree is called an embedding transformation. There is now a need to delete the second John. A transformation which deletes identical noun phrases would do so. To convert "Someone found John lurking in a culvert" into "John was found lurking in a culvert by someone" makes use of a passivizing transformation; and finally, "by someone" is deleted by a transformation which deletes agents. The same sequence of transformations would apply to the right side of the tree, yielding structure (22).

(22)

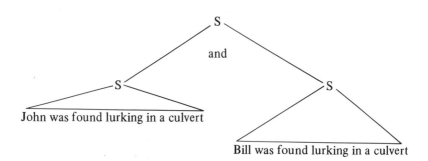

At this point a transformation would conjoin the sentences to yield a surface-structure tree of the form

(23)

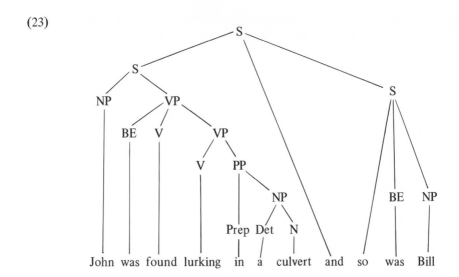

This surface-structure tree is a poor representation of all the syntactic relations and conceptual structures in the sentence. However, it does indicate the superficial order of the elements and provides certain information which is necessary for assigning stress and intonation. Unlike the surface-structure trees of the preceding section, this tree was not directly generated by a phrase-structure grammar. Furthermore, the labels on the nodes do not necessarily represent classes of items which may be interchanged without destroying the acceptability of the sentence.

The transformational model of grammar postulates a deep structure in which the meaning of a sentence and the relationship among its parts are more clearly represented than they are in the surface tree. This deep-structure tree is converted into a surface-structure tree by the transformational component of the grammar. Two of the important theoretical issues in transformational grammar concern the nature and origin of the deep structure and the form of the transformations which convert the deep to the surface structure.

By now many transformations have been fairly thoroughly studied and justified (Jacobs and Rosenbaum, 1968). Less, however, is known about deep structure. Chomsky (1965) proposed that deep structures were generated by the base component of the grammar. Chomsky's base consisted of the type of phrase-structure rules discussed in the illustrations above and a lexicon (a dictionary). The phrase-structure rules are used to generate labeled trees into which lexical items can be inserted by lexical transformations. Syntactic properties are associated with these lexical items to prevent them from being inserted into the wrong types of nodes in a tree.

Chomsky proposed that the semantic component of the grammar relates the deep structure to some kind of semantic representation. The deep structure is generated by the syntactic component. In Chomsky's view, both semantics and phonology are interpretive; semantics interprets deep structure (assigns a meaning to it), and phonology interprets (pronounces) surface structure.

The more deep structure is studied by linguists, the greater the similarity between deep structures underlying equivalent sentences in different languages. Furthermore, proposed deep structures reflect more and more of the meaning of a sentence. Thus it has been suggested that the deep-structure tree is a direct representation of the meaning or conceptual structure of a sentence and is not too closely tied to the structure of the particular language.

Regardless of the outcome of current investigations, however, two points about syntax seem well established. First, there is a superficial syntactic organization for every sentence and this organization is signaled, at least in part, by patterns of function words and morphemes. Second, the information in a sentence is organized into interconnected elementary sentences or propositions, each of which contains a single verb. Whether a verb occurs as a main verb, as a verb embedded within a verb phrase, or as a noun derived from a verb, it retains most of the properties which it has when it occurs alone. Therefore, understanding a sentence involves breaking it up into elements headed by verbs and then finding the nouns and sentences which are related to each of these verbs. The centrality of verbs and their associations with nouns and elementary sentences seem to be a part of most current linguistic theories.

SEMANTICS

Semantics is concerned with meaning and the way in which sentences are related to other sentences and to the world. The purpose of talking is to communicate: to refer, to assert, to promise, to sympathize, to lie, and so forth. Speakers are far more capable of answering questions about the semantics of their language than questions about syntax or phonology. In spite of the abundance of data and the importance of the area, linguists have had little of significance to say about semantic structure. The difficulty is not lack of data or interest, but lack of models or theories for organizing the data.

One approach to semantics starts with the observation that language names or refers to things. More precisely, people in using the sentences of their language name or refer to things. It thus might appear that the meaning of a term is what it refers to. Sentences, of course, do not name. However, many declarative sentences appear to describe or refer to a relationship among things and to assert that this relationship does, in fact, hold. The theory that words refer and that a sentence describes a state of affairs may be called the name-describe theory of semantics.

The view that naming-describing forms the basis for semantics has been widely held. However, it cannot be maintained without some modification. For example, *Richard Nixon* and *the current president of the United States* refer to the same person but do not mean the same thing. Therefore, reference does not capture the meaning of *meaning*.

Two technical terms—extension and intension—have been introduced to differentiate between reference and meaning. The *extension* of a term is the set of things which it refers to or *denotes*. The *intension* or *connotation* of a term is the set of properties which something must have in order to be referred to by the term. *Calvin Coolidge* and *the current president of the United States* had the same extension in 1925, but they did not have the same intension. The intension of the first is the property of being named Calvin Coolidge, and the intension of the second is the property of being president at the time of utterance.

Recognizing that intension is an important part of meaning does not solve the problem of semantics. Words such as *which, seem,* and *been* do not refer. Even with words such as *receive, run,* and *expect,* it is not exactly correct to say that they refer. Noun phrases, in fact, appear to be the smallest units which can refer. However, noun phrases can be arbitrarily complex and can even have whole sentences embedded within them. Therefore, it will be necessary to have complex rules for deriving the meaning or intension of a noun phrase from the dictionary definition of the words which it contains. The deep structures of transformational grammar appear to be a first step toward specifying these rules.

Some sentences do fit the name-describe theory of semantics. The subject and the objects of the verbs and prepositions name things, the verbs and prepositions describe a relationship, and the sentence would normally be used to assert that the description is true. For example:

(24)   a. The ashtray is on the table.
        b. John met Mary in her garden.

Many sentences, however, are not like these. For instance, in the following sentences the meaning does not come entirely from their true description of some state of affairs:

(25)   a. I promise to take you home.
        b. I apologize for hitting you.
        c. You haven't been elected yet.

The first two sentences in (25) do not really describe or refer to an act; they are best analyzed as actually performing the speech acts of promising and apologizing, respectively. Such utterances are called *performatives* (Austin, 1962). The meaning of (25c) is either a warning not to be overconfident or an insinuation that the election will be lost. Almost never would (25c) be used just to describe a state of affairs.

Analyzing sentences in terms of the speech acts which they may be used to perform is important for understanding their meaning. One result of this analysis has been the recognition of the preconditions or *felicity* conditions which are necessary for the successful use of an utterance. For example, a person who used sentence (25b) when he had never hit the person in question would be violating the felicity conditions of the act of apologizing.

The proper use of most sentences requires that certain felicity conditions be satisfied. Looked at the other way, the use of certain sentences presupposes that certain things are true. Two classic examples are

(26)   a. Have you stopped beating your wife yet?
        b. She's dumb, even for a blond.

These sentences assume or presuppose that you beat your wife and that blonds are dumb. A complete semantic theory will need to specify the relationships between sentences, the situations which they presuppose, the felicity conditions for their proper use, and the speech acts which they may be used to perform. Actually there are many types of acts which are performed by a speaker when he utters a sentence. At one level he is merely making noises or saying English words with a certain sense and reference. In making these noises or uttering these words, he is also promising, requesting, reporting, admitting, predicting, thanking, describing, apologizing, and so on. These acts which a speaker performs in saying something have been called *illocutions* (Austin, 1962). By uttering a sentence, a speaker may also be affecting his listener. In fact, he may be embarrassing, persuading, inspiring, boring, encouraging, frightening, or impressing him. These effects on a listener which a speaker achieves are called *perlocutions*. The relationship between an utterance and an illocutionary act is part of linguistics. The relationship of an utterance to a perlocutionary effect is part of psychology.

Not to know the presuppositions and felicity conditions of an English utterance is not to know part of the semantic relationships between words and sentences. For example, the literal interpretation of each of the following sentences violates some aspect of English semantics:

(27)   a. John hoped the team would win but he didn't want them to.
         b. While he expected Bill to go, John didn't think he would.
         c. Harry is a bachelor who is married to a school teacher.
         d. If he's not married, how can he be a bachelor?

The oddness of sentences (27a) and (27b) is not due to a peculiarity in John's psychological makeup. *Hope, expect, think,* and *want* do not just refer to psychological "states." Logically, it is not possible to hope for something and yet not want it to happen. Part of knowing English is knowing the relationships between *hope* and *want, expect* and *think,* and *bachelor* and *married.*

Semantic relationships such as the one between *bachelor* and *married* look very much like the deductive relationships which are studied in traditional logic. In fact, presuppositions and other meaning relationships do constitute a kind of logic which is part of the semantic structure of a language. While current studies in syntax and semantics recognize the need for a deductive component, its final form is still unclear.

The intension of a term is the set of properties which something must possess in order to be referred to by the term. This suggests that the meaning of a term might be analyzed as a combination of elementary meanings. For instance, the following words could be analyzed as shown in (28).

(28)   man   = adult + human + male
         father = male + parent
         son   = male + offspring
         brother = male + sibling
         sister = female + sibling

The terms on the right side of the equations in (28) are the semantic elements (or components) which constitute the meanings of the terms on the left. In general, the meanings or ranges of applicability of the words in one language do not match those of the words in another language. However, it is claimed that semantic elements which result from a componential analysis [as in (28)] of the words of a language are similar, even in unrelated languages. The similarity of these semantic elements suggests that there may be a small set of universal semantic components which underlies the vocabulary of every language. However, there is little solid evidence to support the postulation of such a universal semantic structure for all languages.

In some semantic domains such as kinship terms, an analysis into semantic components seems quite appropriate. Anthropological linguists have made extensive cross-cultural studies of the semantic components in kinship systems. However, it has been argued that components are not adequate to represent the meaning of every word. For instance, Wittgenstein (1953) argues that with words such as *game*, there is no list of properties which can define them exactly. He suggests that we recognize that something is a game, not by checking a list of properties, but by noticing a "family resemblance" between the new instance and previously encountered games.

Many people conceive of meanings as some kind of mysterious objects which may someday be discovered, rather as new atomic particles are discovered. A good antidote for this view is the realization that different kinds of words are meaningful in quite different ways. For instance, in the following sentence each word expresses a meaning of a different type:

(29)   Give me five hot potatoes.

This sentence instructs the listener to find a potato, measure its temperature to see if it is hot, bring the potato to the speaker, and repeat this action five times. The meaning of *five* involves the notion of counting, the meaning of *hot* involves the measurement of temperature, the meaning of *potato* involves the recognition of a particular plant, and so forth. These meanings are not objects and they are certainly not all the same kind of object. It is only when we think in abstract terms about meanings in general that we become confused. The best that can be said about the meanings of words in general is that meanings are rules which specify the situations in which a word can be used.

The discussion up to this point has been concerned only with *literal* meaning; there are several other levels of meaning which might be recognized. In the sentence

(30)   He is a pig.

the literal meaning is that the object referred to by *he* has four legs, a tail, and says *oink*. If the object is a person, the sentence is false in its literal meaning. The *figurative* meaning of this sentence, however, would be that the object referred to had some of the characteristics of a pig. Figurative uses such as *metaphor* are certainly a rule-governed part of the structure of a language. However, it is necessary to separate the figurative level of meaning from the literal to avoid confusion.

The listener might be revolted by pigs or enraged by the suggestion that his friend had the characteristics of one. For him, sentence (30) would have a personal *emotive* meaning. Such an emotional response is not a rule-governed part of linguistic structure; emotional meaning is not part of linguistic meaning.

Up to this point, meaning has been treated in terms such as intension, extension, and semantic rules. Another approach is to analyze meaning as a psychological term related to the word associations and stimulus-response patterns of language users.

A word such as *strawberry* or *vomit* can produce a strong mental image. The listener's response to such a word bears at least a slight resemblance to his response to the object named by the word. Furthermore, words which in the speaker's mind are associated with a particular word are generally related to that word in meaning. For these reasons, most psychological studies of meaning have been based on the assumption that the meaning of words and sentences is connected to the overt or covert responses which an utterance elicits in a listener.

The theory that meaning is related to a listener's response to an utterance is part of the psychological theory of learning and concept formation. It is important to recognize the essential difference between such a theory and the more linguistic, nonpsychological discussion of meaning presented in this chapter. The difference between these approaches can be illustrated by example (31).

(31)   a. Every square is an equilateral rectangle.
          b. Every square is an equilateral triangle.

A linguistic theory of meaning would mark (31a) as *tautologous*: a sentence whose truth follows logically from the meanings of its words. Sentence (31b) would be marked as contradictory. However, there is a strong association between the words *equilateral* and *triangle*. Therefore, a psychological theory of meaning might note that (31b) is more compatible with the associations and responses of many English speakers than is (31a). In general, a theory of meaning in terms of a listener's response deals with the emotive level of meaning rather than with the literal or figurative levels. It describes what a word means to a particular person, but it does not describe the literal meaning of the word.

PHONOLOGY

Phonology is concerned with the relationship between linguistic elements and their physical realizations. While phonology was the first aspect of language to be studied in modern linguistics, changing theories of syntax and advances in electronic instrumentation have led to many revisions in phonological theory.

Viewed as a physical event, an utterance is a continuous movement of the vocal tract. Viewed as a linguistic event, an utterance is a discrete sequence of morphemes, words, or phrases. On the linguistic level, the speaker and listener can almost always agree about which units of the language were present in a particular utterance. Since the division of an utterance into a series of discrete units is so easy for humans, it is difficult to realize how complex the relationship between the physical and linguistic events actually is. Only with the development of modern electronic instrumentation has the full complexity of this relationship been appreciated.

Phonetics

A phonetic description of an utterance is a description which could be obtained, in principle, by a machine without any consideration of the particular language to which the utterance belongs. A phonetic description is generally a sequence of symbols, each of which can be related to some aspect of the physical event. However, this description is very abstract when compared to a purely physical description such as a high-speed X-ray movie or a tape recording.

Speech originates as neural impulses. These impulses produce tension in the muscle of the face, tongue, larynx, and respiratory system. The muscle tensions cause the organs which are involved in articulation to follow trajectories according to the laws of mechanics. The flow of air resulting from the positions and movements of the vocal tract generates vibratory, hissing, or explosive sounds. These sounds are then modified by the resonance characteristics of the vocal tract, which result from the positions assumed by the articulators.

The modified sound is transmitted through the air to the listener's ear. Here it is converted to displacements of points along the basilar membrane. These movements, which are related to the frequency components of the sound wave, finally result in neural impulses to the VIIIth cranial nerve.

An utterance could be described physically at any point along this speech chain. For example, the neural impulses to the articulators, the sequence of articulatory positions, the acoustic wave, or the neural impulses from the ear are all physical descriptions of an utterance. Traditionally, however, the articulatory description of an utterance has formed the basis for phonetic description.

There are two principal ways to relate a physical description to a phonetic transcription. Most typically, an utterance is segmented according to some criteria such as a minimum in the velocity of the articulators. Each segment is then classified according to some taxonomic system. Peterson and Shoup's (1966a) approach is perhaps the most elaborate and consistent attempt to specify such a taxonomic system.

An utterance appears to consist of a sequence of articulatory target positions, most of which are never attained. This fact suggests that a phonetic description might better be the sequence of target positions rather than the sequence of positions of minimal articulator velocity. Such a phonetic description would be very abstract when compared with a physical description but it might more accurately reflect the production of speech.

Systems for classifying articulatory positions generally propose a number of features or parameters for specifying different articulations. For instance, Peterson and Shoup (1966) propose primary phonetic parameters of horizontal place of articulation, vertical place of articulation, and manner of articulation. Secondary parameters such as laryngeal action, air release, tongue shape, and lip shape provide a finer classification for articulatory positions. Prosodic phenomena such as stress, tone, intonation, and duration are described by the primary prosodic parameters of phonetic duration, average laryngeal frequency, and average speech power. While the classification system of Peterson and Shoup is quite closely tied to speech physiology, any classification system must ultimately be based on the significance of the parameters in the linguistic structure of various languages. For instance, a difference in horizontal place of articulation—labial as opposed to alveolar—is used by many languages to signal the difference between words—*me* /mi/ as opposed to *knee* /ni/. Furthermore, within a language all labial sounds are likely to have similar properties. These facts about linguistic structure are evidence that horizontal place of articulation is an important phonetic parameter.

The phonetic classificatory system of Chomsky and Halle (1968) contrasts strongly with that of Peterson and Shoup. Their system is based primarily on the structure of languages and only secondarily on speech physiology. In spite of this difference, both systems have many points in common. Whether the description is in terms of actual positions or target positions and whether the classification is based on physiology or linguistic structure, the science of phonetics provides a system for describing the physical aspect of any utterance as precisely as necessary, independent of the language to which it belongs.

Phonological Units

The problem with phonetics is that the more precise the phonetic transcription of an utterance is, the less useful it is for representing the nonphonetic aspects of the utterance. Therefore, one of the most important discoveries of modern linguistics was that for each language it is possible to specify just those aspects of the phonetic description which are necessary to distinguish the different messages or sentences of the language.

Phonemes are the smallest segmental units of a language. They have the property that an utterance may be transcribed as a sequence of phonemes without ever losing any linguistically significant information. While phonemes are related to the pronunciation of an utterance, they are abstract units and not just a phonetic category. For example, the pronunciation of a given phoneme can change dramatically during the history of a language. On the other hand, a phoneme at a particular time is generally associated with a group of similar sounds.

The primary property of phonemes is that they are adequate units for encoding the utterances of a particular language. However, they are also units of some psychological importance. It is generally easy to teach native speakers of a language to use an alphabet based on phonemes. It is very difficult to teach speakers to use an alphabet which distinguishes sounds that belong to the same phoneme unless there is a nonphonetic basis for the distinction. In other words, native speakers of a language seem to classify sounds into phoneme-sized units automatically.

Since the phonemes of a language are important for transcription, a great effort has been made to develop techniques for phonemic analysis. One way to identify the phonemes of a language is to construct *minimal pairs*—pairs of words which can be phonetically similar except in one segment. For example, *hid, head, had, hood* identify four different vowel phonemes /ɪ, ϵ, æ , ʊ/. Since different messages must be represented by different phonemic spellings, the contrast between minimal pairs is an important technique for recognizing phonemes.

The minimal-pair technique can show that two phonetic units or *phones* must belong to different phonemes. An additional assumption is usually made that if a phone represents a phoneme in one place, every occurrence of that phone will represent the same phoneme. This assumption is equivalent to the claim that phonemes are sets of sounds or phones. Unfortunately, there are certain facts which contradict this claim. The words *spin, pin,* and *bin* would normally be represented phonemically as /sp ɪn, p ɪn, and b ɪn/. Phonetically, however, they are [spɪn, pʰɪn, p ɪn] since both /p/ following /s/ and /b/ are phonetically [p]. As another, more difficult example, the word pairs Adam-atom, bidder-bitter, ladder-latter are often pronounced the same way, at least in conversational speech. Since they are phonemically different, the same sound [ɾ] can represent either of the phonemes /t/ or /d/. Therefore, a phoneme is not always a nonoverlapping set of sounds.

The difficulties cited above have been recognized for 40 years. In spite of such marginal cases, however, a phonemic analysis can be made under the assumption that phonetic overlap will not occur very often. The resulting phonemic alphabet will be useful for transcribing the utterances of the language.

Phonemes are phonological units, but unlike letters of the alphabet, they are systematically related. The phonemes /p, t, k/ contrast in manner of articulation with /m, n, ɔ/; among themselves /p, t, k/ are distinguished by their horizontal place of articulation. It has been suggested that phonemes are not really units of phonology but that, instead, they are themselves composed of the features of parameter values which distinguish them from the other sounds of the language. The relationship between phoneme and feature might be considered analogous to the relationship between a chord and the individual notes which constitute the chord. Under this conception of phonology, an utterance is a matrix in which certain feature or parameter values are specified. For example:

(32)

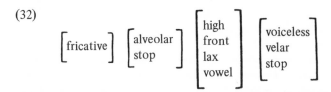

Values for unspecified features can then be added by the phonological rules until a fully specified sequence of phonological parameters is obtained.

(33)

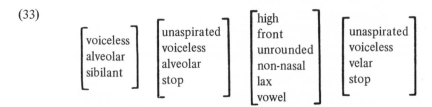

The resulting matrix represents the pronunciation of the utterance "stick." This conception of phonology is most fully presented in Chomsky and Halle (1968).

Phonological Rules

The rules which relate the surface structure of a sentence to its representation as a sequence of phonemes, a matrix of feature values, or a phonetic transcription are quite complex. For example, a noun phrase such as *the red hoúse* normally has its strongest stress on the final word. Contrastive emphasis, of course, can move the stress to almost any other word in the noun phrase. However, when *red house* is a noun or noun compound similar to whíte house or gréen *house*, the stress is on the first part; the second word is weaker than in the corresponding contrastive noun phrase *the réd hoùse*. Thus the stress pattern of a sequence of words is determined both by their syntactic structure and by their meaning.

Within a word, the placement of stress is determined by factors such as the types of morphemes in the suffix. The placement of stress itself determines the pronunciation of the word. For example:

(34)

telegraph   / t é l ə g r ǽ f /

telegraphy   / t ə l é g r ə f ì /

democrat   / d é m ə k r ǽ t /

democracy   / d ə m á k r ə s ì /

While proposed phonological rules for English are quite complex (Chomsky and Halle, 1968) and still open to question, the following example is illustrative. When a morpheme beginning with a high front vowel such as /i, ɪ / is suffixed to a morpheme which ends in an alveolar or voiceless velar stop /k, t, d/, the stop becomes an alveolar sibilant /s, z/.

(35)

/o p e k/ # / ɪ t i/ ⇒ /o p ǽ s ɪ ti/ opacity

/p a ɪ r ə t/ # /i/ ⇒ /p a ɪ r ə s i/ piracy

This rule may be represented as

(36)

$$
\begin{bmatrix} \begin{Bmatrix} \text{voiceless velar} \\ \text{or alveolar} \end{Bmatrix} \text{stop} \end{bmatrix} \rightarrow \begin{bmatrix} \text{alveolar} \\ \text{sibilant} \end{bmatrix} \ / \underline{\quad} \# \begin{bmatrix} \text{high} \\ \text{front} \\ \text{vowel} \end{bmatrix}
$$

where # represents a boundary between morphemes and a → b /__ c means replace the features *a* with the features *b*, when in the environment *c*.

Another rule is that alveolar sibilants followed by high front vowels become palatal sibilants /ʃ, 3/ when followed by a vowel.

(37)

/res/ # /iəl/ ⇒ /reʃəl/ racial

/laǰɪk/ # /iən/ ⇒ /laǰɪsiən/ ⇒ /laǰɪʃən/ logician

(38)

$$\begin{bmatrix} \text{alveolar} \\ \text{sibilant} \end{bmatrix} \begin{bmatrix} \text{high} \\ \text{front} \\ \text{vowel} \end{bmatrix} \rightarrow \begin{bmatrix} \text{palatal} \\ \text{sibilant} \end{bmatrix} /\underline{\qquad} \text{vowel}$$

Finally, a voiced alveolar sibilant /z/ becomes voiceless /s/ before the morpheme /ɪv/.

(39)

/əbiyuz/ # /ɪv/ ⇒ /əbiyusɪv/ abusive

/prsued/ # /ɪv/ ⇒ /prsuezɪv/ ⇒ /prsuesɪv/ persuasive

(40)

$$\begin{bmatrix} \text{voiced} \\ \text{alveolar} \\ \text{sibilant} \end{bmatrix} \rightarrow \text{voiceless} \quad /\underline{\qquad} \# \text{ ɪv}$$

These rules are also used in the pronunciation of the words

logicism	democracy	expression
erasure	enclosure	revision
relation	ignition	presidential
persuasion	corrosive	corrosion
decisive		

The relationship between phonology and syntax should now be apparent. The syntactic rules define surface-structure trees. The bottom nodes on the trees are matrices of features which represent the morphemes that make up the sentence. Redundant features have been added by the phonological rules to the features present in the lexicon. The higher nodes in the tree represent the superficial syntactic information which is necessary to determine stress placement.

The phonological rules operate on the surface structure, assigning stress and changing feature values until a fully specified matrix is derived. This matrix, which is the output of the phonological rules, specifies the pronunciation of the utterance.

LANGUAGE STRUCTURE AND ITS RELEVANCE TO LANGUAGE DISABILITIES IN CHILDREN

The foregoing sections offer a basis from which to view some aspects of language disabilities in children. It was our intent to describe the structure of language as seen by the linguist. Such a description avoids any consideration of the applications that might be made of the information provided. It is obvious that the linguist (even the psycholinguist) has only an indirect interest in language disabilities in children. On the other hand, the speech pathologist, reading specialist, educator, and other professionals have such applications as their primary interest.

Several points are of significance. First, the study of language structure reveals the complexity of language as a means of communication. Second, while it is possible to focus on the phonological, syntactic, and semantic aspects of language, they are not separate in the reality of the language user. Thus, what might appear as "simple" articulatory errors may be a reflection of the child's inability to use a particular morphemic rule appropriately. Such an "error" may not be an error at all, but an aspect of the dialect spoken by the child. Third, language occurs in a social climate, not in isolation from the environment. The child's vocabulary and its use in sentences often must be interpreted in the light of the linguistic community. Words which have one meaning in one subgroup in the society may have a very different meaning in another. Fourth, it must be kept in mind that factors such as intelligence, perceptual abilities, memory capacity, and learning potential all have a bearing on how language is used. It is essential that the distinction between a theory of language and a theory of a language user be maintained when applications of the study of the structure of language are made to children with language disabilities. Knowledge of the structure of language will permit the construction of evaluative instruments which can tap various aspects of language use. Such instruments could well focus on discerning whether a child demonstrated a disability in the application of linguistic competence or in the ability to efficiently use the competence he has. Each of the areas of language structure must be assessed as part of a total evaluation. In addition, the interactions of the various components of the language as used by the child must be examined. New developmental scales will have to be developed which take into account the knowledge we have concerning the structure of language. This will be necessary for evaluation and treatment.

Those concerned with language disabilities in children must know how and why language is the way it is before they can fully appreciate how it is disabled. There is still much that the theoretical linguist must tell us, but he has provided a starting point. We have the map; how far we can travel is still unknown.

REFERENCES

Alston, W. P. 1964. Philosophy of Language. Englewood Cliffs, N. J., Prentice-Hall.

Austin, J. L. 1962. *In* Urmson, J. O., ed., How To Do Things with Words. New York, Oxford University Press.

Bach, Emmon. 1964. An Introduction to Transformational Grammars. New York, Holt, Rinehart and Winston.

Bolinger, Dwight. 1968. Aspects of Language. New York, Harcourt Brace Jovanovich.

Chomsky, Noam. 1957. Syntactic Structures. The Hague, Mouton and Co.

——— 1964. Current Issues in Linguistic Theory. The Hague, Mouton and Co.

——— 1965. Aspects of the Theory of Syntax. Cambridge, Mass. The MIT Press.

——— 1968. Language and Mind. New York, Harcourt Brace Jovanovich.

——— and Morris Halle. 1968. The Sound Pattern of English. New York, Harper & Row.

——— and G. A. Miller. 1963. Introduction to the formal analysis of natural languages. *In* Luce, R. D., R. Bush, and E. Galanter, eds., Handbook of Mathematical Psychology, Vol. 2:269-321. New York, John Wiley & Sons.

Deese, James. 1965. The Structure of Associations in Language and Thought. Baltimore, Johns Hopkins Press.

Denes, P. B., and E. N. Pinson. 1963. The Speech Chain. Murray Hill, N. J., Bell Telephone Laboratories.

Fant, Gunnar. 1960. Acoustic Theory of Speech Production. The Hague, Mouton and Co.

Fodor, J. A., and J. J. Katz, eds. 1964. The Structure of Language: Readings in the Philosophy of Language. Englewood Cliffs, N. J., Prentice-Hall.

Gleason, H. A. 1961. An Introduction to Descriptive Linguistics, 2nd rev. ed. New York, Holt, Rinehart and Winston.

Goodenough, W. H. 1956. Componential analysis and the study of meaning. Language, 32:195-216.

Greenberg, Joseph, ed. 1963. Universals in Language. Cambridge, Mass., The MIT Press.

——— 1966. Language Universals. (Janua Linguarum, Series Minor, 59.) The Hague, Mouton and Co.

Harms, R. T. 1968. Introduction to Phonological theory. Englewood Cliffs, N. J., Prentice-Hall.

Hockett, C. F. 1958. A Course in Modern Linguistics. New York, Macmillan.

Jacobs, R. A., and P. S. Rosenbaum. 1968. English Transformational Grammar. Waltham, Mass., Xerox (Blaisdell).

Jakobson, Roman, Gunnar Fant, and Morris Halle. 1952. Preliminaries to Speech Analysis. Cambridge, Mass., The MIT Press.

——— and M. Halle: 1956. Fundamentals of Language. The Hague, Mouton and Co.

Ladefoged, Peter. 1962. Elements of Acoustic Phonetics. Chicago, University of Chicago Press.

Lamb, S. M. 1966. Outline of Stratificational Grammar. Washington, D. C., Georgetown University Press.

Langacker, R. W. 1968. Language and Its Structure. New York, Harcourt Brace Jovanovich.

Langendoen, T. 1969. The Study of Syntax. New York, Holt, Rinehart and Winston.

Lashley, K. S. 1951. The problem of serial order in behavior. *In* Jeffress, L. A., ed., Cerebral Mechanisms in Behavior. pp. 112-136. (The Hixon Symposium.) New York, John Wiley & Sons.

Lenneberg, E. H. 1967. Biological Foundations of Language. New York, John Wiley & Sons.

Luce, R. D., R. R. Bush, and E. Galanter. 1963. Handbook of Mathematical Psychology, Vol. 2. New York, John Wiley & Sons.

Lyons, John. 1968. Introduction to Theoretical Linguistics. New York, Cambridge University Press.

Malmberg, Bertil, ed. 1968. Manual of Phonetics. Amsterdam, North-Holland Publishing Co.

Peterson, G. E., and J. Shoup. 1966a. A physiological theory of phonetics. J. Speech Hearing Res., 9(1):5-67.

———— and J. Shoup. 1966b. The elements of an acoustic phonetic theory. J. Speech Hearing Res., 9(1):68-120.

Postal, P. M. 1964. Constituent Structure: A Study of Contemporary Models of Syntactic Description. Bloomington, Ind., Indiana University Publications in Folklore and Linguistics.

———— 1968. Aspects of Phonological Theory. New York, Harper & Row.

Potter, R. K., G. Kopp, and H. G. Kopp. 1966. Visible Speech. New York, Dover Publications.

Reibel, D. A., and S. S. Shane, eds. 1969. Modern Studies in English. Englewood Cliffs, N. J., Prentice-Hall.

Searle, J. R. 1969. Speech Acts: An Essay in the Philosophy of Language. New York, Cambridge University Press.

Vendler, Zeno. 1967. Linguistics in Philosophy. Ithaca, N. Y., Cornell University Press.

Wallace, F. C., and J. Atkins. 1960. The meaning of kinship terms. Amer. Anthropol., 62:58-80.

Wittgenstein, L. 1953. Philosophical Investigations. Oxford, Basil Blackwell & Mott.

2: The onset of language

Orlando Taylor and David Swinney

While there are numerous definitions of language disorders, most state, in one form or another, that such disorders are deviations from normal language expectations. These definitions implicitly require knowledge of normal language behavior in order that valid judgments can be made about pathological language. Since, among other factors, linguistic "normalcy" is a function of age, the topic of language disorders must be viewed from a developmental framework.

Although a substantial number of language pathologists have articulated a recognition of the importance of language acquisition data to the diagnosis and management of language disorders, few have attempted to transfer recognition into specific application. Even worse, many language pathologists have approached their missions with little contemporary information on language acquisition. This situation is related, in part, to the abundance of language acquisition research being done in disciplines outside of speech and language pathology, especially in linguistics, psycholinguistics, and sociolinguistics.

As stated elsewhere in this book, linguists are interested in writing theoretical grammars for an idealized language system which will account for all grammatical and novel sentences of a language. Psycholinguists are interested in determining the psychological principles which permit human beings to do such things as acquire, comprehend, produce, store, and perceive a language. Sociolinguists are interested in the interaction between language and culture and, therefore, in the nature and history of linguistic variations within a specified sociocultural setting.

Before presenting the status of research and theory on the acquisition of American English, it should be noted that the topic has almost always been approached from the context of the vocalizations of white, middle-class children. The importance of this point is obvious in light of contemporary sociolinguistic theory which supports the legitimacy of all variations (dialects) of American English. These dialects, which result from the history and culture of their speakers, are realized as identifiable ethnic, regional, and social markings on the English language. Thus, if one is to make valid judgments about linguistic pathologies in children, the judgments must be made in the context of the language system of the child's linguistic community.

33

LANGUAGE ACQUISITION DATA

Philosophies and Methodologies

During the past half century there has been an abundance of research on language acquisition. Prior to the late 1950s, most of this research focused on the establishment of developmental milestones for a predetermined set of linguistic categories in the areas of phonology, lexicology, and grammar. In general, the research was designed without regard to a particular theory of language or language learning. Results were frequently rationalized in a post hoc manner by employing such arguments as experience, learning, and biological maturation.

In addition to theoretical insufficiencies of the more traditional types of language acquisition research, there were several other shortcomings. First, most of this research focused on linguistic production, not comprehension—the aspect of linguistic perform- ance which (1) precedes and exceeds production, and (2) may provide a clearer insight into users' linguistic competence than production. Second, there were substantial variations in experimental design. For example, some of the research was of a laboratory type in which language behavior was elicited and recorded from a cross section of carefully controlled children with respect to such variables as intelligence, age, geography, and so on. These data were typically generalized into a normal developmental sequence. Other researchers observed and recorded spontaneous language of a small number of children (frequently one) over a specified time period. Examples of the former type of work are seen in the research of Irwin and his colleagues (1948) and Templin (1957). Research of the latter type is exemplified by Weir (1962). Because of variations in such areas as sampling techniques, experimental designs, measurement criteria, and dialectic differences, many differences are observable in data generated from traditional language acquisition research.

The emergence of transformational generative theory in the form of Chomsky's (1957) *Syntactic Structures* had a great influence on language acquisition research. Fundamental to the theory was the assumption that language users operate with a set of rules which permit production and comprehension of a nearly infinite number of grammatical sentences of a specified language system. This theory, and its more recent refinements, has caused most contemporary language acquisition scholars to raise serious questions about the importance and validity of traditional language development research which failed to focus on the underlying grammatical rules children must use to produce and comprehend increasingly complex sentences.

The use of a model of language which might be applicable to explanations of how human beings actually use linguistic symbols has resulted in significant improvements in the understanding of language acquisition processes. Data derived from experimental designs based on the model have also been useful for evaluating the "psychological reality" of rules posited by transformational grammarians. Further, they contribute to the broader goals of psycholinguistic theory, i.e., development of a theory of language use with respect to production, comprehension, memory, perception, and so forth.

Though contemporary research in language acquisition has profited from developments in linguistics and psycholinguistics, there has been a continued tendency to study only white, middle-class subjects. As a result, the work has a definite Standard English orientation. There has also been a continued overemphasis on language production (rather than comprehension) as a valid indicator of underlying linguistic competence. (Distinctions among competence, performance, production, and comprehension are presented in Chapter 1 of this book.)

Most recent psycholinguistic work in acquisition has been longitudinal and observational in character, rather than of a laboratory type. Relatively few subjects have been used, although this tendency may not be much of a problem since there seems to be great similarity among acquisition patterns observed in children studied.

Data on Phonological Acquisition

In studying phonological maturation in children, distinctions should be made between sound productions during early life which appear to have a nonsocial purpose (i.e., babbling) and sound production following the onset of language.[1] In other words, the process should be viewed as development from a general phonetic to a language specific phonemic system. Obviously, there is a point at which these two systems overlap. The most frequently articulated generalities about the acquisition of the entire system by American children (white, middle-class) are as follows. [Data on phonological acquisition are presented in more detail by McCarthy (1954), Wood (1964), and Winitz (1969).][2]

1. Type and frequency of phoneme production increase with age, with the number of different phonemes increasing from 7 during the first 1 or 2 months of life, to 27 by age 30 months. ("Phoneme" in this context has almost always been from the framework of the phonemic system of adult Standard English.)

2. In early life, vowels are more common than consonants. After the first year of life, the pattern shifts until approximations of adult vowel-consonant patterns are reached.

3. Newborn infants utter three front vowels, primarily: /i/, /e/, and (∧/. With increasing age, the proportion of back vowels increases while the proportion of front vowels decreases. Middle vowels maintain a stable level. Adult vowel approximations are reached around age 2½.

4. Infants produce a preponderance of back (mainly glottal) consonants, presumably related to reflexive chewing, sucking, and swallowing activity. Progressively fewer back consonants are produced with advancing age. Postdentals, labials, and labiodentals increase with age. Velars and dentals remain relatively unaffected by age.

---

[1] In the present context, sound productions in the language period include echolalia (the repetition of a verbal stimulus), jargon (simulations of mature verbal behavior with recognizable intonational contours and some distinguishable articulatory features), single words, and sentences.

[2] These general patterns show an obvious shift from nonsocial vocal play to increasingly more accurate approximations to the language of the child's environment. For this reason, the phenomena which have been reported are, indeed, expected.

5. Stops, mainly /k/ and /g/, and fricatives, generally /h/, are the major manners of articulation of young children. Glides, semivowels, and nasals appear around the fourth month of life. With advancing age, the latter three categories show increases, while the proportion of fricatives decreases.

Despite many differences in experimental procedures and measurement criteria, research on speech sound development after the onset of language has produced extremely stable results. In general, data reported by researchers such as Wellman et al. (1931), Poole (1934), and Templin (1957) reveal that maturation for the Standard English phonological system occurs between the third and seventh years of life. Further, analysis of speech sound acquisition data as a function of age clearly shows that certain sounds tend to reach adult levels before other sounds.

Winitz (1969) notes that it is difficult to make generalities on the maturation of Standard English phonemes by traditional notions of place and manner of articulation. For example, because of inconsistencies in the acquisition pattern, stops (with the exception of /t/) are acquired before the development of other sounds. Conversely, continuants (with the exception of /f/ and /h/) are mastered relatively late. Voicing elements for cognate sounds are typically separated by 2-year intervals, but the patterns are inconsistent. In some cases, the voiced parallel is mastered initially (e.g., /d/ before /t/), while in other instances the devoiced element is acquired first (e.g., /s/ before /z/).

Jakobson and Halle (1956) assert that there is an identifiable hierarchy of distinctive, phonological features which are acquired by children. (Sounds are characterized as groups of distinctive features, whereby each sound is distinguishable from every other sound on the basis of at least one feature.) The most generic distinctions are presumed to occur in early life with differentiation occurring with age. Thus, Jakobson and Halle argue that the consonant-vowel distinction is the first to be made by children.

Winitz (1969) has summarized in Fig. 1 Jakobson and Halle's claims on the development of distinctive features. Winitz's pictorial representation suggests the following hierarchy of feature acquisition:

1. nonvocalic vs. vocalic
2. consonantal vs. nonconsonantal
3. nasal consonants vs. oral consonants
4. acute consonants vs. grave consonants
5. narrow vowels vs. wide vowels
6. narrow vowels (diffuse): palatal vowels vs. velar vowels
7. wide vowels (compact): palatal vowels vs. velar vowels
8. compact consonants vs. diffuse, grave diffuse, and acute diffuse consonants
9. interrupted consonants vs. continuant consonants; tense consonants vs. lax consonants; and mellow consonants vs. strident consonants

Menyuk (1969) has also commented on the role of distinctive features in phonological acquisition. Her observations of five features in both American and Japanese children revealed a remarkable degree of similarity among the children, the order of feature acquisition being nasal, grave, voice, diffuse, continuant, and strident. The work, though admittedly preliminary, suggests some universal aspects of phonological acquisition, at least on the production side.

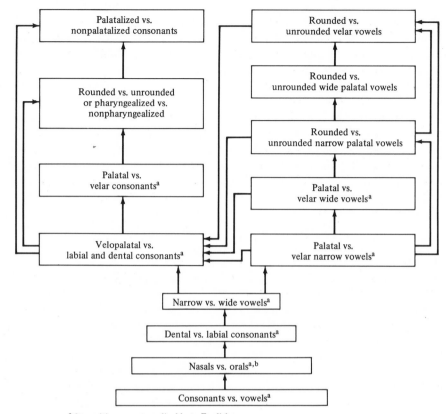

Figure 1. Pictorial representation of Jakobson and Halle's model for the development of phoneme contrasts. Some contrasts are prerequisites for other contrasts. These prerequisites are indicated by an arrow. For example, the fourth contrast, narrow versus wide vowels, cannot occur until the first three contrasts are learned. After the narrow versus wide vowel contrast is learned, one of two contrasts is learned: either velopalatal versus labial or dental versus velar narrow vowels. From here on the reader can trace the phoneme splits that can occur, using the arrows to direct himself and remembering that not all contrasts occur in every language. Adapted from R. Jakobson and M. Halle (1956). Source: Winitz, H., Articulatory Acquisition and Behavior, © 1969, p. 91. By permission of Appleton-Century-Crofts, Meredith Corporation, New York.

Menyuk has argued further that the acquisition of features in children is different from adult norms on frequency of feature usage, the adult order being diffuse, nasal, voice, continuant, strident, and grave. This observation gives rise to a suspicion that imitation alone cannot explain the pattern of phonological acquisition by children.

Traditional research in phonemic acquisition often focused on speech sounds outside the context of other developmental aspects of language. Transformational theory suggests that the phonological component of the grammar is best understood and rationalized on the basis of the strings generated by the syntactic and semantic components. In other words, phonological rules are applied to the surface structures generated by the grammar. Thus, it seems reasonable to postulate that phonological development is related to grammatical development. It is also reasonable to argue that sound elements must be psychologically real, at least from a perceptual standpoint, in order for syntax to develop. Since comprehension precedes production, as will be shown later, serious questions can be raised as to when a phoneme becomes a psychological reality. One could easily make the argument, for example, that a phoneme becomes a reality when it is used as a perceptual unit. Winitz (1969, p. 122) states this position as follows:

> In this treatment of phoneme acquisition, no clear distinction has been made between the child's passive understanding of the adult phoneme system and the active use of his own phoneme system. His understanding of the adult phoneme system, or portion thereof, no doubt antedates any attempt by the child to utter language units. When a child begins to talk he has some understanding of the adult phoneme system but at the present time we do not know the level of passive development, either phonological or grammatical, that is necessary before attempts to talk are made.

A final point is that phonemic development is obviously influenced by the language being acquired. It should be obvious, therefore, that the same phonemes will not necessarily develop in all linguistic communities. For example, most American children do not develop the /x/ phoneme (the final sound in the German pronunciation in the word Bach). Likewise, some black children do not develop a medial /θ/ phoneme in words like "bathtub" and some Spanish children do not use a /z/ phoneme in words like "zebra." In all these instances, phonological differences are related to legitimate linguistic patterns, not pathologies.

Data on the Development of Spoken Vocabularies

Research on vocabulary acquisition in children has suggested that words first make their appearance sometime between months 12 and 18. There is a great variation in this aspect of verbal measurement because of differences in determining when a word attains psychological reality. Some experimenters have used a fairly loose definition, stating that a child's utterance need only approximate real words in adult language. Others have used word imitations as a criterion. Still others require spontaneous use of an utterance to denote a specified referent. Practically all definitions focus on linguistic *production*, not comprehension. Since several researchers have noted that comprehension precedes production in most phases of language growth, it is reasonable to postulate that words are actually acquired *before* their actual production. Thus, most developmental norms on vocabulary are probably conservative.

After the onset of the first words, vocabulary appears to increase rather slowly at first, quite rapidly throughout the preschool period, and then more slowly during later mental maturity. Vocabulary growth never ceases since the individual constantly learns new words and new usages of familiar words throughout life.

Some quantitative studies of vocabulary have focused on size. Smith (1941), for example, gives a typical set of figures for vocabulary growth, suggesting that the average vocabulary of first-grade, middle-class children is 23,700 (ranging from 6,000 to 48,000) words, while twelfth-grade, middle-class children frequently have vocabularies of 80,300 (ranging from 36,700 to 136,500) words. While there are numerous other figures, it is clear that children's vocabularies grow very rapidly and that their actual sizes are probably related to such factors as motivation, experiences, and, of course, the tools used to measure vocabulary.

Qualitative aspects of vocabulary growth are reflected in traditional research on "parts-of-speech" analyses. Since words have little meaning outside their grammatical context, it is very difficult to make statements about parts of speech without making statements about grammar. For this reason, parts-of-speech analyses in children can best be made by discussing child grammars.

Data on the Acquisition of Grammar

As stated earlier, much of the traditional work on the acquisition of grammar was done without sophisticated theoretical notions about natural languages. The result was that many of the measurement categories used in this research focused on surface and, in some cases, trivial aspects of linguistic performance. Perusal of this literature reveals, for example, an overabundance of data on such topics as mean length of response, amount and rate of talking, and sentence "complexity." Of course, judgments in the above areas are related to implicit assumptions about "normal" sentence length, quantity, and complexity. Readers with interest in these approaches to grammatical maturity are referred to McCarthy (1954).

Irrespective of methodological or philosophical orientation, practically all researchers agree that most children begin to form two- and three-word utterances (sentences) sometime between months 18 and 24. In addition, most contemporary writers have demonstrated that children's utterances are not random, but have underlying grammatical rules which permit generation of a large number of sentences.

Berko (1958) was among the first writers after the publication of Syntactic Structures (Chomsky, 1957) to document the fact that children operate with grammatical rules which appear to result from inductions from linguistic data provided by the environment. In a study of the ability to control certain elements of English inflectional morphology in the environment of nonsense "words," Berko found a definite hierarchical sequence for the acquisition of morphological rules. The rules, many of which were not completely acquired by first-grade children, seemed to be associated more with grammatical than with phonological factors. For example, the /s/ and /z/ allomorphs were used more correctly in the context of possessive and plural nouns than in the third-person singular of verbs, despite phonological similarity.

Berko's work was important in the sense that it demonstrated that children operated with a substantial amount of linguistic competence. The major criticism of it, however, might be that it was done from the framework of an adult grammar, rather than from a unique child grammar.

Besides Berko, other early linguistically oriented researchers of language acquisition used adult grammar orientations. For example, Ervin (1964) reported that children's grammars were reductions[3] of adult grammars where, within memory constraints, (1) the most recent and stressed words (mainly content words) are maintained, and (2) word order is preserved. Nevertheless, these researchers recognized two important aspects of child language. First, children have more advanced grammars than they demonstrate in their productions (Fraser et al., 1963). Second, sentence reductions, if they in fact exist, require some knowledge (competence) of the most important portions of sentences. For these and other reasons (e.g., children's utterances include linguistic features which they have probably never heard), several researchers (see Ervin, 1964) began to question the long-believed notion that imitation plays an important role in the acquisition of grammar. Ultimately, research was designed which made no a priori assumptions concerning the relationship between child and adult language.

Brown and Fraser (1964a, b), Ervin (1964), Braine (1963), McNeill (1966a, b), Klima and Bellugi (1966), and Menyuk (1969) are among those who have reported some of the most extensive data on early child grammars from a nonadult perspective. Though several rules have been advanced to rationalize the grammatical characteristics of these constructions, McNeill (1966a, 1967) argues that the child's first grammar can be explained adequately by the following rule:

$$\text{Sentence} \longrightarrow (P) + 0 \quad (\text{rule 1})$$

[P = optional pivot word

0 = mandatory open word]

Pivot-word classes typically have fewer members than open-word classes; however, each pivot word is used more frequently than individual open words. Further, pivot-word classes are relatively slow to take in new members. As Braine (1965) observed, pivot words have characteristics similar to function words (e.g., prepositions, articles) in adult grammar. [Open-class words behave more like adult content words (e.g., nouns, adjectives, and so on).] However, the actual class of words which are used as pivot words apparently contains many members which are not typically a part of the function-word category for adults. Indeed, many words children use as function words are similar to adult content words. This observation leads one to again raise serious questions as to whether the grammatical rules children use could be imitations of what they have heard from adults.

[3] Children's oral reductions of language are thought to be followed by oral expansions by the adult environment in which *suspected* missing elements are supplied. Reductions, and subsequent expansions, are thought by some scholars to be important aspects of child language growth (see Brown, 1964; Slobin, 1964). The precise role of reductions and expansions, especially with respect to how close they have to be to the child's intended message, is unclear.

The S ——→ (P) + 0 rule asserts that children's first sentences are constructed by optionally producing a pivot word plus a mandatory open-class word. This means that pivot words cannot stand alone, although open-class words can. In short, the rule permits production of both one- and two-word sentences by children, e.g., *shoe, green boot, here baby,* and so on.

Brown and Bellugi (1964) report that open-class words seem to be established before month 18. However, pivot-class words seem to undergo a differentiation process which does not begin until month 18. Approximately 2½ months after the onset of pivot words, articles (e.g., *a,* and *the*) and demonstratives (e.g., *that* and *this*) have differentiated from the remainder of the pivot category. At this time it is possible for sentences to occur with an optional demonstrative, plus an optional article, plus an optional pivot word, plus a required noun (rule 2). Five months after the onset, adjectives and possessives separate from the pivot class to form independent classes. This additional differentiation permits sentences by using either:

1. An optional article, plus an optional adjective, plus a required noun (rule 3).

2. An optional pivot word, plus a required noun; or an optional possessive, plus a required noun; or an optional demonstrative, plus a required noun (rule 4).

3. An optional article, plus a required noun, plus an optional adjective (rule 5).

The whole process of pivot class differentiation is presented in Fig. 2.

McNeill (1966a) has also summarized data from other sources to generate three additional early grammatical rules[4]:

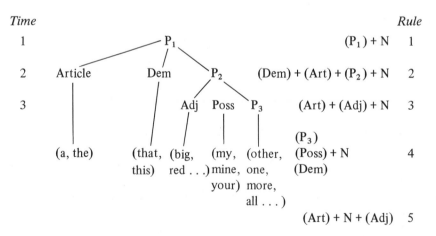

Figure 2. Differentiation of the pivot class. Abbreviations are as follows: N = noun (i.e., one of the open classes); Art = articles; Dem = demonstrative pronouns; Adj = adjectives; Poss = possessive pronouns; P_1, P_2, and P_3 = pivot class at times 1, 2, and 3, respectively. Reprinted from "Developmental Psycholinguistics" by D. McNeill. In Smith, F., and G. Miller, eds., The Genesis of Language, by permission of The MIT Press, Cambridge, Mass. Copyright © 1966, by the Massachusetts Institute of Technology.

[4] Reprinted from "Developmental Psycholinguistics" by D. McNeill *in* Smith, F., and G. Miller (eds.), The Genesis of Language, by permission of The MIT Press, Cambridge, Mass. Copyright © 1966, by the Massachusetts Institute of Technology.

1. S ⟶ N + N   rule 6

```
          S
         / \
        N   N
        |   |
      Adam  Coat
```

2. S ⟶ (P) + NP   rule 7

    NP ⟶ { (P) + N }
          { N + N   }

```
              S
            /   \
           P     NP
           |    /  \
         that {P}   N
              {N}   |
               |   Coat
               my
             Adam
```

3. S ⟶ Pred P   rule 8

    Pred P ⟶ (V) + (NP)

    NP ⟶ { (P) + N }
          { N + N   }

```
             S
             |
           Pred P
           /    \
          V      NP
          |     /  \
        want  {P}   N
              {N}   |
               |   coat
             that
             Adam
```

Menyuk (1969) added the intonational component of child language and the notion of the "sentence topic" to write rules for early child utterances. She asserts that children's earliest sentences frequently contain a single morpheme. They are "sentences" in that they reflect a competence for the concept of a sentence. They typically utilize a specific topic in the form of a phonetic or phonological string (usually a word), plus one of three available intonational markers (question, declarative, or imperative) (rule 9). Later, sentences add such components as (1) adverbial and adjectival optional modifiers (rule 10) and (2) morphological replacements for intonational markers in the form of NP, wh, or negative morphemes (rule 11).

Menyuk's early grammatical rules are as follows[5]:

---

[5] Reprinted from Sentences Children Use by P. Menyuk by permission of The MIT Press, Cambridge, Mass. Copyright © 1969 by the Massachusetts Institute of Technology.

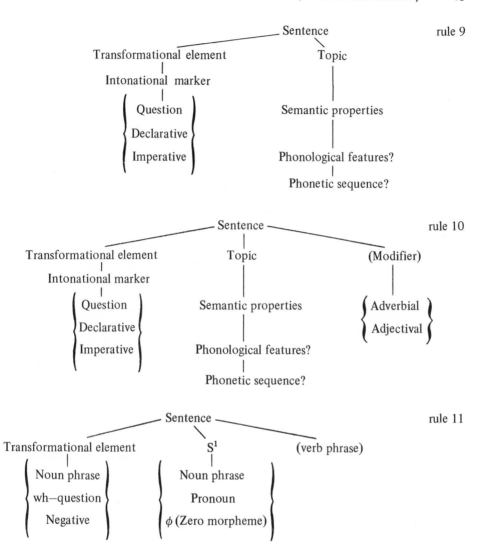

In making a case for the legitimacy of early child grammars, it should be pointed out that an argument is not being made that there is no relationship whatsoever between the kinds of sentences adults produce and those produced by children. Though different, there are certain universal features of both grammars. The notion of universals in language acquisition has been discussed by Chomsky (1964) in the form of an hypothesis which states that the first stages of linguistic development are sensitive to universal hierarchies of syntactic categories. Chomsky (1961, 1965) and Katz (1966) discuss the universal features in the form of something called a Language Acquisition Device (LAD). LAD can be imagined as being an innate structure which contains all the language universals. Linguistic data from the child's environment are fed into LAD, which has the task of selectively filtering out all the universals it contains which are unnecessary for acquiring the particular language the child will ultimately use. Thus, the child's task is to move from a set of general grammatical rules to a set of rules specific for his language. In other words, he must induce a grammar. This notion will be discussed further in a later section.

On the basis of these early two- and three-word grammars, both McNeill (1966b, c) and Menyuk (1969) argue that the early grammars of children are characterized by universal elements of the basic grammatical relations of the deep structure. McNeill asserts that the following basic grammatical relations appear in children's earliest utterances: the concepts of subject and predicate of a sentence; main verb and object of a verb phrase; and a modifier and head of a noun phrase. Menyuk supports the claim and has added that the basic grammatical elements cited by McNeill, plus others, are typically acquired by the age of three years. Slobin (1966) and McNeill (1966b) have presented data from Russian and Japanese children to support the universality of the claim. For Menyuk and McNeill these elements must be established before more complex operations (transformations) can occur.

Among other things, the above notions suggest that every word which is acquired by the child must be acquired in the context of some grammatical function, as each word is capable of assuming more than one grammatical role in a sentence. For example, a given word might assume the role of head of a noun phrase in one sentence and object of a verb phrase in another sentence.

After establishment of basic grammatical relations, children begin to apply transformational rules to generate more complex sentences. These rules either rearrange, delete, or add elements to the basic grammatical relations just discussed. Their application permits generation of a number of new, more complex sentences. The use of transformations may be related to establishment of left cerebral dominance for language. Bever (1968) suggests, however, that the shift of cerebral laterality for language from a bilateral to a left-sided function may result from changes in linguistic performance, not the reverse.

On the whole, there has been little work on the growth of transformations in children. This failure is related, in part, to the fact that a large amount of language acquisition research has focused on the language of very young children. Also, until the last few years there has been no adequate linguistic model of syntax or vocabulary, a fact which left much doubt concerning what a valid language acquisition theory need rationalize. For whatever reason, the fact is that much language acquisition research (especially in the area of grammar) has overlooked developmental patterns in children after the first 4 or 5 years of life. There have been three exceptions to this trend: the work of Klima and Bellugi (1966), Menyuk (1963, 1964b, 1969), and C. Chomsky (1968).

Klima and Bellugi's research focused primarily on the acquisition of the negative transformation. The negative transformation, in its various forms, is one of the more difficult to explain linguistically. Nevertheless, negative sentences, in one form or another, are present in children's language almost from the outset of sentence generation. Klima and Bellugi suggested four stages in the acquisition of negatives. The first stage, which is pretransformational, occurs early in the acquisition process and involves a grammatical rule similar to one of the early rules described by Menyuk (rule 11). At this stage, there are no negatives within the sentence and there are no auxiliary verbs. Negation is signaled by the presence of a *no* or *not* outside the nucleus of a sentence. Further, there is no evidence to suggest that the child even understands the negative embedded in the auxiliary of adult speech. The rule for stage I negation can be written as follows:

(rule 12)[6]

$$\left[\begin{Bmatrix} no \\ not \end{Bmatrix} \text{———Nucleus} \right] \quad S \quad \text{or} \quad \left[\text{Nucleus ——— no} \right] \quad S$$

Examples of negative sentences generated by this rule are *no singing song; not a teddy bear; wear mitten no.*

Stage II, which appears 3 to 6 months after the onset of negatives, still shows no use of transformations. However, auxiliaries (*don't* and *can't*) are used uniquely before nonprogressive main verbs in negative constructions; i.e., they are not used elsewhere in the grammar. It is also clear that children understand the negative embedded in the auxiliary at this stage. Stage II negation can be considered as follows:

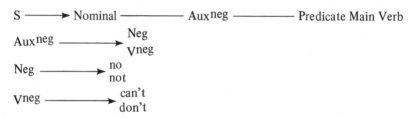

Examples of stage II negative sentences are *That no mommy, He not little, he big, I can't talk,* and *I don't want it.*

In stage III, another 3 to 6 months later, modal auxiliaries *can* and *will, do* and *be* appear in negative sentences, as well as in declarative and interrogative sentences. In these sentences *be* is optional, but restricted to predicate and progressive. *Can* and *do* are restricted to nonprogressive main verbs. Stage III negation can be considered as follows:

S ⟶ Nominal ——— Aux ——— Predicate Main Verb   (rule 13)[6]

Aux ⟶ Tense ——— Vaux ——— (Neg)

Vaux ⟶ Modal (will or can) do / be

[6] Figures from Klima, E., and U. Bellugi. Syntactic Regularities in the Speech of Children. *In* Lyons, J., and R. Wales (eds.), Psycholinguistic Papers, The University Press, Edinburgh, 1966. By permission of The University Press, Edinburgh, Scotland.

Examples of stage III negatives are as follows: *You didn't caught me, I can't see it, That was not me,* and *I gave him some so he won't cry.*

At the fourth stage, two main types of transformations are reported. They are

Optional *be* deletion   (rule 14)[6]

$$NP \text{———} be \Longrightarrow NP$$

Do deletion

$$do \text{———} V \Longrightarrow V$$

At this stage, negative auxiliaries are no longer limited to *don't* and *can't.* Further, auxiliary verbs now appear in other kinds of sentences and, therefore, can be considered as being separate from the negative element of sentences. Another feature of this early transformational stage is the appearance of indeterminates in affirmative and negative sentences, e.g., *I want some supper* and *I don't want some supper.*

Klima and Bellugi have discussed the development of the interrogative transformation in a manner similar to the one used to describe negation. In fairly great detail, they trace the growth of questions from an early stage in which yes/no and wh-*like* (e.g., *See hole?, Where milk go?*, etc.) questions are produced through the acquisition of interrogative proposing, interrogative inversion, and *do* deletion transformations.

Menyuk (1969) has made observations similar to those of Bellugi concerning transformational growth. While recognizing that sentences requiring transformations are generally not produced until the establishment of deep structures, Menyuk notes that even the earliest utterances of children have some elements to which transformations would apply, although they are not used in production. For example, in the growth of negatives it seems as though the negative transformation concept is recognized by the child even though his production of negation is marked only by intonation on a deep structure string. Thus, one might postulate a competence for certain transformational elements, even when oral performance does not necessarily reveal it. This point reinforces the need for data on comprehension acquisition in order to induce valid judgments of child linguistic competence.

Carol Chomsky (1968) has also addressed herself to the topic of late grammatical development. Though her work focused on comprehension, the results show that some grammatical constructions are not acquired until the fifth year of life. In view of the lead comprehension has over production, it is probable that production of these same constructions will not appear until after the age of 5. Chomsky's work will be discussed in the following section.

Data on the Acquisition of Linguistic Comprehension

Most authorities agree that comprehension of a specific linguistic unit precedes the ability to produce that same unit. (In fact, comprehension is thought to remain superior to production throughout life.) McNeill (1966a) argues that this phenomenon should be expected since passive control (comprehension) of a given linguistic unit has less obstructing and distorting factors separating it from competence than active control (production). For example, motor programming and execution are not possible sources of "noise" during comprehension, though they are during production. This assumption, if correct, provides support to the notion that data on comprehension acquisition might provide more valid insights into children's linguistic competence than production.

Despite general agreement with the above assertions, few researchers have reported data on the acquisition of linguistic comprehension. This dearth of research may be related to the absence of adequate psycholinguistic models and experimental paradigms for assessing comprehension in any group of subjects, irrespective of age.[7] Obviously, it will be difficult if not impossible, to obtain valid data on comprehension acquisition during childhood until these problems are resolved. One of the most complete studies of linguistic comprehension is reported by Fraser et al. (1963).[8] They presented paired sentences representative of 10 grammatical contrasts (e.g., *the sheep is jumping/the sheep are jumping*) to a group of twelve 3- to 3½-year-old boys and girls. Subjects were required to (1) imitate the sentences, (2) point to appropriate pictures to indicate comprehension of the sentences, and (3) produce sentences from the same pictures to indicate active control of the contrasts.

Fraser, Bellugi, and Brown's results provide formal support for many of the theoretical notions stated throughout this chapter.

Specifically, they show that imitation ability exceeds comprehension, which, in turn, exceeds production. The data also suggest a performance hierarchy for grammatical complexity. The grammatical hierarchy for comprehension, shown in comparison with imitation and production, is presented in Table 1.

Gaer (1969) has also studied comprehension in terms of modern grammatical theory. He reports that children's relative abilities to comprehend certain transformations vary as

---

[7] A major exception is the "decoding" hypothesis (see Gough, 1965). It states that linguistic comprehension involves the inverse of the processes used to generate sentences. Thus, comprehension is achieved by (1) perceiving the phonological representation of an utterance by assigning appropriate phonological rules to it; (2) assigning appropriate surface structure to phonological information; (3) discovering the transformational rules which were obviously necessary to generate the surface structure; (4) assigning the proper deep structure to the surface structure, based on the application of (3); and (5) assigning the appropriate semantic and conceptual categories to the basic grammatical relations of the deep structure. Obviously, memory and perception influence the efficiency with which the entire system operates.

[8] There has been work (mainly of the normative type) in acquisition of vocabulary comprehension (e.g., Peabody, 1959; Templin, 1957) and the comprehension of grammatical form classes (e.g., Wolski, 1962; Carrow, 1968). This research has been based generally on Standard English expectations. Obviously, the data generated from research of this type should not be generalized or considered "normal" for children from all linguistic communities in the United States.

Table 1. Grammatical Hierarchy for Imitation, Comprehension, and Production.

	Feature	Comprehension rank	Imitation rank	Production rank
1.	Affirmative/Negative	1	5	1
2.	Subject/Object, in active voice	2	4	2
3.	Present Progressive tense/future tense	3	2	5
		3	2	5
4.	Singular/Plural, of 3rd-person possessive pronouns	4	1	3
5.	Present progressive tense/past tense	5	6	6
6.	Mass noun/count noun	6	8	9
7.	Singular/Plural, marked by is and are	7	3	4
8.	Singular/Plural, marked by inflections	8	7	10
9.	Subject/Object, in passive voice	9	9	8
10.	Indirect object/direct object	10	10	7

a function of age. At age 3 they seem to understand active, passive, question, and negative transformations more or less equally well, performing at about 58 percent accuracy. By age 4 active sentences are understood better than questions, which, in turn, are better understood than passives and negatives. For 5- and 6-year-old children actives, questions, and passives show no difference, all being understood better than negatives. Adults, on the other hand, tend to understand all these transformations at about 95 percent accuracy.

Carol Chomsky (1968) has reported an experiment on late grammatical acquisition which focused primarily on comprehension. Her task required a group of children to manipulate dolls, pictures, objects, and so on, to indicate comprehension, and in some cases production, of a set of sentences of the following structural types:

Structure	*Category*
1. John is easy to see.	Easy to see
2. John promised Bill to go.	Promise
3. John asked Bill what to do.	Ask/tell
4. He knew that John was going to win the race.	Pronominization

Chomsky's data show that syntactic development continues until at least the ninth year of life. While there were individual variations in the exact time children seemed to acquire the above structures, as well as differences in the acquisition pattern for each structure, the following developmental hierarchy emerged:

1. Pronominization—about 5.6 years

2. Easy to see; promise—between the ages of 5.6 and 9 years

3. Ask/tell—often past year 10

Though incomplete, data presently available on comprehension provide some very important insights into the process of language maturation. Unfortunately, not enough data are available. Specifically, all structures have not been studied, all ages have not been assessed, and dialectic considerations have largely been ignored. Therefore, application of these data must be done with caution.

SUBSYMBOLIC SYSTEMS RELATED TO LANGUAGE ACQUISITION

A crude, but topically comprehensive, model of the total communication system is displayed in Fig. 3. The model is relevant to language acquisition research in that it

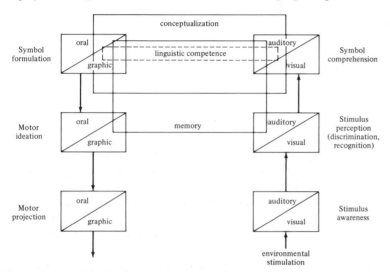

Figure 3. Model of a human communication system based, in part, on models of Osgood (1953) in Osgood, C., and M. Miron, Approaches to the Study of Aphasia, © 1953. Permission for publication of adaptions by University of Illinois Press, Urbana, Illinois.

indicates the several sensory, cognitive, and motor systems necessary for normal linguistic performance (i.e., symbol comprehension and production). These prerequisite systems can be called "subsymbolic" in that they are required for normal symbolic behavior though, in and of themselves, they are not symbolic. Their status and acquisition can affect the child's development of language. Some general information in these areas will be summarized.

Memory

Some comprehension research has been based on a theoretical model which suggests that sentences are understood by assigning appropriate deep structures to surface structures through inverse application of the transformational rules used to generate them (e.g., Gough, 1965). It is assumed that grammatical structures must be coded into some storable unit(s) and retained in memory so as to make comprehension possible (see Miller,

1962; Savin and Perchanock, 1965). Presumably, sentence decoders retain sentences in their short-term memory and subject them to linguistic rules stored in their long-term memory, [Evidence is given for this dichotomization of memory in Milner's (1959) research on hypocampal lesions. She reports that there is apparently a breakdown of both retrieval and input to long-term store, but that short-term store remains intact.] Production does not seem to require the short-term memory aspect, but depends on a long-term memory process which permits appropriate selection of linguistic symbols and grammatical rules.

Atkinson and Shiffrin (1968) have offered one of the most comprehensive theoretical models of human memory. Their model suggests a memory which consists, among other things, of permanent structural features, which include

1. A sensory register in which information is first perceived but, thereafter, decays rapidly (within several hundred milliseconds).

2. A long-term memory which stores information relatively permanently.

3. A short-term store into which information can be selectively shifted from either the sensory register or long-term memory. Thus, short-term memory is the "working" component of memory. Short-term stored information decays in about 15 to 30 seconds, but a control process called "rehearsal" can maintain a limited number of information units as long as desired. Regardless of the form of sensory input, most information in short-term storage appears to be coded in an auditory-verbal-linguistic form.

Rohrman (1968), among others, has postulated that transformational rules may be stored in long-term memory. Thus, language comprehension requires (1) a sensory register scan of auditory inputs which allows them to be "chunked" into usable, storable sequences in short-term memory and (2) comparison and interpretation of "chunked" materials on the basis of basic grammatical relations and transformational rules stored in long-term memory.

Perusal of the literature reveals little research on memory development as it relates to language acquisition. Zinchenko's work (1969) is an exception. He has described research on memory development which suggests that involuntary memory plays a more important role than voluntary memory in language acquisition. McNeill (1966a), in related research, has suggested three progressively longer memory spans (those for grammatical production, grammatical comprehension, and phonological production) to account for the relative order of accomplishment of children in imitation, comprehension, and production tasks. The concept, however, appears to be totally ad hoc and insufficient in light of known data on memory. The facts appear more easily explained by a concept of perceptual set or expectancy.

Perception

Memory is linked directly to perceptual aspects of cognition. It has been shown by Smirnov (1969) and Zankov (1969), for example, that the form of preattentive set influences the orientation to material that is being remembered in terms of its content, structure, and oral form. For instance, Mishkin and Forgays (1952) have found a left-to-right perceptual set important to recognition of English words and, thus, to the processing of written language. Neisser (1967) suggests that speech perception is accomplished by analysis-by-synthesis. Basically, auditory synthesis can produce units of varying size. A person can ask "What was meant?" or "What sounds are uttered?" and synthesize accordingly. Neisser (1967) discusses a "preliminary analysis of the signal," or a preattentive perceptual process, which guides and chooses the units the person uses in analysis.

The elements of language that are perceived, perhaps as determined by the hypothesized preattentive process, have long been a point of contention for researchers in the area of speech science. The International Phonetic Alphabet has been used to describe the total *sound* system of languages. In this research, phonemes have been hypothesized as being the raw perceptual materials of language. Speech sounds are classified by manner of production and by the position of the articulators in making the sound. These classifications, and others, e.g., voicing classifications, have been shown by Jakobson and Halle (1956) and Jakobson, Fant, and Halle (1967) to represent a group of distinctive features in which each separate sound can be classified and distinguished by at least one feature from every other sound. All features are defined in physical terms by the amount and concentration of energy in the frequency spectrum and by time. These physical correlates correspond roughly to the sensory perceptions of loudness of voice, pitch of voice, and subjective judgments of duration.

Acceptance of the phoneme as the basic unit of language perception has often been challenged. It is difficult to explain, for example, how allophones can be perceived as being the same or similar when the acoustic characteristics of each differ greatly (Carroll, 1964). Perhaps it is the phonemic environment, in addition to the phoneme under discussion, which is actually the perceived unit of speech. If the child depended only on phonemic discrimination, he would have to possess an enormous amount of innate knowledge concerning sound wave analysis to comprehend a language.

Jakobson and Halle (1956) suggest that the phonemic syllable appears to be the perceptual unit of language. This hypothesis follows from evidence which shows that syllables have rule-like determinability and predictability. Vowel-consonant contrasts often render the syllable prominent and permit predictions of subsequent syllables, although there are other important cognate contrasts.

Although this argument will not be pursued further, it should be noted that the syllable is by no means the universally accepted perceptual unit of speech. There are excellent arguments, using evidence of suprasegmental phonemes (e.g., stress, pitch, juncture), which indicate that the word, phrase, or even the underlying grammatical structure may well be the units of perception the human senses use in comprehending and, ultimately, in acquiring oral production (see Fodor and Bever, 1965). Obviously, further research is needed to determine the actual unit(s) of speech perception.

Three final observations concerning perception merit some discussion in relation to language acquisition. The first concerns evidence that the suprasegmental phonemes appear to be learned, or perceived, by the child in advance of some of the other patterned phonemic and syllabic units. Weir (1962) has discussed this fact in terms of the child learning the intonational contours of his language.

Second, Bever (1970) has pointed out that certain strategies basic to all perceptual processes are innate while others undoubtedly grow out of linguistic experience. Thus, perception changes with age and experience. In fact, Bever (1968) suggests that cerebral dominance for language may develop, in part, in response to external language experiences. That is, dominance for speech may be related to the behavioral strategies used by individuals in listening to sentences.

Third, Whorf (1956) has shown through the example of Indo-European languages that different linguistic communities perceive reality in different ways and that the language spoken by a community aids in structuring the cognitive processes of those speaking that language. Given that the child utilizes data provided by his environment in acquiring language, this point suggests that the language the child acquires will be molded by the perception of the world that his parents and his community share. This postulation forms the basis for a substantial amount of contemporary sociolinguistic theory.

Motor Speech Development

Motor development, much like perceptual development, appears to be largely a process of maturation. Lenneberg (1967) has indicated that the pattern of general motor development corresponds with the onset of speech and that speech is dependent upon this coordination. Miller (1951), for example, specifies that Broca's area (the part of the brain which controls motor speech) does not typically develop until the month 17, although other cortical motor centers are differentiated by month 11. In considering motor development in terms of speech development, there appear to be corresponding "stages" of motor development for each "stage" of speech development. These "stages" are really not separate, distinct steps. Rather, they are distinctive points on a developmental continuum. The physiological correlates of these speech development stages are related to changes in size and structure of the articulating and resonating apparatus, as well as to development of motor coordination.

The earliest sounds of the child appear to be a part of nondirected bodily reflex responses to new physical environments. During the first month of life the child uses crying, whimpering, and contented vocal behavior, which are believed to serve as prerequisites for later phonetic development. [Van Riper (1963) has itemized the phonetic sounds that occur during the earliest period of differentiation.] At about 8 weeks of age, the child usually begins to engage in babbling (nonsocial sound production). These random sounds are governed by the maturation of the motor mechanisms which control the movements of the lips, tongue, and so on. For instance, few, if any, back vowels are produced during this period because of the apparent difficulty in coordinating the musculature well enough to lower the tongue in the back of the mouth.

Following babbling, vocal play (social sound productions) appears around the sixth to eighth month. This activity generally includes echolalia, which Van Riper (1963) discusses as occurring in month 10 to 11, and contouring (utilization of correct adult inflection patterns with nonsensical articulatory utterances). Contouring has been discussed as one of the first linguistic features of adult language that a child acquires. Weir (1962) discusses two forms of stress and four separate distinct pitch patterns as occurring prior to articulatory features, at about the eighth month. Vocal play overlaps into the stage of purposive utterances, in which appropriate use of words or syllables occurs. This stage begins sometime near or before the end of the first year.

Theories of First Language Acquisition

Several theories of language acquisition have been advanced to rationalize the reported "facts" surrounding language development during childhood. In varying degrees, these theories take into account certain anthropological, sociological, biological, and psychological principles. The more recent ones attempt to explain assumptions implicit in contemporary linguistic (transformational) models. Regardless of viewpoint, however, a theory has not yet been presented which sufficiently accounts for both the theoretical assumptions of contemporary linguistics and the large body of empirical data on language development. Perhaps the answer will come from more descriptive data on patterns of linguistic maturation, or, possibly from refinement or restructuring of some of the present theories. Most likely, however, both are needed. Nonetheless, within the total range of present theories, attempts have been made to explain both the necessary process and the facts associated with language growth.

Loosely speaking, there are three basic postures concerning first language acquisition. (In-depth expositions of many of these theories are found in numerous sources; see Jenkins, 1967; McNeill, 1966c; and Staats, 1968.) All deal primarily with linguistic production, not comprehension. In light of some of the points discussed in preceding sections of this chapter, this fact is unfortunate since comprehension seems to always exceed production and is probably a more valid indicator of linguistic competence.

One theory might be categorized as having an empiricist or *learning* theory orientation. The term empiricist is derived from the manner in which data used to construct behavior models are collected. Only empirical, or observable, data are considered in the building of learning theories of language growth. These theories have the most extensive history and corpus of data. They are derivatives of performance learning models of observed behavior in animals and include various systems of stimulus-response contiguities. The theories in this classification range from single-stage chaining (conditioning) of stimuli and responses to complex combinations of all learning theories (see Staats, 1968). In nearly all the learning-oriented theories, the single word and its acquisition of "meaning" has been the basic linguistic unit examined and explained. Grammatical elements of the language have generally been relegated to secondary considerations by these theories (DeCecco, 1967). In essence, learning theorists assert that language is acquired through pairing of verbal behavior with proper reward situations, thus ensuring continued usage of these verbal behaviors.

The second posture concerning language acquisition is a derivative of transformational generative grammar. The theory appears to have developed out of a belief that human language behavior cannot be sufficiently expressed by descriptions of observable environmental events alone. Further, this reaction against learning theories also involves rejection of generalizations from lower animal species to humans. Close analysis of the writing of these theorists, who advocate a *nativist* or "innate propensity" orientation, reveals a preponderance of speculative and logical arguments which attempt to refute various points of learning theories. Nativists argue that the "facts" of a complex language system of linguistic rules which generate a nearly infinite number of sentences and which develops over a short number of months can only be explained by a *competence* or *innate propensity* for language. A major portion of this assumption is based on the fact that many grammatical elements the child produces are never heard by the child and, therefore, have never been reinforced.

Finally, there is a posture which represents a mixture of the above two stances. While the theorists discussed in this regard may feel more attached to one or the other of the above viewpoints, their arguments include combinations of the learning and nativist viewpoints—utilizing the most logical and persuasive points of each.

A more detailed summary and review of the principles of the above-mentioned theories follow.

Learning Theories

Learning theories of language acquisition range from simplistic to complex and have a lengthy history of development. They arose from the great need for psychology to extract itself from "mentalistic" reasoning and to evade the necessity for introspection in which much of human behavioral research was entrenched until the turn of the twentieth century. In order to implement this change, many psychologists postulated that behavioral processes should be studied in organisms less complex than man, that is, in animals. Since the origin of the empirical era in psychology, some of the extreme reaction against mentalism has changed, but present-day learning theories still tend to reflect this posture of antimentalism. In this section, we will examine learning theories in order of increasing complexity of the major stimulus-response mechanisms held as responsible for first language learning. This order of classifications does not necessarily reflect upon the quality of the explanations used to substantiate a particular model, or its ability to account for known linguistic "facts."

Markov Processes   The simplest of the learning theories, and perhaps potentially the most appealing to many psychologists (as it comes closest to molding information theory[9] with behavior theory), is one which holds that any word in an utterance is dependent upon and determined by those words which have preceded it.[10] This model is derived from the area of *Markov processes*. The process consists of the occurrence of left-to-right *chaining* of words through conditioned S-R connections. Each word has a simple, theoretically determinable, probability of occurrence based on the strength of previous associations (habit formation) between any one word and those words preceding it. Thus, based on previous experience, any word has a certain probability for eliciting future words. The following model is an example of a possible set of words elicited by preceding words:

[9] Information theory discusses transfer of information by means of reducing uncertainty (probability) through binary sampling techniques.

[10] The learning theories presented in this chapter are examples of behavior theories.

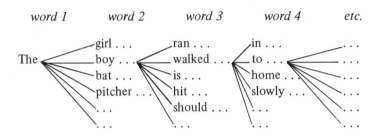

Thus, the sentence "The boy walked to . . ." could be generated in the manner illustrated above. In this model, there is no *plan* by which words might occur in the future (it is a nonanticipatory grammar), only probabilities of future developments. This structure has been demonstrated to be an insufficient model of language behavior and of syntactic acquisition on several grounds (see Miller et al., 1966). For example, the left-to-right generator only has the "grammatical" rule that once a word (or group of words) is produced, the next word(s) is chosen from a set of probabilistically related words. Chomsky (1957) has shown that English sentences are not generated through serial dependencies, but through nested dependencies (for example, think of the sentence *The dog the boy saw bit the mailman.*). This "fact" eliminates Markov processes from serious consideration as an explanation of syntactic development. Further, since both the lexicon and syntax arise only through previous experience, a speaker (or listener) would obviously have to hear *each* variation of word combinations at least once to establish sufficient contingencies to enable him to speak the potentially unlimited set of sentences he has been shown to be capable of producing. Miller et al. (1966) have shown that it would take over 100 years of continuous listening to be exposed just once to all the word combinations necessary for a man to produce all variations of sentences up to 20 words in length. Finally, the Markov process would generate many drastically ungrammatical utterances, a fact which does not occur in reality, and for which the Markov model provides no controls.

It has been noted, however, that, in contrast to the transformational model, the Markov model does provide a potentially useful theory of decision making processes for language. As will be discussed later, the transformational model only explains decisions in terms of selecting "optional" transformations, a basically mentalistic concept which imparts no predictive information.

Operant Conditioning Skinner (1957) discusses language acquisition in terms of extensions of the principles of instrumental (operant) conditioning which he and others

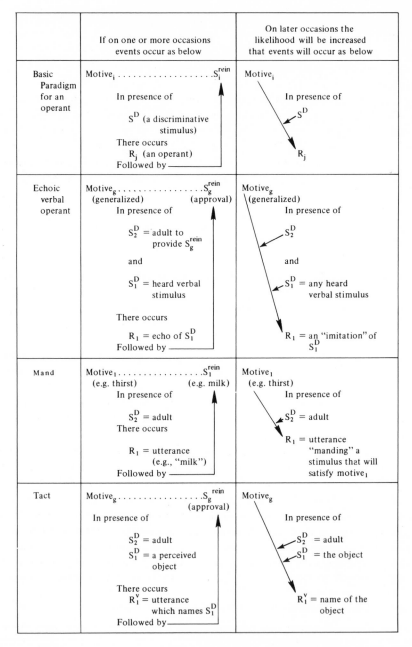

Figure 4. Operant paradigms for the learning and maintenance of verbal responses. Source: J. Carroll, Language and Thought, © 1964. By permission of Prentice-Hall, Inc., Englewood Cliffs, N. J.

developed through laboratory research with animals. Operant conditioning consists of a model wherein responses are first emitted and then rewarded. This reinforcement contingency assures further occurrence of the rewarded response. The emitted response, for which there is no observable stimulus, is termed an *operant*. Skinner classifies verbal operants into different functional categories.

A *mand* is a verbal operant wherein the response is reinforced by a characteristic consequence and is therefore under the control of relevant conditions of deprivation or aversive stimuli. Mands include such utterances as commands and questions. A *tact* is a verbal operant wherein the response is evoked (or at least strengthened) by a particular object (or part of an object). In other words, this response is under stimulus control. A tact is the response a child might emit when he sees an object, say a dog, in his room. *Echoic* operants are those wherein the response is under the control of prior verbal stimuli. Thus an echoic operant is a response which generates a sound pattern similar to that of a prior stimulus. In essence, this accounts for the occurrence of imitation. Each of the above points is shown schematically in Fig. 4. In addition to these operants, Skinner reports

1. *Textual* operants, which are verbal responses to a written stimulus (e.g., reading).

2. *Intraverbal* operants, which are verbal responses to verbal stimuli (e.g., the response "four" in answer to the verbal stimulus "two plus two").

3. *Autoclitic* operants, which are highly complex manipulations of verbal "thinking" which include assertions and various sentence structures.

Operants are subject to processes and manipulations such as response shaping (a change in behavior caused through selective reinforcement), stimulus discrimination ("shaping" of a response so that it is only emitted in the presence of a particular stimulus), secondary reinforcement (reinforcement by association of a stimulus, perhaps a word, with an already reinforcing stimulus, e.g., food), and response strength (the probability of emission of a response).

The basis of Skinner's approach to language acquisition is contiguity between response and reward (reinforcing stimulus). Laws of operant behavior stress that the strength of an operant is increased if the operant is followed by a reinforcing stimulus and, if not, it decreases. The frequency of response-reward pairing determines the magnitude of its probability of occurrence in the future. Thus, Skinner's system, in many ways like a Markov process, specifies the verbal unit with greatest response strength in a particular situation. In this system, lexical and phonological acquisition are presumed to result from verbal (or physical) rewarding of the child for saying a word-like sound(s). Rewarding, again, gives the word a certain probability of future occurrence. Mass undifferentiated verbal responses of a child are basically seen as being shaped by appropriate stimulus reinforcment.

Operant principles can account for the development of syntax through the use of "chaining" of operants, where each operant is induced by its own specific cue. These cues may be inherent in previously spoken words. In effect, succeeding words are emitted in the form of discriminate operants which have been rewarded in the presence of these stimulus situations. The hypothesis is enhanced by the argument that when an operant has been conditioned in one stimulus situation, it may occur, without further conditioning, in another stimulus condition by the process of generalization. Generalization may presumably occur with sentences as well as with words.

Chomsky (1967), in his review of *Verbal Behavior* (Skinner, 1957), criticized Skinner on many levels, both specific and general. He asserted, for example, that verbalizations cannot be adequately discussed in terms of response strength as Skinner described it. Skinner's response strength was defined as "probability of emission" and was determined primarily by frequency of occurrence of the R-S association. Chomsky noted, however, that response frequency is directly attributable to the frequency of occurrence of the controlling variables and, thus, there is no "probability" involved in response strength—rather, each response is uniquely determined by occurrence of variables. In short, Chomsky argues that the term "response strength" is merely used to give the appearance of objectivity to Skinner's theory. Fodor (1965) discusses the operant principles and points out pitfalls as related to language. He asserts, for instance, that according to R-S theory there is a nonverbal response, R, such that presentation of X (a physical item) increases the probability of R and the probability of the utterance of a word, W (standing for physical object). There are no data, however, to indicate that the name of an object which is present in the room where a person is speaking will be spoken with any greater frequency than the name of an object not present. Fodor also notes that one cannot know whether any two behavioral acts are part of the same response or not because there is no way of determining if two verbal utterances are functionally equivalent. Chomsky summarizes his criticism of Skinner by stating that the operant model has yet to explain the fact that all normal children acquire essentially comparable complex grammars in a very short period of time and that the operant model does not adequately account for novel utterances. Further, the model fails to account for the acquisition of comprehension of syntax.

Mediation The apparent insufficiency of a single stage S-R theory has led theorists to attempt to adapt two-stage learning models, as suggested by the research of Hull (1943), to the topic of first language acquisition. The result is the *mediation* model.

A major proponent of Hullian theory as applied to language is Osgood (1967). He has proposed and defended both two- and three-stage mediation to explain language acquisition. Expansion of the two-stage model to a three-stage model was done to accommodate perceptual and motor behavior. The three-stage model is based, however, on the two-stage model and for this reason, and the reason that it must face most of the basic objectives a two-stage model faces, only a discussion of a two-stage model will follow. The basic two-stage model involves the following:

1. $\boxed{A}$ —an originally neutral stimulus (sign).

2. $\textcircled{A}$ —another stimulus which will occur contiguously with $\boxed{A}$ and which regularly elicits R_t (significate).

3. R_t —a total response which is elicited regularly by $\textcircled{A}$.

4. r_m —some portion of the total response, R_t, which will become associated with $\boxed{A}$ (r_m is the mediating response).

5. s_m —a mediation stimulus which can become associated selectively (under self-control) with various instrumental acts.

6. R_x—instrumental acts with which s_m becomes associated.
The entire mediation process can be diagrammed as

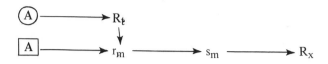

The overall process is one similar to single-stage conditioning, the difference being that the mediating reaction to the sign, $\boxed{A}$, is not identified with the reaction of the significate to the total response, R_t, but rather consists of the conditioning of the most effortless and least interfering components of the total reaction, R_t. Thus, the mediating response is a part of the total response. The self-stimulation, s_m, then becomes associated with various instrumental acts, R_x, which are theoretically relevant to the significate, $\textcircled{A}$.

In reality, mediation theory is a combination of two single-stage S-R models; "s_m" is seen as self-stimulation, and "r_m" may be part of. the total response. Any sign, $\boxed{A}$, conditioned contiguously with an object may come to trigger a reaction (the mediating response, r_m) which then leads to a linguistic response through self-stimulation. Thus, the presence of a cow ($\boxed{A}$) might come to elicit a response of "desire for milk" (r_m) similar to the total response (R_t) which occurs in the presence of milk ($\textcircled{A}$). The s_m, related to the r_m, may then elicit a reaction, R_x, such as the linguistic utterance "milk." The sign, $\boxed{A}$, may also be a verbal unit.

Obviously, the explanatory power of the mediation model appears to be much increased over that of the single-stage model. Specifically, the model can account for the production of an appropriate linguistic response in the absence of an overt stimulus. This process is particularly useful in accounting for the acquisition of "word meaning."

Criticism of mediation models has dealt primarily with specifiable behaviors for which mediation theory appears unable to account. Fodor (1965) has posed the most direct threat to mediation theory by showing that a distinct mediator (r_m) must be postulated for each distinct total response (R_t). This assertion appears logically correct; otherwise there is no method for determining which R_t is being anticipated by a particular r_m. If true, the significate ($\textcircled{A}$) is only redundant information, as the total response (R_t) is unequivocally specified. With the R_t and r_m in apparent one-to-one correspondence, the only difference between single-stage and mediation theory is that some members of the S-R chain in mediation are unobserved. [Osgood (1966) has countered this argument by asserting that the difference in observability is important because it accounts for the fact that conditioned responses have been shown to transfer across words of similar content with no observable r_m.] Thus, there appears to be essentially no difference between single-stage and mediation theories. Fodor (1965) further states that mediation theory is insufficient in that the components of the R_t most likely to become the r_m are the broad but distinctive overt responses common to all mankind. Thus, it would appear impossible to determine a one-to-one correspondence between each R_t and r_m, a fact violating a necessary law of the theory just discussed. [Osgood (1966), however, sees the r_m as multicomponental (a number of patterns linked into a code) where only one feature difference in the code is necessary to differentiate it from other r_m's. This argument, however, still must concede a one-to-one correspondence such as Fodor (1965) has suggested.]

Other authors have also cited behaviors which the mediation model does not explain. In general, they are topics which single-stage theories also fail to handle, e.g., comprehension, novel utterances, and the development of grammatically complex sentences.

Imitation (autism) Model   Mowrer (1954, 1966) presents an S-R theory of language acquisition based on imitation and derived from behavior observed in animals. The theory, based on behavior of so-called "talking birds," postulates the following learning procedure. First, in order for a sound to be learned for production, the sound has to be repeatedly produced in an agreeable, pleasant context (such as linking it with a food reward). When this situation occurs, the bird, during babble play, will make sounds similar to the word and hear himself saying it. Imitation then takes on secondary reinforcement properties, and, more important, the reinforcer is "built in" to the bird itself. The secondary reinforcement (originally conditioned to the words the trainer utters) generalizes to the word stimuli the bird utters. The better the imitation of the trainer's words, the stronger the reinforcement and consequent continuation of the behavior. If one replaced "bird" with "child" and "trainer" with "parent" in the above discussion, the reward contingencies can be seen which, by Mowrer's reasoning, account for language acquisition. (For Mowrer, words acquire *meaning* by second-order conditioning. In first-order conditioning some part of the total reaction gets shifted to the word, and in second-order conditioning this same part of the reaction gets shifted to another word in context with the first conditioned response.) Generally, Mowrer feels that through reinforced practice, muscular and neural patterns are established and, later, the motion of saying words triggers self-satisfying reinforcement. It is for this latter reason that the theory may be termed *autistic*. Mowrer further states that for learning to take place the child does not even have to be reinforced for producing the words—though he may be—since secondary reinforcement only requires a pattern of stimulation occurring contiguously with a primary reinforcer.

While imitation models are open to many levels of criticism, the most obvious and important is that the models by themselves provide no means of accounting for comprehension and novel utterances. A sentence may be imitated orally but, obviously, comprehension cannot be imitated. Further, children's spontaneous productions cannot be explained by an imitation model, since children's utterances have been shown not to be precise replications of adult sentences.

Contextual Generalization   Braine (1963, 1965) has explored contextual generalization as an explanation of the acquisition of grammatical structure. The basic premise of this theory is that when a segment of a sentence has been experienced in a certain position and context, it will later be placed in the same position in other contexts on the basis of S-R generalization (where the mediating property is the temporal location of an utterance). The theory grew out of the recognition that while mediational properties in

S-R generalization are usually *intrinsic*, this occurrence is not mandatory. [Miller (1951) described *extrinsic* properties of contextual constraint as appearing in controlled word-association tests.] Braine (1963) sees the 2-year-old as using two sets of cues to define borders which indicate segment or phrase position in language. One set is intonation patterns (pitch, stress, juncture, etc.). The second is "closed-class" morphemes (articles, prepositions, etc.). For example, in a sentence such as *The boy rides his bike*, presumably two things occur in the listener who recognizes the fact that the subject or noun phrase frequently comes first in a sentence and the verb phrase follows it. The closed-class morpheme *The* and the intonational stress on the verb serve to indicate the boundaries of the noun phrase, while the verb stress and intonational pattern indicating the end of the sentence provide cues for discrimination of the verb phrase. With larger or more complicated sentences a process of binary fractionation may occur. That is, a child may learn the location of a unit within the next larger containing unit of a hierarchy of units. For example, a child may learn that within a verb phrase, the verb and its modifiers frequently occur first, followed by the object and its modifiers. Such a hierarchy of positions is learned for each of the transformations. (Braine sees each transformation as having fairly standard word order, and claims that simple declarative sentences are the "kernels" of Chomsky's 1957 grammar.)

Bever et al. (1965), in a critique of Braine's position, have argued the following major points:

1. A theory of syntax should explain the fact that no one language appears harder to learn than any other language. Russian and German, for example, appear no harder to learn than English, yet because they have less constrained surface ordering of words, the contextual generalization model would suggest they are harder to learn.

2. Braine's (1965) use of suprasegmental cues as a delineating factor for position boundaries of phrases fails to account for the extreme problems in learning that should occur from listening to everyday, nonfluent speech with its accidental acoustic gaps and incorrect stress.

3. Simple declarative sentences are not the underlying form in the production of sentences. Rather, a generative grammar produces only abstract structures (basic grammatical relations of the deep structure), which are then transformed into sentence types. Thus, in failing to distinguish between surface and underlying structure, Bever et al. (1965) feel that Braine loses the mechanism accounting for rapid acquisition of comprehension and for easy transformation of one structure to another. [Braine (1965), in replying to this last argument of Bever, Fodor, and Weksel, asserts that the looseness of transformational rules and their consequent lack of empirical validity prevent him from accepting the "necessary properties" of natural language that transformational grammars demand.]

Integrated Theories of Learning As the traditional learning models have failed to explain all aspects of language acquisition, several theorists, notably Staats (1968) and Jenkins and Palermo (1964), have felt that an integration of many of the learning principles is necessary. In these cases the authors have not attempted to postulate a total theory of verbal behavior but, rather, have been content to describe which learning principles work best for various aspects of language behavior. In general, researchers and reviewers (see Kagan, 1964) have found fault with these positions much as they did with individual learning positions—on the basis of insufficiencies. For example, adequate use has not been made of known features of verbal behavior (such as loudness contours) and, further, there has been no reasonable explanation of comprehension behavior or of *grammatical* novel sentence production.

It should be noted in concluding a discussion of learning theories that recent learning theories have expressed disapproval with the "mentalistic" proposals of generative grammarians concerning language acquisition and behavior. Staats, for one, makes the point that linguistic theory cannot make explanatory statements, as it does not have sufficient contact with data on the conditions which determine behavior. For example, the linguistic assumption that there are cognitive structures corresponding to phrase-structure rules is weak, as it can only be validated through bioneurological observations which, presently, do not exist. Staats (1968) also provides one of the few learning arguments which account for the fact of language universals. (Nativists use these universals as a foundation for their arguments against learning theory, as well as for the existence of innate structures.) Staats states that languages, after all, should have commonalities in that they have evolved to relate to essentially the same world of events, a world common to all men. [Some scholars (see Whorf, 1956) have argued, however, that different cultures view reality differently.]

Nativist Theory

In general, nativist theories of language acquisition hold that language maturation must be explained in terms of certain innate properties of the human organism, not on the basis of experience and learning.

Chomsky (1965, 1967) asserts that the induction learning paradigms advanced by empirical psychologists are insufficient for producing grammars within the constraints of time, access, and uniformity which data have shown to exist. Instead, he holds that a rationalist approach, i.e., one which assumes an innate system capable of handling language, is more tenable. A major problem with this assumption is found in developing an hypothesis about acquired structure that is able to account for both the universals and diversities of language. Chomsky's basic hypothesis is that children have no more control over the processes governing the development of linguistic rules for generating sentences than they have for, say, their visual perception. As stated earlier, Chomsky (1965) and Katz (1966) have assumed the existence of a Language Acquisition Device (LAD) as one component of a total system of intellectual structures. LAD is presumed to have various formal universals as its intrinsic properties. These universals provide a schema that is applied to data so as to determine, in a highly restricted way, the general form and feature of the grammar that emerges upon presentation of language samples from the environment. Obviously, the grammar can change over time since the child continues to receive new linguistic data.

Lenneberg (1964), using some data from Greenberg (1966), has listed many traits of language which, to him, totally and sufficiently categorize language as being a species-specific trait, based on a number of biologically given and genetically transmitted mechanisms.

To support this claim, Lenneberg cites the following facts:

1. The onset and development of speech in the child is a regular, fixed sequence (McCarthy, 1954).

2. All languages of the world seem to conform to a set of universal semantic, syntactic, and phonological features.

3. Any child is capable, at birth, of acquiring any language in the world.

4. Man has anatomic and physiologic correlates with language activities, e.g., cerebral dominance and coordination centers for motor speech.

5. Propensity for language is a specific and genetically founded capacity, as demonstrated by the fact that language acquisition is independent (beyond minimal levels) of what is currently labeled intelligence.

McNeill (1966a, 1966b, 1968) also argues that the child must bring both formal and substantive linguistic universals to the language acquisition situation.[11] As stated earlier, these universals are representations of basic grammatical relations and of hierarchical classification systems. McNeill advances this hypothesis on the basis of the apparent fact that one must know the deep structure of a sentence in order to comprehend its meaning. Surface structure alone will not supply the referents necessary for comprehension. For example, in the constructions *John is easy to please, John is eager to please,* meaning is only *easily* determined by reference to the deep structure of these similar surface constructions. Occurrence of contextual generalization or S-R habit formations would cause difficulty in distinguishing that *John* is an object in the first sentence, while *John* is the subject of the second sentence. Thus, for McNeill, a theory of language acquisition must explain development of deep structures and the transformational rules which transform them into more complex surface structures. He also postulates that a comprehensive theory of language acquisition must account for both comprehension and production. For these reasons, McNeill also uses Chomsky's LAD in his theory of acquisition. According to McNeill, the universals of LAD are such that verbal behavior is comprehended or generated at the deep-structure level according to one of the six basic universal grammatical relations discussed earlier (see page 43). What is then "*learned*" by the child are the basic transformations needed to produce grammatical sentences. This process occurs presumably as a result of LAD taking a corpus of utterances and creating a grammatical system (the transformations) according to the innate universals it already has.

McNeill's assumptions permit prediction of what will constitute a future grammatical utterance (verbal behavior). Further, it accounts for the fact that (1) the child's acquisition is rapid and regular, and (2) language performance is realized as both comprehension and production.

[11] McNeill makes this argument on the basis of claims advanced by Chomsky (1965). Chomsky defines substantive universals as the fixed linguistic classes from which all items of a particular language must be drawn. For example, all languages select phonemes from a small set of fixed, universal phonetic features. Formal universals are certain abstract features (i.e., they do not exist in an empirical sense) which presumably characterize all language systems. For example, the syntactic component of all grammar must contain certain transformational rules which translate semantically interpreted deep structures into phonologically interpreted surface structures.

While expressing an interest in McNeill's assertions, Fraser (1966) feels that they fail to account for some important aspects of verbal behavior, the role of primary and secondary reinforcement. In making this case, Fraser cites the work of a Japanese linguist on the speech of a Japanese child. He found the child began to speak not as a result of hearing normal adult conversation, but by imitating words and short utterances produced clearly by adults. (The child failed to learn Tata, a rapid conversation language used by the mother, but acquired the type of "Japanese" that was explicitly and clearly presented.)

Even if innate structures account for the facts of syntactic development, the mechanisms by which this occurs must be specified. Lenneberg (1964) has even argued that innate models of language acquisition must include specific anatomical and physiological correlates for language. To date, little progress has been made in discovering such correlates.

Fodor (1966) also believes that the child is born with an innate propensity for learning specific principles and with some intrinsic structure for language. He views the child as receiving an enormous sample of grammatical and ungrammatical utterances from his environment from which he must induce and extrapolate the correct subset which constitutes grammaticalness. In other words, the child must *induce* deep structures for various sentence types. Fodor has shown this concept to be necessary for a theory of language acquisition inasmuch as there is no way to learn *simple* rules or S-R contingencies for transforming, for example, an active sentence to a passive sentence. Fodor argues that the only way to resolve the apparent conflict between the relatively easy *act* of transforming such a sentence and the theoretically large number of rules S-R theory requires to perform such a transformation is to postulate an underlying deep structure from which these sentence types are specified. However, the child never actually hears deep structures. If this hypothesis is true, learning theories for the acquisition of syntax are rendered useless. Fodor posits that the child innately has the rules to assure that (1) only a small number of possible analyses is performed on a corpus of data (to fit with time considerations) and (2) the correct analysis is *among these*. Thus, the child is thought to have many rules for analyzing surface structures and changing them to their corresponding deep structure. With them, the child is able to select syntactic descriptions which maximize the probability of determining the underlying and derived structural relationship.

Thus, Fodor's "innate mechanism" is in the form of *specific inference rules* that work in specific cases, rather than a list of total solutions to all language data. In this sense, Fodor is a part of the final group of first-language acquisition theorists who will be discussed—the mixturists.

Mixture Theories

Recently, various authors have attempted to bridge the gaps between the nativist and learning viewpoints. DeCecco (1967, p. 309), for instance, states:

If Chomsky and Skinner could accept the *cue function* of words as external stimuli that mediate internal processes, and if they could accept the possibility of behavior chains capable of both horizontal and vertical arrangements, their positions would not be as opposed as they now seem to be.

Fodor et al. (1967, p. 198) feel that

> ... the question about innateness is sometimes raised not in terms of the evidence for or against some particular theory about what is innate, but rather in terms of whether anything need be innately contributed at all. The answer to this question must be obvious. Any organism that generalized its experiences at all must, on pain of infinite regress, have some unlearned principles for extrapolation. The dispute between associative theories of language learning and the kinds of theories we have been discussing [nativist] is not over whether there are some innate principles, it is only over the content and complexity of the innate endowment."[12]

Slobin (1966), in commenting on McNeill's position, agrees that a LAD is necessary for a viable approach to language acquisition. However, he prefers a "process approach" (i.e., whereby generalized cognitive processes induce language universals) to LAD, while McNeill prefers a "control approach" (i.e., where universal characteristics of language are part of the innate structure). Slobin feels further that McNeill's idea of giving the child credit for having all the rules with which it is necessary to process language has flaws shown by empirical behavioral data. For instance, McNeill's work suggests that the child would innately have an *entire* hierarchy of adult word classes, whereas evidence from Miller and Ervin (1964) indicated otherwise (in that subjects placed adjectives in *both* their pivot and open classes). A control approach to LAD would account for this data discrepancy, since the structure would consist of a set of procedures and inference rules used to process data. Thus, there would be progressive definement of word classes as the inference rules had an increasingly larger corpus of data on which to work. The use of these innate rules on the corpus of linguistic data presented the child could develop the linguistic universal—as well as produce an appropriate grammar. Slobin postulates that the semantic nature of words and word classes would then specify the hierarchy of word classes which McNeill posits as innate. For instance, if the inductive rules develop a sense of the universal class of nouns, the semantic nature of the nouns would, by these same processes, subdivide into animate-inanimate, masculine-feminine-neuter, and so forth. Slobin suggests that learnable semantic features develop the underlying grammatical categories which the innate LAD inferred, and thus Slobin bridges the gap of nativist and learning theorist.

[12] From Fodor, J., J. Jenkins, and S. Saporta. Psycholinguistics and Communication Theory. *In* Dance (ed.), Human Communication Theory, (C) 1967, by permission of Holt, Rinehart and Winston, Inc.

Some Closing Remarks

Analysis of the above theories shows many favorable and unfavorable features. The major criticism of learning theories of language acquisition is that they do not explain the child's potential for generating and comprehending an enormous number of novel grammatical sentences. Further, learning theories do not satisfactorily explain language universals. Learning theories rarely, if ever, deal with the fact that comprehension of linguistic units seems to be acquired before production, or why items which have been comprehended are not immediately producible. The only way in which comprehension might be handled appears to be through assertion of an innate (unlearned) mechanism for decoding and manipulating verbal output. On the other hand, learning theories appear adequate for describing acquisiton of meaning for words, short phrases, and phonological rules.

Nativist theories tend to suffer from a lack of specificity in their explanations. In their most extreme form, they fail to explain the occurrence of certain overt linguistic phenomena (e.g., imitation). To claim that phenomena such as these are unimportant is purely judgmental and denies explanations of many features of linguistic performance. Nativists are also in the precarious position of losing explanatory power by positing too much as innate. Without neurologically supportive data, they are in the position of having all their arguments dismissed as being good imagination or sophisticated opinions. Obviously, more developmental neurolinguistic data are needed of the type being generated by Bever and associates in New York (1970).

For these, and other reasons it seems most profitable to consider the case presented in a mixture point of view. Here the universals of language are accounted for by means of innate mechanisms and the principles of S-R conditioning, with all its varieties, are seen as aiding in the child's acquisition of an intricate language system. In this regard, Slobin's ideas appear to be quite reasonable and exciting. Positing a general organization of the mind which allows for inductive reasoning, and which can be applied specifically to language (among other things), appears to be the most parsimonious organization of such a varied, all-pervading, integrated organ as the human brain.

CONCLUSION

The goals of linguistic, psycholinguistic, and sociolinguistic approaches to the study of first language acquisition have not been oriented toward the language pathologist. In general, the goals, which were discussed in the introduction to this chapter, have been to develop theories of language and language use. If the data are to assume relevance for language pathologists, they themselves must determine the implications. In so doing, language pathologists can possibly make contributions to the understanding of human language systems. The present authors believe that data and theories on language maturation have important implications for the study, diagnosis, and management of language disorders in a number of areas.

First, utilization of language acquisition data should improve the validity of norms used to determine the presence or absence of language pathology. Present information on acquisition suggests that norms must be established for both comprehension and production of language at increasing levels of phonological, lexical, and syntactic complexity within the context of the various linguistic communities of the United States. This point cannot be overemphasized since application of a single set of normative data to all speakers, irrespective of their dialectic communities, may result in erroneous judgments of language pathology when, in reality, only legitimate differences exist.

Second, normative data on language acquisition should be used by language pathologists to develop valid and dialectically unbiased test instruments to assess the aspects of language discussed above.

Further, application of these tests to nonstandard speakers is likely to yield invalid judgments about their true linguistic competence (see Gerber and Hertel, 1969). Resolution of this problem is not to be found by simply translating existing tests into the various dialects of American English. Legitimate answers can only be secured by developing tests based on normative language and cognitive information secured from speakers of the linguistic communities for which the tests are intended.

Third, language acquisition data and theory, together with normative data and valid tests, can be used to determine the characteristics of various types of language disorders. This information can be helpful in the diagnosis, prognosis, and management of language disorders.

Finally, innovative approaches to language therapy might ensue from application of language acquisition data and theory. In general, therapy should probably focus, depending on degree of neurological and linguistic integrity, on the following items, in the order presented: (1) memory/perceptual/motor systems, (2) comprehension, and (3) production. Function in these levels should progress through increasingly complex control of phonology, lexicon, and syntax. It is logical to argue that teaching of these features in therapy situations should occur in an integrated way: the teaching of phonology and vocabulary in the context of increasingly complex grammatical units.

REFERENCES

Atkinson, R., and R. Shiffrin. 1968. Human memory: a proposed system and its control process. *In* Spence, K. W., and J. T. Spence, eds., The Psychology of Learning and Motivation, Vol. 2. New York, Academic Press.

Bellugi, U. 1958. The emergence of inflections and negation systems in the speech of two children. Paper presented at New England Psychol. Assn., 1964.

Berko, J. 1958. The child's learning of English morphology. Word, 14:150-177.

Bever, T. 1968. The nature of cerebral dominance in the speech behavior of the child and adult. Paper presented at CIBA Foundation, May 1968.

————1970. The cognitive basis of linguistic structures. *In* Hayes, J. R., ed., Cognition and the Development of Language. New York, John Wiley & Sons.

————J. Fodor, and W. Weksel. 1965. On the acquisition of syntax: a critique of contextual generalization. Psychol. Rev. 72:467-482.

Braine, M. 1963. On learning the grammatical order of words. Psychol. Rev., 70:323-348.
———1965. On the basis of phrase structure: a reply to Bever, Fodor, and Weksel. Psychol. Rev., 72:483-492.
Brown, R. 1964. The acquisition of language. In Rioch, D. M., and E. A. Weinstein, eds., Disorders of Communication. Res. Publ. Ass. Nerv. Ment. Dis., 42:56-61.
——— and U. Bellugi. 1964. Three processes in the child's acquisition of syntax. Harvard Educ. Rev., 32:133-151.
——— and C. Fraser. 1964. The acquisition of syntax. Monographs of the Society for Research in Child Development, 29:43-79.
Carroll, J. 1964. Language and Thought. Englewood Cliffs, N. J., Prentice-Hall.
Carrow, Sister M. 1968. Development of auditory comprehension of language structure in children. J. Speech Hearing Dis., 33::99-111.
Chomsky, C. 1969. The acquisition of syntax in children from 5 to 10. Research Monograph No. 57. Cambridge, Mass. The MIT Press.
———1961. Some methodological remarks on generative grammar. Word, 17:219-239.
Chomsky, N. 1957. Syntactic Structures. The Hague, Mouton and Co.
———1964. Degrees of grammaticalness. In Fodor, J., and J. Katz, eds., The Structure of Language. Englewood Cliffs, N. J., Prentice-Hall.
———1965. Aspects of the Theory of Syntax, pp. 47-62. Cambridge, Mass., The MIT Press.
———1967. Review of Skinner's Verbal Learning. (1959). In Jakobivits, L., and M. Miron, eds., Readings in the Psychology of Language, pp. 142-171. Englewood Cliffs, N. J., Prentice-Hall.
DeCecco, J. 1967. The Psychology of Language, Thought, and Instruction, pp. 306-309. New York, Holt, Rinehart and Winston.
Dunn, L. 1969. Peabody Picture Vocabulary Test. Minneapolis, Minn., American Guidance Service.
Ervin, S. 1964. Imitation and structural change in children's language. In Lenneberg, E., ed., New Directions in the Study of Language, pp. 163-190. Cambridge, Mass., The MIT Press.
Fodor, J. 1965. Could meaning be an r_m? J. Verb. Learn. Verb. Behav., 4:73-81.
——— 1966. How to learn to talk: some simple ways. In Smith, F., and G. Miller, eds., The Genesis of Language: A Psycholinguistic Approach, pp. 105-122. Cambridge, Mass., The MIT Press.
——— and T. Bever. 1965. The psychological reality of linguistic segments. J. Verb. Learn. Verb. Behav., 4:414-420.
———J. Jenkins, and S. Saporta. 1967. Psycholinguistics and communication theory. In Dance, F. ed., Human Communication Theory, pp. 191-198. New York, Holt, Rinehart and Winston.
Fraser, C. 1966. Formal discussion of the creation of language by children. In Lyons, J. and R. Wales, eds., Psycholinguistic Papers. Edinburgh, The University Press.
———U. Bellugi, and R. Brown. 1963. Control of grammar in imitation, comprehension, and production. J. Verb. Learn. Verb. Behav., 2:121-135.
Gerber, S., and C. Hertel. 1969. Language deficiency of disadvantaged children. J. Speech Hearing Res., 12:270-280.
Gough, P. 1965 Grammatical transformations and speed of understanding. J. Verb. Learn. Verb. Behav., 4:107-111.
Gray, G., and C. Wise. 1959. The Bases of Speech. New York, Harper & Row.

Greenberg, J., ed. 1966. Universals of Language. Cambridge, Mass., The MIT Press.

Hull, C. L. 1943. Principles of Behavior. New York, Appleton-Century-Crofts.

Irwin, O. 1948. Infant speech: the effect of family occupational status and of age on use of sound types. J. Speech Hearing Dis., 13:224-226.

Jakobson, R., C. Fant, and M. Halle. 1967. Preliminary to Speech Analysis. Cambridge, Mass., The MIT Press.

—— and M. Halle. 1956. Fundamentals of Language. The Hague, Mouton and Co.

Jenkins, J. 1967. Learning Theories. In DeCecco, J., ed., The Psychology of Language, Thought, and Instruction, pp. 310-317. New York, Holt, Rinehart and Winston.

—— and D. Palermo. 1964. Mediation processes and the acquisition of linguistic structure. The Acquisition of Language, pp. 141-168. Child Development Monographs. Lafayette, Ind., Purdue University.

Kagen, J. 1964. Formal discussion of mediation processes and the acquisition of linguistic structure. In Bellugi, U., and R. Brown, eds., Acquisition of Language. Monogr. Soc. Res. Child Develop., 29(1):169-173.

Katz, J. J. 1966. The Philosophy of Language. New York, Harper & Row.

Klima, E., and U. Bellugi. 1966. Syntactic regularities in the speech of children. In Lyons, J., and R. Wales, eds., Psycholinguistic Papers. Edinburgh, The University Press.

Lee, L. 1966. Development sentence types: A method for comparing normal and deviant syntactic development. J. Speech Hearing Dis., 31(4):311-330.

——1970. Screening tests for syntactic development. J. Speech Hearing Dis., 35:103-112.

Lenneberg, E. 1964. A biological perspective of language. In Lenneberg, E., ed., New Directions in the Study of Language, pp. 65-88. Cambridge, Mass., The MIT Press.

——1967. Biological Foundations of Language. New York, John Wiley & Sons.

McCarthy, D. 1954. Language development in children. In Carmichael, L., ed., Manual of Child Psychology. New York, John Wiley & Sons.

McNeill, D. 1966a. The creation of language by children. In Lyons, J., and R. Wales, eds., Psycholinguistic Papers. Edinburgh, The University Press.

——1966b. Developmental psycholinguistics. In Smith, F., and G. Miller, eds., The Genesis of Language: A Psycholinguistic Approach, pp. 15-84. Cambridge, Mass., The MIT Press.

——1966c. Theories of language acquisition. Stud. Lang. Lang. Behav., 3:1-40.

——1967. The development of language. Stud. Lang. Lang. Behav., 4:429-463.

——1968. The creation of language. In Oldfield, R., and J. Marshall, eds., Language, pp. 21-31. Baltimore, Penguin Books.

Menyuk, P. 1963. Syntactic structures in the language of children. Child Develop., 34(2):407-427.

——1964a. Comparison of grammar of children with functionally deviant and normal speech. J. Speech Hearing Dis., 7:109-121.

——1964b. Syntactic rules used by children from pre-school through first grade. Child Develop., 35:533-546.

——1968. The role of distinctive features in children's acquisition of phonology. J. Speech Hearing Res., 11:138-146.

——1969. Sentences children use. In Research Monograph No. 52. Cambridge, Mass., The MIT Press.

Miller, G. 1951. Language and Communication. New York, McGraw-Hill.

——1962. Some psychological studies of grammar. Amer. Psychol., 17:748-762.

———— E. Galanter, and K. Pribram. 1966. Plans and the Structure of Behavior, pp. 139-158. New York, Holt, Rinehart and Winston.

Miller, W., and S. Ervin. 1964. The development of grammar in child language. *In* R. Brown, and U. Bellugi, eds., Acquisition of Language. Monogr. Soc. Res. Child Develop. 29:9-34.

Milner, B. 1959. The memory defect in bilateral hypocampal lesions. Psychiat. Res. Rep., 11:43-52.

Mowrer, O. 1954. The psychologist looks at language. *Reprinted in* Jakobivitz, L., and M. Miron, eds., Readings in the Psychology of Language, pp. 6-50. Englewood Cliffs, N. J., Prentice-Hall.

————1966. Learning Theory and the Symbolic Process, Chap. 3. New York, John Wiley & Sons.

Neisser, U. 1967. Cognitive Psychology. New York, Appleton-Century-Crofts.

Osgood, C. 1966. Meaning cannot be rm? J. Verb. Learn. Verb. Behav., 5:402-408.

————1967. On understanding and creating sentences (1963). *Reprinted in* Jakobivitz, L., and M. Miron, eds., Readings in the Psychology of Language, pp. 104-127. Englewood Cliffs, N. J., Prentice-Hall.

———— and M. Miron. 1963. Approaches to the Study of Aphasia. Urbana, University of Illinois Press.

Poole, I. 1934. Genetic development of articulation of consonant sounds in speech. Elem. English Rev., 11:159-161.

Rohrman, W. 1968. Role of syntactic structure in recall of English nominalizations. J. Verb. Learn. Verb. Behav., 7:904-912.

Savin, H., and E. Perchanock. 1965. Grammatical structure and immediate recall of English sentences. J. Verb. Learn. Verb. Behav., 4:348-353.

Skinner, B. 1957. Verbal Behavior. New York, Appleton-Century-Crofts.

Slobin, D. 1964. Imitation and the acquisition of syntax. Paper presented at Second Research Planning Conference of Project Literacy.

————1966. Comments on developmental psycholinguistics. *In* Smith, F., and G. Miller, eds., The Genesis of Language: A Psycholinguistic Approach, pp. 85-92. Cambridge, Mass., The MIT Press.

Smirnov, A. 1969. Problems in the psychology of memory. *In* Cole, M., and I. Maltzman, eds., A Handbook of Contemporary Soviet Psychology. New York, Basic Books.

Smith, M. 1941. Measurement of the size of general English vocabulary through elementary grades and high school. Genet. Psychol. Monogr., 24:311-345.

Staats, A. 1968. Learning, Language, and Cognition, Chap. 10. New York, Holt, Rinehart and Winston.

Taylor, O., and C. Anderson. 1968. Neuropsycholinguistics and language retraining. *In* Black, ed., Proceedings of the Conference on Language Retraining for Aphasics. Columbus, Ohio State University.

Templin, M. 1957. Certain language skills in children: their development and interrelationships. Institute of Child Welfare Monograph Series, No. 26. Minneapolis, University of Minnesota Press.

Van Riper, C. 1963. Speech Correction. Englewood Cliffs, N. J., Prentice-Hall.

Weir, R. 1962. Language in the Crib. The Hague, Mouton and Co.

Wellman, B., I. Case, I. Mengert, and D. Bradbury. 1931. Speech sounds of young children. University of Iowa Studies in Child Welfare, Vol. 5:2.

Wepman, J., L. Jones, R. Bock, and D. Pelt. 1960. Studies in aphasia: background and theoretical formulations. J. Speech Hearing Dis., 25:323-332.

Whorf, B. 1956. *In* Carroll, J., ed., Language, Thought and Reality: Selected Writings of Benjamin Lee Whorf. Cambridge, Mass., The MIT Press.

Winitz, H. 1969. Articulatory Acquisition and Behavior. New York, Appleton-Century-Crofts.

Wolski, W. 1962. Language development of normal children four, five and six years of age as measured by the Michigan State Language Inventory. Doctoral dissertation. Ann Arbor, Mich., University of Michigan.

Wood, W. 1964 Delayed Speech and Language Development. Englewood Cliffs, N. J., Prentice-Hall.

Zankov, L. 1969. Memory. *In* Cole, M., and I. Maltzman, eds., A Handbook of Contemporary Soviet Psychology. New York, Basic Books.

Zinchenko, P. 1969. Problems in the psychology of memory. *In* Cole, M., and I. Maltzman, eds., A Handbook of Contemporary Soviet Psychology. New York, Basic Books.

Part 2: Disabilities in children viewed etiologically

3: The general problem of language disabilities in children

Michael Marge

Language is essential to contemporary human life in its broadest sense. It is the chief mode of communication between and among humans. It facilitates learning, stores and transmits the culture, enables one to attain his needs in an efficient and expeditious manner, and provides a mechanism by which one enters and maintains membership in his society. In his treatise on verbal behavior, Skinner (1957, p. 459) states: "The history of science is the history of the growth of man's place in nature . . . . [Men] have extended their power to alter and control the physical world with machines and instruments of many sorts. A large part of this achievement has been verbal." Furthermore, an individual's language ability is one of the most significant variables which determines his level of social and economic attainment. Finally, language plays a meaningful role in the development of emotional maturity and appropriate social behavior.

Language behavior may be divided into four components: listening, speaking, reading, and writing. Of these four, Hall (1960) perceives human language as primarily an oral-aural system of signaling, implying that listening and speaking represent by far the main activities in communications. If these activities of language behavior, especially oral expression and/or aural reception, have not developed to a level where they can be meaningfully utilized or have been developed and then become seriously impaired, it is understandable that an individual would be profoundly handicapped.

In terms of the age when problems with language result in handicaps for the individual, a language disability is no less critical in children than it is in adults. A child

The author wishes to express his appreciation to Laura Lee (Northwestern University), Donald Harrington (Childrens Bureau, Washington, D. C.), James J. Gallagher (University of North Carolina), Robert Mulder (Fresno State College), and Philip J. Schmitt (Gallaudet College)—all of whom reviewed the manuscript for this chapter and offered many valuable suggestions.

75

may suffer from the effects of language disability in many ways, initially in the area of oral-aural modalities and later in activities of reading and writing. The child realizes quite early the pervasiveness of his language handicap in all aspects of his life. First, the development of a child's overall learning capacity may be hindered. Failure to attain skill in language usage results in immeasurable handicaps for a child's general intellectual and cognitive development. Numerous experiments demonstrate the paramount importance of language in concept formation, problem solving, thinking, and learning (Carroll, 1961; Mussen, 1963). Second, and a corollary to the first, he may experience profound and prolonged academic retardation in classrooms which place a great deal of value on the child's ability to use language and in which much of the classroom time from the primary to the midelementary grades is devoted to formal and informal discussion between the teacher and the students and among the students (Bangs, 1968). Third, the child may develop problems in emotional and social adjustment as he is faced daily with communicative situations with peers and adults which result in failure and frustration (Frostig and Maslow, 1968; McCarthy, 1954a). And fourth, when the parents or guardians of the child seek appropriate professional assistance, they discover that there is noticeable difficulty in obtaining effective service which incorporates comprehensiveness and continuity of programming for the child. The realization that their child is handicapped generally presents a deep-felt strain on the family. But the further realization that effective and sufficient professional services are difficult to obtain compounds the problem presented by the child's disability.

The role of language and its related disorders in the emotional, social, and educational growth and development of the child, therefore, is of considerable consequence. To better understand the significant influence of language on the child's behavior and the problems arising from language disability, it will be necessary to review the current theories of language acquisition in children, causes of language disability, the issue of definition and classification, and the scope of the national problem of language disability in children, including the difficulties and limitations in the provision of necessary diagnostic and training services.

LANGUAGE ACQUISITION IN CHILDREN

During the past two decades we have seen a dramatic change in the study of language behavior in children. At one time the scholar assumed that child language developed according to a series of stages which were, on the one hand, deviations of the adult norms and, on the other hand, approximations toward those norms (McNeill, 1966.). Studies of language acquisition focused upon speech-sound development, vocabulary growth, and, in a narrow sense, the acquisition of sentence structure and knowledge of grammar. His study of grammatical development, as McNeill (1966) points out, was based on the supposition that he knew the child's grammar in advance and that it was reasonable to use categories of adult grammar to describe child language. But, today, a number of researchers approach the study of child language from a new perspective with the following points in mind:

1. The fundamental question is: how do children acquire language in a remarkably short time span? For example, beginning before 1½ years of age and completed by 3½ years, a span of 24 months, most children acquire grammatical speech and possess a basis for the development of adult grammar.

2. In the minds of many scholars, the study of language restricted to the traditional items of the development of speech sounds, vocabulary, and adult grammar has been relatively unproductive. Drawing from the theoretical constructs and methodologies of linguists and psychologists, the new approaches divide the study of language into three main branches: (a) sound, (b) form, and (c) meaning, their acquisition and their interrelationships. Under form and meaning fall the study of grammar, which has become to many the principal object of interest. It has been observed that language acquisition in children progresses in a series of unique stages from very short, telegraphic utterances to complex sentences which approximate the speech of adults. Changes in the successive grammars of children have provided a means by which to record and analyze growth in language.

3. Whereas the traditional approach to the study of language acquisition stresses verbal performance, a number of researchers have turned to the study of the development of linguistic competence. "Competence" refers to the knowledge which a native speaker of a language must possess in order to produce and understand any of the infinitely many grammatical sentences of his language (McNeill, 1966). "Performance," as defined by linguists, is the overt expression of competence in the linguistic activities of listening, speaking, reading, and writing. Before performance can be understood, we must comprehend the development and operations of competence.

4. Environmental stimulation, once assumed to be the most significant variable in the development of language in children, cannot satisfactorily explain how language is acquired in a surprisingly short time. Despite the significant differences in child-rearing habits (including language stimulation) throughout the world, almost all children acquire language at about the same time. From cross-cultural studies of the effects of parental management on the linguistic achievement of children, one could conclude that a universal of language is that all normal children learn language by simply being exposed to it, without formal teaching (Houston, 1968). This suggests a biological predisposition for the acquisition of language, which may be described as an innate capacity for language learning. Through maturational development and in the milieu of an "adequate" language-stimulating environment, a series of states of readiness within the child—his innate capacities—leads to a sequence in language acquisition at relatively constant chronological ages (Lenneberg, 1966).

Theories of Language Acquisition

The explanation for man's unique facility of speech, which, more than any other behavior, separates him from animals, has been the subject of study for centuries. In recent years two major schools of thought—structural linguistics and transformational linguistics—have emerged to provide substantial arguments in favor of their positions.

Structuralism was introduced with the publication of Bloomfield's *Language* (1933), which dominated linguistic thought for two decades. The structuralists claim that language is a *habit* which a child acquires by imitating the adults in his environment. The proper study of language acquisition is the analysis of sounds and how they are manipulated to form words and sentences.

In contrast with the structuralists' theory, some transformationalists contend that language is an innate, instinctively acquired facility and the proper study of child language is to begin with sentences and the rules by which they are formed. The term "transformationalists" refers to proponents of the linguistic system based on the tenets of transformational-generative grammar. Noam Chomsky (1957, 1965), the prime contributor to the theory of transformational linguistics, argues that the fruitful study of language centers on the characterization of grammar. Further, he and his collaborators (Lenneberg, 1967) propose that though the child must hear someone speak before he can speak meaningfully himself, adult speech only serves to trigger the child's biological endowment for learning language.

Though both approaches have generated research and analyses which resulted in a rich literature with many significant items of information, each approach leaves many questions about child language development unanswered. For example, some transformationalists place little stress on the importance of the environment in shaping linguistic performance. They hold that environment only "triggers" innate language-learning mechanisms. This contention is not necessarily supported by all proponents of the Chomsky school of thought. Some have recently reported evidence which underscores the significance of the influence of adult speech modeling and other contextual variables in the child's environment (Ervin, 1964; Brown and Bellugi, 1964; Cazden, 1965).

A Theoretical Synthesis

The two most popular theories of language acquisition in children contain elements which when combined provide a more credible explanation of the process of acquisition than each theory taken individually.

There are three major variables which affect the acquisition of language in children—heredity, maturation, and environment (see Table 1).

Heredity   A child is born with anatomical and physiological endowment, intellectual propensity, and an assumed innate capacity for language learning which, to a substantial extent, determines the rate and level of language skills development. It is not enough to speak only of a biological endowment for language acquisition to explain the onset of linguistic behavior; we must include the state of the anatomy and physiology of the speech and hearing mechanism. Before oral language can be attempted, the child must possess certain fundamental organs and organic functions which allow for the production of speech. The innate capacity for language learning is very strongly related to the fact that language is normally learned acoustically (Fry, 1966). Comprehension of language precedes the development of expressive language. Comprehension of oral language is the result of the child's ability to hear, i.e., to perceive the speech of others. Therefore, the

Table 1. Significant Variables in Language Acquisition

1. Heredity
   a. Anatomical and physiological factors
   b. Innate capacity for language learning (assumed)
   c. Intelligence
2. Maturation
   Emergence of "readiness" stages for language acquisition
3. Environment
   a. Adult language used with the child
   b. Child-rearing practices
   c. Peer-group language used with the child

receptive-expressive language concept implies a time sequence in language acquisition as well as the necessity of the receptive component for the development of expressive language.

Also, intelligence certainly plays a role not only in the rate of acquisition but at early stages in the quality and quantity of linguistic performance (Carroll, 1961; Irwin, 1952). Intelligence is classified under heredity only to indicate that at birth a child possesses a potential intellectual capacity which is subsequently influenced by environment. Experiences after birth could prevent, retard, or facilitate the attainment of his full potential.

Each of the three variables should be perceived as a continuum from "poor" to "good" with a critical point below which the child's language development is seriously affected. With regard to anatomical and physiological factors, the absence of a functioning hearing mechanism will interfere with the child's reception of the oral language of others. Unless some compensatory action is taken, i.e., to provide the child with a hearing aid if appropriate, to place him in a highly stimulating language environment, and to train the child to compensate for the hearing loss, he may acquire only the most rudimentary language skills. With regard to intelligence, children with extremely low intellectual potentials may never acquire language.

It should be noted that the factor of innate capacity for language learning is qualified by the term "assumed." Though the arguments by some linguists in support of the notion that man is born with a biological predisposition for language acquisition are compelling, the fact remains that there is no scientific evidence to substantiate this belief. Furthermore, psychologists have shown that language acquisition and linguistic proficiency are related to intelligence, and one wonders whether language learning is a component of intelligence rather than a separate biological mechanism.

Maturation The emergence of language behavior is probably paced by the innate mechanism for language learning. It has been repeatedly proposed that language cannot begin to develop until a certain level of physical maturation and growth has been attained (Lenneberg, 1966). Carmichael (1964) observes that though the receptor mechanisms and motor mechanisms of speech are functional at birth and even before birth, and though some postnatal development of these mechanisms does take place, it is clear that the development of language is largely dependent on the maturation of specific brain mechanisms which are known to be essential in adult speech. He further indicates that the rate and character of the maturation of the different parts of the brain are largely determined by heredity (Carmichael, 1964). Normal acquisition of language is the result of a gradual unfolding of capacities in a series of more or less well-circumscribed events that take place between birth and 3½ years of age. The regularity in the sequence of appearance of given milestones is correlated with age and other concomitant developmental factors. The maturation of certain brain centers is necessary to produce a state of *speech readiness* in which the child realizes rapid and facile development of oral language. According to Carmichael (1964), the readiness is most likely not a characteristic of the total brain, but rather of quite specific brain mechanisms referred to earlier. In a study of the effect of premature birth on the development of language, de Hirsch et al. (1964) report that premature children are generally inferior to maturely born ones in important aspects of oral language development. The investigators hypothesized that the findings result from the premature children's lingering neurophysiological immaturity. Most investigators agree that heredity and maturation account for the appearance of coos and chuckles at age 4 months and babbling behavior at ages 6 to 9 months. These behaviors would occur even in the absence of any linguistic stimulation in the child's environment. The appearance of the next milestone—the first word at approximately one year—is the result of the addition of the third major variable affecting language learning, environmental stimulation.

Environment   Environmental factors play a significant role in the linguistic development of children during and after the babbling stage, though the amount and type of stimulation critical for maintaining the process of maturation is not known. The significant effect of the environmental variables on language development has been documented in the literature. The summary of the evidence by McCarthy (1954b) supports the contention that the quality of a child's early linguistic environment has significant influence on the rate and level of language development. The influence of factors in the home environment on language development is by no means a simple process. Recent research has challenged the commonly accepted direct causal relationship between environment and language by revealing that the relationship is complex and much more subtle than once believed (Marge, 1965a).

Since the early linguistic environment has been found to be a function of socioeconomic status (SES), we can account for the findings of many studies which conclude that language development is faster and quantitatively and qualitatively superior in the upper socioeconomic levels (Templin, 1957; Deutsch, M., 1964; Deutsch, C., 1964; Hess et al., 1965; Olim et al., 1965; Bernstein, 1962; Brainin, 1964; Irwin, 1948; Dave, 1963; McCarthy, 1930). A note of caution is in order in the use of SES as a predictor of language skills development in children. SES as an intervening variable in the relationship between specific characteristics of family patterns and subsequent language behavior in children cannot explain all the variation found among families. It is more important and meaningful to study the effects of parental speech (or the speech of the adults who manage the child), peer-group speech, and type and quality of child-rearing practices on the rate and level development of linguistic skills.

Parental speech appears to provide the child with (1) a basis for developing a repertoire of appropriate phonemes, (2) a criterion against which the child measures the correctness of his linguistic utterances, and (3) a means by which, in certain circumstances, he may be stimulated to acquire language more rapidly than normally expected. Evidence seems to support the observation that children whose parents "expand" a great deal, i.e., repeat the speech of small children and, in so doing, change the children's sentences into the nearest well-formed adult equivalent, show more rapid acquisition of language than children whose parents expand little (Brown and Bellugi, 1964).

Type and degree of child interaction with others represents another environmental variable which may influence the rate and level of language development. Degree of association with adults appears to be the significant factor which, to some extent, is related to the number of siblings in the family, twinning, and parental attitudes toward adult-child verbal interaction. Studies by McCarthy (1930), Day (1932), Davis (1937), and Smith (1935) corroborate the observation that children who associate chiefly with adults use longer and more complex sentences than those who associate chiefly with their peers. These studies imply that peer-group speech is not as beneficial as adult speech in the development of proficient language in the child.

Marge (1965a) studied the effects of certain child-rearing practices and parental attitudes on child language development. Permissive mothers were found to have children who attained higher levels in language maturity than those from restrictive homes.

As a result of the three major variables of heredity, maturation, and environment operating simultaneously, the following milestones are noted (see Table 2).

Summary of Language Acquisition

The process of the acquisition of language in children is the result of three major factors: heredity (anatomy and physiology, intelligence, and an innate capacity for language learning); maturation (a gradual unfolding of states of readiness within the child for linguistic performance); and environmental stimulation. The onset of linguistic behavior from birth through 6 to 9 months is most likely triggered by heredity and maturational factors. At that stage in development and thereafter throughout life, the environment becomes one of the major factors in the rate and level of language skills attainment. Most children begin to say their first word by approximately 1 year. By the age of 36 months, most children have mastered the complex syntactical structure of the language sufficiently well to be able to produce all major varieties of English simple sentences up to a length of 10 or 11 words. And by 4 to 5 years, most children have attained almost completely correct usage of the sounds and language forms used by the adults in the community. Therefore, whereas the onset of language is made possible by inherited capacities, the normal attainment of mature language skills is impossible without linguistic stimulation from the environment. Furthermore, heredity and maturation factors held constant, the quantity and quality of child-rearing practices and parental speech explain the difference in rate and level of language skills attainment.

Table 2. Milestones in Language Acquisition

Age (months)	Linguistic characteristics[a]
18-21	20 words at 18 months to 200 words at 21; comprehends simple questions; forms two-word sentences.
24-27	300 to 400 words; forms two- to three-word sentences; uses prepositions and pronouns.
30-33	Fastest increase in vocabulary; forms three- to four-word sentences; word order, phrase structure, grammatical agreement approximate language of surroundings, though many utterances are unlike adult grammar.
36-39	Vocabulary of 1,000 words or more; well-formed sentences up to the length of 10 or 11 words, using complex grammatical rules, though certain rules have not been fully mastered.
48-60	Most English sounds produced accurately; mastered the inflectional rules of English; grammatical usage of adult speech is generally completely mastered; early attempts at reading and writing the native language.

[a] After Lenneberg (1966, p. 222).

LANGUAGE DISABILITIES: DEFINITIONS AND CLASSIFICATION

In the preceding paragraphs we have discussed the normal process of language acquisition in the typical child. But what about the substantial number of children with language disabilities which impair their communications with peers and adults? What factors lead to the difficulties which they possess? This is a most complicated problem which is directly related to the issues of definition and classification.

The common practice in the literature is to relate language disabilities to etiology so that the clinician speaks of congenital aphasia, autism, speech and language of the mentally retarded, and so forth. This practice appears to be no more than a persistent need to follow the medical model of defining disease states or types by describing the *cause* and the *sequela*. The application of this model to personal and social behaviors, such as language, has resulted in a semantic morass of confusion, in which authors have dwelled upon etiologies rather than specific characteristics of the language behavior in need of modification. The search for an etiology has been frequently unsuccessful, and if one is found, the conclusions become highly speculative. The discussion about major variables presented in an earlier section hints at the complexity of factors which separately and/or together explain how children acquire language. To use the medical model which limits the concern for causation to one or a combination of several variables is a fallacy and does not reflect an understanding of the difficulties one faces in analyzing human behavior. In view of these and other arguments, classification schemes built on etiological factors alone are not very meaningful in the management of language disabilities. This in no way attempts to deny the value of exploring etiology and factors which may be maintaining the disability, but an analysis of linguistic behavior should serve as the main focus of the diagnosis and classification. If effective interventional techniques can be applied to remove the causes of a language disability, then by all means appropriate steps should be taken. For example, in cases of hearing impairments which may respond successfully to medical treatment, the results generally lead to considerably improved chances for correcting the language disability, though the hearing impairment alone is rarely the sole cause of the disability. If the language disability were hypothesized to be related to a condition of brain damage, the information, as will be shown later, is of limited value since there is little which can be done to correct the neurological deficit at this time. After a reasonable search for etiologies, the next most important question is: What are the current linguistic characteristics of the child? Specifically, we are seeking answers to three questions about the quantity and quality of child language:

1. Has the child acquired any language by age 4 years when language should be well developed?

2. How delayed is the language usage of a child as compared with his age peers?

3. What is the status of his language usage after the child has acquired adequate language function?

Definitions of Normal Language

Definitions should not be accepted as fixed and immutable statements which describe and/or explain a given term but should be perceived as tentative in nature and subject to continuous change. This is especially true in the case of "language," in which the term refers to an area of knowledge undergoing rapid change and expansion. Language is defined in a number of ways according to the definer's major discipline and point of view. Most definitions of language allude to the purpose or purposes of linguistic units—sounds, forms, and meanings—which together allow for the human communication of ideas, thoughts, and feelings.

The definitions which follow are based on certain assumptions drawn from several theories currently expounded. Essentially, the definitions are a synthesis of prevailing views concerning language and may represent the author's bias (Marge, 1968).

Communications Earlier the term communications was used in connection with language. As a referent to those means by which man interacts with his fellow man, communications is much broader in scope than the term language. Consider the following definition:

Communication(s) is any means by which man transmits his experiences, ideas, knowledge, and feelings to his fellow man. Included under this definition are speech, sign language, gesture, writing, or any other code which permits messages to be converted or transformed from one set of signs to another, e.g., written signs to speech (Denes and Pinson, 1963, p. 1). It should be noted that communications includes "any means" by which humans interact.

Language *Language* (this definition concerns itself only with spoken language and specifically excludes written language) is the most common means of communication. In its broadest sense it is a system composed of *sounds* arranged in ordered sequences to form *words* and *morphemes* (Hockett, 1958) and the *rules* for combining these elements into sequences or strings that express *thoughts, intentions, experience,* and *feelings* (Chomsky, 1967). Thus, language is made up of phonological, morphological, syntactic and semantic components which must be learned to understand and speak a given language. Specific terms in the definition are further defined as follows.

1. Sounds: analyzable as sets of distinctive features (phonemes); and phonology, the laws governing the permitted sequences and selection of sounds in a given language (Chomsky, 1967).

2. Morphemes: The smallest individually meaningful elements in the utterance of language.

3. Rules: ordered ways in which sentences are formed. Syntax refers to rules for placing words in specific order.

4. Thoughts, intentions, feelings: meanings communicated through use of words and sentences. Refers to the semantic aspects of language production.

Though this definition focuses upon spoken language, it can be easily extended to include the other linguistic activities of listening, reading, and writing.

Important to an understanding of language is a distinction between "speech community" and "dialect speech community."

Speech community is that set of people who communicate with each other, directly or indirectly, via a common language as defined above (Hockett, 1958).

Dialect speech community is a set of people who communicate with each other directly or indirectly, using a language (as defined above) which is not typical of that spoken by the dominant dialect group in the particular geographic region. The language used by this subset of the community may differ from the dominant one in terms of its phonological, semantic, or syntactic components or some combination thereof.

Definitions of Language Disabilities

We turn now to a consideration of language disabilities. The attempt to define and classify deviant language behavior in terms of etiology was discussed earlier and judged to be a relatively unproductive approach for a number of reasons. John Irwin (1964) observes that the traditional scheme of classification of communicative disorders has been an unfortunate development. The scheme is not consistent in the manner in which it describes a disorder either in terms of output or in terms of condition. Irwin further observes that the undesirable scheme has had a powerful influence on the development of the field of speech pathology and audiology by shaping speech and hearing training programs, clinical organizations, and their research and therapy throughout the country. There are a number of other reasons for the dissatisfaction with the current classification scheme with its emphasis on etiology. First, the reference to etiology carries the possible implication that there is a primary single cause for the deviant behavior; that once the cause is identified, it may be corrected, resulting in substantial gain in the process to eliminate the disability; that etiology provides the single most significant criterion by which to determine the differences between and among language disabilities; and that the classification by etiology provides a convenient way in which to plan for a program of corrective measures and training.

Let us consider in some detail the reasons for abandoning the classification by etiology and developing a classification scheme with greater utility. In applying the medical model of classifying by etiology, specialists in communicative disorders searched for the primary single cause of language disability, resulting in the following referents: speech and language of the mentally retarded, cleft palate speech, congenital or childhood aphasia, and speech of the cerebral palsied. Even the term "functional" disorders, such as functional articulation disorders and stuttering, imply the absence of a known disease process or anatomical anomaly, but hint that the condition resulted from adverse environmental factors during the process of language acquisition. Though it is possible that specific etiology may be the single most significant factor in the development of a disability, current knowledge about the interrelationships of many significant variables in human development leads us to question the *probability* of such an occurrence. In fact, the myriad of factors within the child and between the child and his environment which come into play when a disease process is initiated create an extremely difficult situation for the diagnostician who starts out to seek the factor(s) creating the disability. The search often ends with the identification of one or many factors and hypotheses about their relationships to the language disability. In some instances the etiological factors may lend themselves to corrective treatment, as in hearing impairment, and thereby eliminate a possible maintaining cause of the language disability. But in most instances the diagnostic process is not so simple. Take the case of brain injury in children. The usual sequelae of brain injury involve certain bodily functions, such as vision, metabolism, and body temperature, and the reduction in language function. Though it is no problem to measure the status of the bodily functions, measuring the effects of the neurological deficit on language is much more difficult. It is important, for example, to determine the time of the injury, and the type, extent, and location of the neurological insult before a causal relationship between the injury and the language disability is established. Because of the large number of factors which could have played some role in the development of an individual's language function, it does not necessarily follow that the existence of brain injury and language disability have a direct causal relationship. In the case of a child who received brain damage before the age of four years, the course of the recovery is very rapid with a sequence of events which roughly correspond to a telescoped normal history of language acquisition (Lenneberg, 1964). In fact, the entire left hemisphere may be excised during the first 2 years of life without interfering with the normal acquisition of language (Lenneberg, 1964). If such a child were found to possess a language disability at age 6 years, the conclusion that the disability was caused by his neurological condition is invalid, though it is generally assumed that the two variables are highly correlated. Even if a child had received a brain injury after the acquisition of language, one still cannot conclude that an observed language disability is related to the brain damage on a one-to-one basis. Lenneberg (1967) compiled 17 published case reports on children who possessed language before suffering a one-sided lesion in the brain. He states that the overwhelming majority of children having sustained aphasia between four and ten years of age recover to a remarkable degree.

With the development of better linguistic instruments which have direct implications for the type and nature of the training program necessary, another classification is sought. Though knowledge of etiology, even hypotheses about causation, may assist in the preparation of the child for a training program by eliminating factors which may be maintaining the disability, e.g., unrepaired cleft of the palate, tense environmental setting, malnutrition resulting in general physical debility, this information alone should not significantly affect the choice of interventional technique.

The metaphoric character of the etiological referents in language disabilities is analogous to the development of certain terms in the field of psychology for the purpose of resolving uncertainty or ambiguity. As an example, anxiety is a term which was introduced as a hypothetical construct in the 1930s to account for behavioral outcomes that could not be satisfactorily explained with existing knowledge (Sarbin, 1968). Once the term became popular, testing instruments were developed to assess the behavior described by the term (e.g., Taylor Manifest Anxiety Scale). Levy's (1961) analysis of entries in *Psychological Abstracts* in which "anxiety" appeared in the title showed a positively accelerated increase in the number of articles following the introduction of the Taylor Manifest Anxiety Scale, with a similar spurt after the introduction of the children's form of the scale. The development of a scientific tool with the name of anxiety led to the spurious conclusion that the term had empirical reference after all. Sarbin (1968) states: "Hundreds of experiments have been done under the belief that the MA (Taylor Manifest Anxiety Scale) measured an elusive mental state, a psychic trait, or both."

Therefore, in addition to etiology, it is more important to obtain information about the child's level of language development according to linguistic milestones for typical children in his speech community. These include the developmental level of speech sounds, vocabulary, concept formation, and, most essential, sentence formation (syntax). Besides a status report of the child's linguistic profile, it is useful for the training program to determine whether the language disability represents a developmental retardation or was acquired after the development of normal language function.

With these factors in mind, definitions and a classification system were sought which represented a simple and meaningful approach to the problems of language. Consider the following classification of language disabilities:

1. *Failure to acquire any language.* Children who by age 4 years have not shown any sign of acquiring the language of their speech community as defined above.

2. *Delayed language acquisition.* Children whose language acquisition is below levels attained by their age peers in their speech community. The delay may occur in all, one, or some combination of the phonological, semantic, and syntactic components of the language of their speech community.

3. *Acquired language disabilities.* Members of a speech community who had at some point in their developmental history acquired the language of their speech community,

who subsequent to such adequate language acquisition suffered a complete loss or reduction of their capacity to use the language common to their speech community.

Little has been said about the communication problems of members of a dialect speech community. The definitions of language disability purposely avoid any reference to dialect as a handicap for several reasons. A language disability either prevents or seriously hinders communication within a speech community. Most students of language agree that a dialect, such as Negro dialect, represents a bona fide language system which allows its speakers to effectively communicate with one another. The determination of whether a dialect speaker has a language disability is a function of (1) deviations in language within the dialect form, and (2) the speaker's desire and capability for social and economic mobility from the dialect speech community to the major language community. Within the confines of the dialect speech community, the speaker of dialect is not at all disabled since his language serves him well in the expression of thoughts and feelings. However, if he has developed a serious deviation in language functioning within his dialect, he may be said to possess a disability. Or, if the speaker of a dialect attempts to move into the greater society and does not possess the linguistic skills necessary for meaningful and effective communication within the major language community, he may be said to possess a disability. Linguists, such as Stewart (1967) and Bailey (1967), emphasize that the study of dialect is unrelated to the question of what constitutes a language problem and when perceived in the context of typical speech patterns within a dialect speech community, this contention would not be disputed. But if the speaker of a dialect wishes to attain social and economic mobility, his dialect alone will most likely not suffice. He must learn the language of the major community, while maintaining his skill in the utilization of the dialect.

Throughout this discussion of definitions and classification of language disabilities, the pertinent relationship between the comprehension and expression of language has not been explored. There is some research evidence to support the view that passive control and comprehension of grammar appears earlier in development than active control and production of grammatical utterances in the child (Fraser et al., 1963). It is entirely possible, therefore, for children to understand the language of others without having acquired any proficiency in the expression of the language. This implies that the semantic development, involving concept formation, precedes the acquisition of expressive language. Once the child understands the meaning of an object or event, he is prepared to apply names or labels to them. Such skill in labeling facilitates concept formation and the acquisition of language (Mussen, 1963). It was proposed earlier that certain factors must be present to some degree before language may be acquired in the child. The most essential factors include normally developing speech and hearing mechanisms which allow for the reception and understanding of the oral language of others and the expression of utterances which continue to approximate and eventually match the utterances of adult speakers, a degree of intelligence which allows for some learning and intellectual functioning, and sufficient environmental stimulation to trigger the readiness stages leading from one plateau of language learning to the next.

Table 3. Continuum of Language Ability

Language disabilities			Language proficiency	
Absence of language ability	Severe disabilities	Mild disabilities	Average language skills development	Superior language skills development
(No language development since birth, type I, or acquired language disability, type III)	(Delayed language development type II, or acquired language disabilities, type III)			

It is also possible that children may not understand the language of others and therefore cannot develop expressive language. The child with a severe hearing loss, who is unable to perceive the oral language of others, may not develop the passive control and comprehension of grammar found in his peers with normal hearing. With this observation in mind, the categories of language disability adopted here refer only to the expression of language and do not attempt to imply anything about the child's ability to comprehend the language in his linguistic environment.

The acquisition of language in the child may be viewed from the aspect of language proficiency, that is, having sufficient skills in the use of the language of his speech community to function effectively in all or most communicative situations. These skills may be divided into the following classes (after Marge, 1964, p. 32):

1. Mechanics of language expression
   a. Voice quality appropriate for age and sex
   b. Fluency of speech
   c. Clarity of articulation
2. Content of language expression
   a. Correct pronunciation and intonation
   b. Appropriate vocabulary to express most thoughts and feelings
   c. Clarity of thought
   d. Wealth of ideas
   e. Correct grammatical usage and complexity of sentence structure
3. Applied skills in communicative situations
   a. Skill in listening
   b. Skill in conversation
   c. Skill in group discussion
   d. Skill in oral reading
   e. Ability to persuade classmates
   f. Skill in impromptu speech

It is to be noted that the classes are descriptive of the expectations for oral language development and reflect the positive end of a scale of language ability. In Table 3, we find a representation of the continuum of language proficiency, covering the broad range from the absence of "oral language ability" to the acquisition of "superior language skills development." Two broad divisions are identified—language disabilities and language proficiency—within which there are varying degrees of language skills development. Under language disabilities, the range from total absence of language to mild language disabilities is represented. Language proficiency varies from language development of the typical child to the high levels of linguistic ability. The continuum demonstrates the great range of variation in the study of language acquisition in children. Even those who have acquired normal language by age 4 years reveal noticeable individual differences in their development and ability to use their linguistic skills.

To understand the relationship between children with language disabilities and children who speak a so-called dialect, such as Negro dialect, or a foreign language which is their native mode of expression, it is suggested that the linguistic proficiencies of the child be applied to the scale in Table 3. If the child cannot at all speak the major language of the society in which he intends to function, he would be classified as a type I disability. If he has some ability, though limited, to communicate in the major language, he would be classified as a type II disability. As mentioned earlier, he also may possess a disability in his native language or dialect and in such a case would be classified in the same manner. The child who proficiently speaks a native language other than the language of the major speech community and the child with limited or no ability in his native language requires different interventional techniques. Though more will be said about this in Chapter 11, it is sufficient now to say that the proficient dialect or foreign language speaker should be taught Standard English as a second language and should not be managed as a child with reduced or no oral language ability.

THE NATIONAL SCOPE OF THE PROBLEM

Problems related to the provision of necessary services to the child with language disabiities may be considered according to the incidence and current prevalence of language disabilities, the status of interventional techniques for language disabilities, the availability of professional services, and the gap between demands for services and current resources.

Incidence and Prevalence of Language Disabilities

There are noticeably few studies of the incidence and prevalence of language disabilities in the total population. The best estimates are based on small population studies that use different definitions of linguistic disability and methodology so that comparisons between and among studies cannot readily be made (Marge, 1965b). And, of course, extrapolations from the findings in these studies to the general population must be done with great caution and tolerance of broad error. At best, the current estimates are only approximations which serve to set some limits to the question of need. As a step to ameliorate this situation, the United States Office of Education has funded a long-term broadband study of the prevalence of speech, language, and hearing problems in school-age children (Hull and Timmons, 1966).

Without any complete national statistics related specifically to the problem of language disabilities, an attempt was made to answer the question of the magnitude of the problem by obtaining estimates of language difficulties among various handicapped populations and by pooling the data under the suggested classification scheme. Table 4 summarizes these data which relate only to oral language disabilities. Several cautions should be heeded in the use of these figures. First, in what may appear to be an obvious contradiction of what was said earlier by the author concerning etiology, the estimates are based on current reports of oral language disabilities among children with specific handicapping conditions, such as deafness, mental retardation, and emotional disturbance. Therefore, data from studies on handicapped populations classified according to primary etiological factors were pooled and reclassified into a different scheme. Such a

practice is subject to serious question and must render the data as only speculat
Second, several assumptions which were used to group the data from the various
traditional categories could easily be challenged. One assumption was that the failure to
acquire any oral language by age 4 years is a rare event. Another assumption was that
almost all acquired language deviations (type III) resulted from conditions of adventitious
hearing impairment and neurological deficits.

A number of comments about Table 4 are in order. Type I language disability refers
to children who fail to show any signs of acquiring the language of their speech
community at age 4 years, when language maturity is normally achieved, to age 17 years,

Table 4. Estimates of Prevalence and Incidence of Oral Language Disabilities by Type (Ages 4-17)

Type of language disability	Current prevalence[a]	Incidence[b] (%)
I. Failure to acquire any language		
A. Age 4	A. 22,854[c]	A. 0.6
B. Ages 4-17	B. 44,745[d]	B. 0.08
II. Delayed language acquisition	3,467,784[e]	6.2
III. Acquired language disability	139,830[f]	0.25
Total	3,652,359[g]	6.53

[a]The total population of children age 4 through 17 years in the United States for 1969 was 55,932,000. (U. S. Government Bureau of the Census, 1969.)

[b]Incidence estimated by dividing the total number of children in the United States, for specific age range, into totals under each type of disability.

[c]Represents total number of children estimated to have failed to acquire any oral language function by age 4. Includes 100% of profoundly mentally retarded, 90% of severely mentally retarded, 10% of congenitally deaf, 25% of emotionally disturbed.

[d]Represents total of children estimated to have failed to acquire any oral language function between ages 4 and 17. Includes the total in footnote c and the following: 100% of children 5 to 17 who are profoundly mentally retarded and 25% of children 5 to 17 who are severely emotionally disturbed. It is assumed that almost all the deaf, all the seriously mentally retarded, and most of the severely emotionally disturbed who were included under footnote c will have realized some language acquisition by puberty and are, therefore, classified under Type II disabilities.

[e]Represents 10% of severely mentally retarded, age 4, and 100% of severely mentally retarded, ages 5 to 17; 100% of moderately mentally retarded and 80% mildly retarded, ages 4 to 17; 90% of congenitally deaf, age 4, and 100% of congenital hard-of-hearing, age 4; 100% of congenital deaf and hard-of-hearing, ages 5 to 17; 10% of emotionally disturbed, ages 4 to 17; 50% of specific learning disabilities, ages 4 to 17; and 95% of the speech handicapped (not included in other categories), ages 4 to 17.

[f]Represents total of 100% of adventitious deaf and hard-of-hearing, ages 4 to 17; 10% of speech handicapped, ages 4 to 17, primarily related to acquired neurological deficits.

[g]Total of (d) + (e) + (f).

which represents an arbitrary terminal age for school children. Of the traditional categories in use, these estimates include a small number of the profoundly deaf, most of the profoundly retarded, and approximately 25 percent of the profoundly emotionally disturbed (autism and schizophrenia). The number of children at age 4 years with no oral language development is reported separately to identify the magnitude of the problem relating to the needs of preschool children. These children will require intensive interventional approaches in order to develop some fundamental communication skills before they receive formal educational programming. It is hypothesized that type I disabilities are more apparent at the age of 4 years when normal language acquisition is expected but that a large number of these children eventually acquire some oral language ability by the midteens, thereby placing them in type II category. Supporting the thesis that most children acquire language despite the severity of handicapping conditions, Lenneberg (1964) observes: "A complete and total absence of speech and language is only seen in the lowest grades of idiocy." The implication of type I disabilities for the development of a program for intervention is the need for intensive programming. Though the prognosis for the acquisition of language proficiency by these children is not at all good as contrasted with those who have acquired some language by age 4 years, limited language ability can be expected.

Type II disabilities refer to children who have developed some language functions but are delayed in their acquisition when compared with their peers. This classification generally includes most children with moderate impairments in hearing, almost all children with mild to severe mental retardation, a small percentage of children with emotional disturbance, and a majority of children with the label "learning disability." Type II problems are, by far, the largest group with significant difficulties in language ability. The difficulties represented by type II vary in range of severity from mild handicapping articulation problems to serious difficulties with syntactic formulation and have implications for the nature and intensity of training. The general rule is the more severely disabled the child, the more intensive and extensive the program of intervention. Prognosis for language acquisition is considerably better for a child with some language development at age 4 years than for a child who has not realized any language acquisition.

Type III disabilities include those children who have acquired normal language function, but who then suffer a reduction in the use of their language. Generally, this category refers to children who have suffered personality disturbance or neurological insult following trauma or disease. The age of onset of language disability and the severity of the disability are the two most significant factors in determining prognosis for type III problems. Specifically, the younger the child, especially before the time of puberty (Lenneberg, 1967), and the less severe the difficulty, the better the prognosis for complete or almost complete recovery.

Table 4 does not provide any information about the number of children who speak either a dialect or a foreign language and have experienced or will experience difficulty in achieving social and economic mobility in the major speech community. Of the entire population of nonwhite children in the United States, it is estimated that approximately 75 percent would fall into the category of those in need of language training in order to function in a society of standard English speakers (R. Shuy, personal communication,

1969). Given a 1967 nonwhite United States population of 6,766,000 children from ages 6 to 17 (U. S. Bureau of the Census, 1968), we estimate a population of about 5,074,500 with current or potential language handicaps. Combining this estimate with the total of children with type I, II, or III disabilities reported in Table 4 results in a grand total of 8.7 million children with oral language disabilities.

THE STATUS OF INTERVENTIONAL TECHNIQUES FOR LANGUAGE DISABILITIES

Interventional techniques currently available for children with language disabilities may be divided into two broad categories: (1) diagnostic approaches, or those methods which assess the status of the child's disability, attempt to determine etiology and prognosis, and suggest appropriate procedures for modifying the child's linguistic behavior; and (2) training methods, or those procedures which assist the child in attaining language function appropriate for his age.

Diagnostic approaches may be described by two factors: (1) *frequency of assessment*—on a continuum, from an examination conducted on a one-time basis to an assessment process which is continuously carried out while the child is in training over a long period of time; and (2) *comprehensiveness of assessment*—on a continuum, from the sole use of the expertise of one discipline, such as speech pathology and audiology, pediatrics, or special education, to an interdisciplinary team approach. The two continua interact at points to represent the philosophy and approach to diagnosis posited by the diagnostician. Most diagnostic efforts include the use of standardized and/or unstandardized tests and personal observation to assess the function of the young child's speech and hearing mechanisms, intellectual capacity, personality characteristics, health and family history, present general health, and oral language skills. In older children there may be an attempt to determine the level of a child's reading and writing skills. Some elements of the examination are often irrelevant for the management process. For example, tests of motility of the tongue, lips, and jaw were once thought to provide essential information about the cause of language disabilities on the assumption that a direct one-to-one relationship existed between articulator motility and speech proficiency. Research evidence indicates, however, that the actions of these structures taken individually reveal a small indirect relationship with the combined and coordinated movements of these structures in speech behavior (Van Riper and Irwin, 1958). Some diagnosticians have begun to review the traditional approaches with an eye toward restricting the examination only to those elements which relate useful information for training. A more complete discussion of the topic of diagnosis is found in Chapters 9 and 10.

The approaches used for modifying and improving the linguistic behavior of children may be classified according to (1) those which emphasize sound-to-language forms, and (2) those which chiefly focus on language forms. In the first approach, children are taught the sounds of the language in isolation, proceeding to nonsense syllables, words, phrases, and sentences. The second major approach is to teach the child syntactic forms in developmental progression. And, there are combinations of both approaches which may teach both sounds and syntax simultaneously. Common to all approaches are the following: meaningful communicative settings in which speech practice takes place, intensive stimulation with speech sounds, words, and sentences, and building of vocabulary and concepts through planned activities in discovering new relationships among objects and events and in labeling these concepts. Whether these activities are conducted with children on an individual or group basis often depends on the educational philosophy of the language trainer, the severity of the language disability, and the client capacity of the agency providing the training.

Not all scholars agree that interventional techniques are absolutely necessary or effective based on the contention that children with delayed language development will eventually acquire language, regardless of the severity of their intellectual and sensory impairments (Lenneberg, 1964). There is sufficient clinical and research evidence to support the efficacy of training programs for children with language disabilities by facilitating language acquisition, by raising the level of the quality of language skills, and by increasing the quantity of language responses (Frostig and Maslow, 1968; Lenneberg, 1964; Monsees, 1968; Schlanger, 1959; Lewis et al., 1960; McGinnis, 1963; Blackman and Battin, 1957; Lent, 1968; and Clawson and Schlanger, 1968). More will be said about educative procedures for linguistically handicapped children in Chapters 11 through 16.

AVAILABILITY OF SERVICES

The national problem of language disabilities in children is compounded by the lack of adequate manpower to provide necessary services of identification, diagnosis, and training to all children in need of them. Excluding professional personnel from medicine and psychology necessary for diagnosis and some aspects of training, Table 5 summarizes the current estimates of available manpower, according to type of services.

The estimates in Table 5 are based on the assumption that the professional personnel listed are sufficiently trained or could be readily trained to manage the various types of language disabilities. Excluded from this summary are an estimated small number of clinical child psychologists and applied linguists who may be currently engaged in the provision of services. Recommended ratios for professional to language disabled children range on a continuum from 1 to 7 for teachers of the deaf to 1 to 40 for speech pathologists and audiologists. But with a professional cadre of only approximately 41,500 to serve 3,652,360 children, resulting in a ratio of 1 professional to 88 language-handicapped children, the problem becomes considerably more acute.

With this limited resource in professional manpower, it can readily be seen that the need for management services is far greater than what is available. Consideration must be given to the necessity of using the services of several specialties in order to conduct an effective program of diagnosis. Medical or psychological treatment may be necessary before the child is introduced to a specific training program or may be offered concurrently with the language management program. The need for team effort is more critical during the identification and diagnostic stage than after a prescribed management program has been instituted.

Another factor which complicates the national problem of language disability is the availability of services in all geographical regions of the United States. Parents and their children from sparsely populated sections may have to travel miles to obtain necessary

Table 5. Estimates of Manpower Resources in the United States

Professional personnel	Number of professional personnel	Types of services provided	Recommended professional-child ratio
1. Speech pathologists and audiologists	21,850[a]	Diagnosis and training for types I, II, III language disabilities	1:40
2. Special education teachers: A. Teachers of the deaf	6,048[b]	Training for types I, II, III language disabilities	1:7
B. Teachers of the hard-of-hearing	4,000[c]	Training for types I, II, III language disabilities	1:20
C. Teachers of specific learning disabilities	9,400[d]	Diagnosis and training for types I, II, III language disabilities	1:20
Total	41,298		

[a]Speech pathologists and audiologists from all job environments who are engaged in providing services. (Source: Estimates provided by American Speech and Hearing Association, January 1971.)
[b]American Annals of the Deaf, Directory of Services for the Deaf in the United States, Vol. 115, No. 3, May 1970. Total of teachers of deaf elementary and secondary children is 6,048.
[c]State Plans for Title VI of the Elementary and Secondary Education Act estimate that the number of teachers of hard-of-hearing children in local public schools is 4,000. (U. S. Office of Education, 1970.)
[d]Personal communication by Corrine Kass, formerly coordinator of Special Learning Disabilities Unit, Bureau of Education for the Handicapped, U. S. Office of Education, Department of Health, Education, and Welfare.

services which are not available in their community. Even in urban areas where the majority of community centers providing services to the linguistically handicapped are located, parents complain of long waiting periods before their children are placed in a management program.

Finally, the comprehensiveness of services—both diagnostic and language training—offered by the agency raises the question of adequacy of programming available to meet the needs of children with language handicaps. The quantity and quality of services in each agency are dependent upon many factors, which include the training and expertise of professional personnel, type of professional disciplines represented, number of personnel, priorities for managing handicapped children, physical facilities, and community need and demand for services. More will be said about the availability and type of management programs in Chapter 11.

REFERENCES

Bailey, B. 1967. Concern for special curriculum aspects: bilingualism. *In* Jablonsky, A., ed., Imperatives for Change: Proceedings of the New York State Education Department Conference on College and University Programs for Teachers of the Disadvantaged. New York, Yeshiva University.

Bangs, T. 1968. Language and Learning Disorders of the Pre-Academic Child. New York, Appleton-Century-Crofts.

Bernstein, B. 1962. Linguistic codes, hesitation phenomena and intelligence. Lang. Speech, 5:31-46.

Blackman, R., and R. Battin. 1957. Case study of delayed language. J. Speech Hearing Dis., 22:381-384.

Bloomfield, L. 1933. Language. New York, Holt, Rinehart and Winston.

Brainin, S. 1964. Language Skills, Formal Education and the Lower Class Child. New York, Mobilization for Youth.

Brown, R., and U. Bellugi. 1964. Three processes in the child's acquisition of syntax. Harvard Educ. Rev., 34:133-151.

Carmichael, L. 1964. The early growth of language capacity in the individual. *In* Lenneberg, E., ed., New Directions in the Study of Language. Cambridge, Mass., The MIT Press.

Carroll, J. 1961. Language development in children. *In* Saporta, S., ed., Psycholinguistics. New York, Holt, Rinehart and Winston.

Cazden, C. 1965. Environmental Assistance to the Child's Acquisition of Grammar. Doctoral Dissertation, Cambridge, Mass., School of Education, Harvard University.

Chomsky, N. 1957. Syntactic Structures. The Hague, Mouton and Co.

——— 1965. Aspects of the Theory of Syntax. Cambridge, Mass., The MIT Press.

——— 1967. The formal nature of language. *In* Lenneberg, E., Biological Foundations of Language. New York, John Wiley & Sons.

Clawson, W., and B. Schlanger. 1968. Oral vocabulary responses of educable mentally retarded adolescent boys in a dyadic situation. Except. Child., 34:761-762.

Dave, R. 1963. The identification and measurement of environmental process variables that are related to educational achievement. Doctoral dissertation, Chicago, University of Chicago.

Davis, E. 1937. The development of linguistic skills in twins, singletons with siblings, and only children from age five to ten years. University of Minnesota Institute Child Welfare Monographs, No. 14. Minneapolis, University of Minnesota Press.

Day, E. 1932. The development of language in twins. Child Develop., 3:179-199.

de Hirsch, K., J. Jansky, and W. Langford. 1964. The oral language performance of premature children and controls. J. Speech Hearing Dis., 29:60-69.

Denes, P., and E. Pinson. 1963. The Speech Chain. Murray Hill, N. J., Bell Laboratories.

Deutsch, C. 1964. Auditory discrimination and learning: social factors. Merrill-Palmer Quart., 10:277-296.

Deutsch, M. 1964. The role of social class in language development and cognition. J. Orthopsychiat., 25.

Ervin, S. 1964. Imitation and structural change in children's language. *In* Lenneberg, E., ed., New Directions in the Study of Language. Cambridge, Mass., The MIT Press.

Fraser, C., U. Bellugi, and R. Brown. 1963. Control of grammar in imitation, comprehension, and production. J. Verb. Learn. Verb. Behav., 2:121-135.

Frostig, M., and P. Maslow. 1968. Language training: a form of ability training. J. Learn. Dis., 1:105-115.

Fry, D. 1966. The development of the phonological system in the normal and the deaf child. *In* Smith, F., and G. Miller, eds., The Genesis of Language. Cambridge, Mass., The MIT Press.

Hall, R. 1960. Linguistics and Your Language. Garden City, N. Y., Doubleday (Anchor Books).

Hess, R., V. Shipman, and D. Jackson. 1965. Early experience and the socialization of cognitive modes in children. Child Develop., 36:869-886.

Hockett, C. 1958. Modern Linguistics. New York, Macmillan.

Houston, S. 1968. A diachronic examination of the linguistic universal. ASHA, 10:247-249.

Hull, F., and R. Timmons. 1966. A national speech and hearing survey. J. Speech Hearing Dis., 31:359-361.

Irwin, J. 1964. Comments. *In* House, A., ed., Proceedings of the Conference on Communicating by Language: The Speech Process. Bethesda, Md., National Institute of Child Health and Human Development, National Institutes of Health.

Irwin, O. 1948. Infant speech: the effect of family occupational status and of age on sound frequency. J. Speech Hearing Dis., 13:320-323.

————1952. Speech development in the young child: 2. Some factors related to the speech development of the infant and young child. J. Speech Hearing Dis., 17:269-279.

Lenneberg, E. 1964. Language disorders in childhood. Harvard Educ. Rev., 34:152-177.

———— 1966. The natural history of language. *In* Smith, F., and G. Miller, eds., The Genesis of Language. Cambridge, Mass., The MIT Press.

———— 1967. Biological Foundations of Language. New York, John Wiley & Sons.

Lent, J. 1968. Mimosa cottage: experiment in hope. Psychol. Today, 2:51-58.

Levy, L. 1961. Anxiety and behavior scientists' behavior. Amer. Psychol., 16:66-68.

Lewis, R., A. Strauss, and L. Lehtinen. 1960. The Other Child. New York. Grune & Stratton.

Marge, M. 1964. A factor analysis of oral communication skills in older children. J. Speech Hearing Res., 7:31-46.

————1965a. The influence of selected home background variables on the development of oral communication skill in children. J. Speech Hearing Res., 8:291-312.

————1965b. A review of incidence studies of speech and hearing disorders: 1936 to present. (Unpublished report.) Washington, D. C., United States Office of Education.

————1968. Annual Report of the ASHA Committee on Language. Washington, D. C., American Speech and Hearing Association. (The author acknowledges the contribution of Dr. Ronald Tikofsky, University of Michigan, in the development of the definitions.)

McCarthy, D. 1930. Language Development of the Preschool Child. Minneapolis, University of Minnesota Press.

————1954a. Language disorders and parent-child relationships. J. Speech Hearing Dis., 19:514-523.

————1954b. Language development in children. *In* Carmichael, L., ed., A Manual of Child Psychology, 2nd ed. New York, John Wiley & Sons.

McGinnis, M. 1963. Aphasic Children. Washington, D. C., Alexander Graham Bell Association for the Deaf.

McNeill, D. 1966. Developmental psycholinguistics. *In* Smith, F., and G. Miller, eds., The Genesis of Language. Cambridge, Mass., The MIT Press.

Monsees, E. 1968. Temporal sequence and expressive language disorders. Except. Child., 35:141-148.

Mussen, P. 1963. The Psychological Development of the Child. Englewood Cliffs, N. J., Prentice-Hall.

Olim, E., R. Hess, and V. Shipman. 1965. Maternal language styles and their implication for children's cognitive development. Presented at the Symposium on the Effect of Maternal Behavior on Cognitive Development and Impulsivity, American Psychological Association Meeting, Chicago, September.

Sarbin, T. 1968. Ontology recapitulates philology: the mystic nature of anxiety. Amer. Psychol., 23:411-418.

Schlanger, B. 1959. A longitudinal study of speech and language development of brain damaged retarded children. J. Speech Hearing Dis., 24:354-360.

Skinner, B. 1957. Verbal Behavior. New York, Appleton-Century-Crofts.

Smith, M. 1935. A study of some factors influencing the development of the sentence in preschool children. J. Genet. Psychol., 46:182-212.

Stewart, W. 1967. Sociolinguistic factors in the history of American Negro dialects. Florida FL Reporter, 5:Spring.

Templin, M. 1957. Certain Language Skills in Children: Their Development and Interrelationships. Minneapolis, University of Minnesota Press.

United States Government, Bureau of the Census. 1968. Estimates of the population of the United States, by age, race, and sex: Jul 1, 1964 to 1967. Population Estimates, Series P-25, No. 385, February 14. Washington, D. C., United States Department of Commerce.

Van Riper, C., and J. V. Irwin. 1958. Voice and Articulation. Englewood Cliffs, N. J., Prentice-Hall.

4: Neurological aspects of language disorders in children

Richard Allen Chase

HUMAN COMMUNICATION

A functioning language system requires shared conventions about the structure of messages and the significance of messages. These conventions must be shared because the recipient of a message must, in some sense, be able to reconstitute the intent of the sender. In some instances the conformity required between the formulation of a message to be sent and the interpretation of a message received is achieved by introducing a high degree of genetically determined constraint into brain structures that mediate communicative functions. This can be observed in the case of language systems used to communicate information essential to survival: information about danger, aggression and submission, location of food, attraction of a mate, and defense of territory. The ability to communicate about such matters is found in the case of animals with brains far less complex than those of primates. These phylogenetically old communication capabilities are also available to the human. In this case, we find them mediated largely by facial expression, head and neck posture, and gestures. In addition, however, man is capable of constructing any number of communication systems that make use of completely arbitrary conventions. Our use of highway signs is a good example of a completely arbitrary system of communication conventions. Any visual shape can be introduced into this system as long as the users of the system agree about the significance of each shape.

The ability to design and use any number of communication systems provides great advantages. We can develop some way of communicating about almost anything we can experience. One of the requirements of this capability is the ability to learn communication conventions. The plasticity of the human nervous system for language learning is, however, accompanied by some real hazards. It is possible to deprive a nervous system of some of the essential experiences necessary for language learning. This fact must be clearly in mind when one surveys the territory of language disorders in children.

It is the purpose of this chapter to review some of the language disorders of children, and to discuss some of the neurological aspects of these disorders. The main body of the discussion will be preceded by a review of some anatomical, physiological, and behavioral observations.

DEVELOPMENTAL NEUROANATOMY AND NEUROPHYSIOLOGY

The major cortical areas that are necessary for language function are the posterior frontal lobe (Broca's area) and adjacent portions of the motor cortex (precentral gyrus) concerned with speech musculature (face area), and the posterior-superior temporal lobe and adjacent portions of the parietal and occipital lobes (Wernicke's area) (Figs. 1 and 2). These areas are connected by the superior longitudinal fasciculus. Some of the fibers of the superior longitudinal fasciculus synapse in the inferior parietal region before connecting with Broca's area, and others go directly to Broca's area. Fibers from Broca's area project onto those portions of the motor cortex in which the speech musculature is represented. Broca's area thereby serves as a way-station between the posterior auditory association cortex and the speech musculature area of the motor cortex. Broca's area, in concert with the speech musculature area of the motor cortex, is concerned with the motor organization of speech. Broca's area, in concert with the arm and hand area of the motor cortex, is concerned with the motor organization of writing. Lesions of these frontal regions result in speech and writing that is slow, effortful, sparse, and

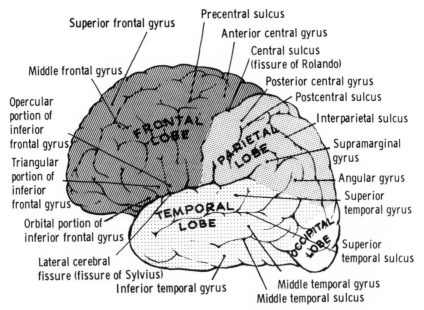

Figure 1. Lateral view of the left cerebral hemisphere. From Chusid and McDonald, Correlative Neuroanatomy and Functional Neurology, 13th ed., Los Altos, Calif., Lange, 1967.

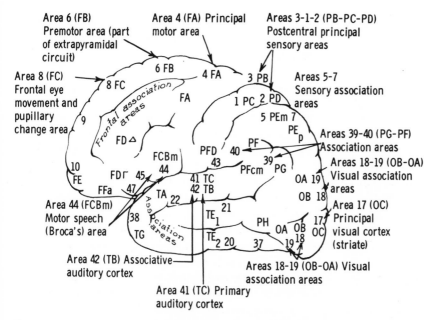

Figure 2. Lateral view of the left cerebral hemisphere showing functional localizations and cortical areas according to Brodman (numbers) and Von Economo (letters). From Chusid and McDonald, Correlative Neuroanatomy and Functional Neurology, 13th ed. Los Altos, Calif., Lange, 1967.

mechanically inexact (Benson, 1967; Geschwind, 1968). Lesions of Wernicke's area result in speech and writing that is more fluent and less effortful with respect to motor organization, but which is very inexact with respect to the way in which words are formulated and used (Alajouanine and Lhermitte, 1964; Benson, 1967; Geschwind, 1968). Substitutions of words that sound somewhat like the intended word, or have a meaning somewhat similar to the intended word, are common. Complete inability to recall many words, and grammatical distortions, are also common. It would seem that Wernicke's area is closely concerned with the ideational organization of language, the auditory organization of the language underlying initial language acquisition, and the exercise of grammatical rule structures that allow additional meaning to be conveyed as a function of the ordering of words (von Bonin, 1963; Penfield and Roberts, 1959; Polyakov, 1966).

It is clear that Broca's area and Wernicke's area (cortical speech areas) do not function in isolation. Large lesions of the dominant parietal lobe that partially isolate these areas result in fluent aphasic speech and marked speech comprehension deficit (Geschwind, 1965; Geschwind, 1968). A patient with such a lesion might also demonstrate echolalia (Denny-Brown, 1963; Geschwind, 1964). Echolalia can be thought of as direct and obligatory transduction of a speech sound input into its speech motor counterpart. This phenomenon is observed in normal infants, possibly as a result of the functional isolation of the speech areas from posterior parietal association cortex due to the disproportionately advanced maturation of the cortical speech areas at that age.

The posterior parietal association cortex is considered to play a very important role in language function (Geschwind, 1965; Geschwind, 1968; Polyakov, 1961; Polyakov, 1966). It is a phylogenetically new structure and it has undergone great expansion in the human brain. It is strategically located between the cortical association areas of the visual, auditory, and somesthetic systems. Intracortical connections with these association systems allow a mixing of information which might well underlie the cross-modal association capability essential to using names in place of objects, and the recognition of the same word whether spoken, written, or traced on the skin.

The posterior parietal association area progresses phylogenetically with the pulvinar of the thalamus (Ojemann, Fedio, and Van Buren, 1968; Polyakov, 1966). This portion of the thalamus projects onto the posterior temporal lobe and the parietal association areas (Figs. 3 and 4). It receives inputs from the lateral and medial geniculate bodies, thereby having access to some of the same information from the highest subcortical stations of the visual and auditory systems that is being simultaneously conveyed to the calcarine cortex of the occipital lobe and Heschel's gyrus in the temporal lobe (Fig. 3) (Crosby, Humphrey, and Lauer, 1962; Truex and Carpenter, 1964). Aphasia has resulted from lesions involving the pulvinar, and electrical stimulation of the pulvinar in the human has produced naming difficulty (Ciemins, 1968; Hermann et al., 1966; Ojemann, Fedio, and Van Buren, 1968; Russell and Espir, 1961).

Focal lesions involving the angular gyrus result in reading and writing deficits, and it has been inferred that this region is importantly involved in visual-auditory association function (Fig. 1) (Geschwind, 1962; Russell and Espir, 1961). Focal lesions involving posterior parieto-occipital cortex may result in writing deficits (Russell and Espir, 1961), presumably due, in part, to disconnection in the visual-somesthetic association system.

Language learning depends upon normal function of the auditory and visual systems. Initially, language is largely an auditory experience, characterized by the perception of speech sounds and motor replication of these sounds (Preston, Yeni-Komshian, and Stark, 1967a; Preston, Yeni-Komshian, and Stark, 1967b). A congenitally deaf infant fails to differentiate his early repertoire of vocalizations, and does not imitate adult speech sounds (Fry, 1966; Whetnall and Fry, 1964). If a profound bilateral hearing loss is sustained during the first few years of life, after language development has started, speech production diminishes markedly. Access to the auditory representation of language is also necessary for the development of normal grammatical competence. Bright deaf individuals show altered grammatical structure that is probably the result of restricted early experience in the use of spoken language, impoverished language models, and disproportionate use of sign language (Mendelson et al., 1964; Stokoe, 1964). The auditory experience of a language may be thought of as the scaffolding upon which other dimensions of language function are organized. The entire auditory system is, therefore, of critical importance to the acquisition of language. High-frequency hearing losses that interfere with the discrimination of consonants will significantly impair the process of speech learning (Hirsh, 1966; Morley, 1965). However, normal pure-tone hearing acuity does not ensure normal speech perception. Auditory pattern recognition probably

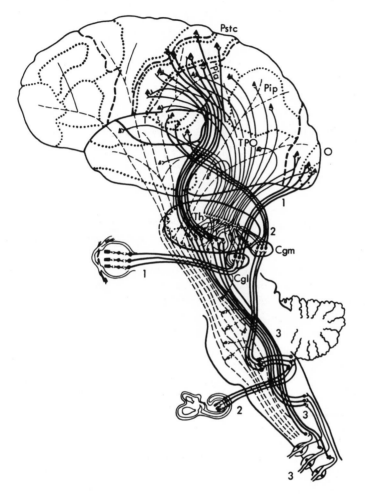

Figure 3. Auditory, visual, and somesthetic pathways. (1) visual, (2) auditory, and (3) somesthetic system transducers. (T) temporal cortex; (O) occipital cortex; (Pstc) postcentral gyrus; (Pip) angular gyrus; (Pia) supramarginal gyrus; (TPO) temporo-parietal-occipital junction; (Th) thalamus; (Cgm) medial geniculate body; (Cgl) lateral geniculate body. From Polyakov, G. I., Modern data on the structural organization of the cerebral cortex. *In* Luria, A. R., ed., Higher Cortical Functions in Man. New York, Basic Books, 1966.

requires preprocessing operations involving the nuclei of the central auditory pathways, and computational capabilities of the auditory cortex and auditory association cortex (Bocca and Calearo, 1963; Deutsch, 1967; Neff, 1964; Whitfield, 1967).

The visual system plays a role in early vocabulary acquisition, so much of which consists of attaching sounds to objects seen. More complex visual system capabilities underlie the pattern recognition and spatial orientation functions essential to the acquisition of reading and writing.

How does a child learn the speech code when no two speakers make the same sound in exactly the same way? How does a child learn to read cursive script when no two authors write the same letter in exactly the same way? How does a child acquire the use of grammatical rules in early life when he is only exposed to generalizations about these rules many years later? Efficiency and accuracy in language usage requires the recognition of common formal features of language despite a great deal of individual differences in speech and writing. The nervous system must extract the common features that constitute the language system from a diversity of spoken and written samples (Carne, 1965; Chase, 1967b; Deutsch, 1967; George, 1962; Sholl, 1967; Taylor, 1964; Uhr, 1966). The necessary critical feature extraction and generalization operations have not yet been localized.

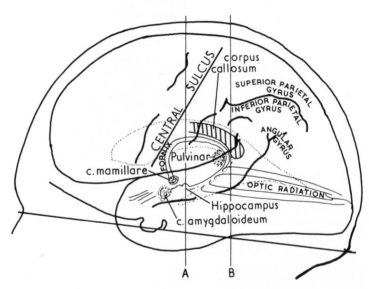

Figure 4. Diagram showing medial brain structures (corpus callosum, fornix, mammilary body, pulvinar, amygdala, and
hippocampus) mapped onto a lateral view of the left
cerebral hemisphere. From Russell, W. R., and M. L. E.
Espir, Traumatic Aphasia. New York, Oxford University
Press, 1961; after Delmas and Pertuise, Topométrie
cranio-encéphalique chez l'homme, Paris, Masson et Cie,
1969.

The plan of a spoken sentence must be formulated and held in some form during the complete time course of the serial utterance. Similarly, we receive speech in serial order, and must hold long strings of sounds until the sample is sufficient to allow interpretation. The demands on an auditory memory system are therefore heavy both for speech production and speech perception (Brain, 1961). Lesions of Wernicke's area disturb these memory functions (Russell and Espir, 1961). Bilateral lesions of the hippocampus and hippocampal gyrus impair long-term memory for all events, including language (Fig. 4) (Barbizet, 1963; Green, 1964; Koikegami, 1964; Milner and Teuber, 1968; Richter 1966).

The acquisition and use of language is an integral part of larger systems of behavior (Luria, 1961; Luria, 1967a). Language serves as an instrument for exchanging information with other people and with the physical environment. Lesions that profoundly alter motivation and the expression of affect also alter the pattern of language acquisition and use. It is in this context that the limbic system and the frontal association areas become of concern to the student of the neurology of language (Luria, 1967b; Russell and Espir, 1961).

In the full-term infant some areas of the cerebral cortex are far more advanced in morphologic maturation than other areas (Altman, 1967; Himwich, 1962). The most advanced development is found in the motor cortex and projection areas for the visual, auditory, and somesthetic systems. Myelination of the cortical end of the auditory projections is protracted beyond the first year, whereas myelination of the cortical end of the visual projections is completed soon after birth (Yakovlev and Lecours, 1967). There is a comparable discrepancy in the rate of myelination of the geniculotemporal and the geniculocalcarine radiations (Yakovlev and Lecours, 1967). The association cortex immediately surrounding these areas is morphologically less mature, and the large frontal and posterior parietal association areas are least mature (Fig. 5) (Altman, 1967; Bronson, 1965; Polyakov, 1961; Polyakov, 1966). The myelination of thalamic projections to these cortical areas shows a similar gradient of differential maturation (Fig. 6) (Yakovlev and Lecours, 1967). That portion of parietal association cortex that is located between the association cortices of the visual, auditory, and somesthetic systems (inferior parietal lobule) is said to receive relatively few thalamic projections—most of its input being provided from the association cortices of the primary sensory systems (Geschwind, 1965). Myelination of the inferior parietal lobule continues to progress well into the fourth decade (Fig. 6) (Yakovlev and Lecours, 1967).

The gradients of maturation of cortical regions known to be related to language function, and the thalamic projections to these cortical areas, can be roughly correlated with some of the major behavioral aspects of language development (Sloan, 1967). Initially, language is almost exclusively an auditory experience. Adults produce copious vocalizations directed toward infants. During the second half of the first year of life the vocalization repertoire of the infant shows some of the segmental and suprasegmental features of the adult language system (Brown, 1965; Ervin and Miller, 1963; Fry, 1966). Imitative vocalization is common during this period. Adults speak to infants in a manner that is perceptibly different from the way they speak to other adults, and it would be interesting to know more about the acoustic characteristics of the speech of adults that is directed to very young infants. It is quite clear that exposure to acoustic representations

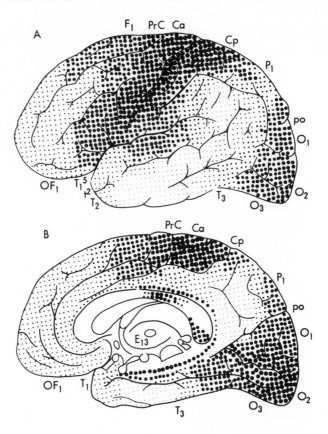

Figure 5. Lateral view of the left cerebral hemisphere
(top) and medial view of the right cerebral
hemisphere (bottom). The large dots indicate
cortical regions that become myelinated first,
and the small dots indicate cortical regions
that become myelinated last. From Polyakov,
G. I., Modern data on the structural organization of the cerebral cortex. *In* Luria, A. R.,
ed., Higher Cortical Functions in Man. New
York, Basic Books, 1966; from Vogt, C., and
O. Vogt, Allgemeine ergebnisse unserer
hirnforschung. J. Psychol. Neurol., 25
(1919-1920).

of adult speech is essential to the normal development of speech motor capability (Fry,
1966; Whetnall and Fry, 1964). It would appear that the earliest stage of language
learning consists of the analysis of incoming acoustic signals, and the derivation of a
motor plan that allows replication of the sounds heard. The essential components
necessary for this rudimentary stage of language learning are auditory cortex, the face

area of the motor cortex, and connections between these cortical areas. These components are disproportionately mature at birth. The progressive development of motor association cortex for the face area (Broca's area) and posterior auditory association cortex (Wernicke's area) may well underlie the progressive stabilization of the phonological system and the ability to learn longer and more complex sound sequences. At about 1 year of age most normal infants have a vocabulary of one or more words—usually names for objects seen (Brown, Darley, and Gomez, 1967; Ervin and Miller, 1963). This stage of language development requires the ability to mix information from the visual and auditory association areas. Sufficient maturation of the inferior parietal lobule must be required for naming, and it is quite possible that the extreme immaturity of this region in the term infant assists the earliest stages of phonological development by

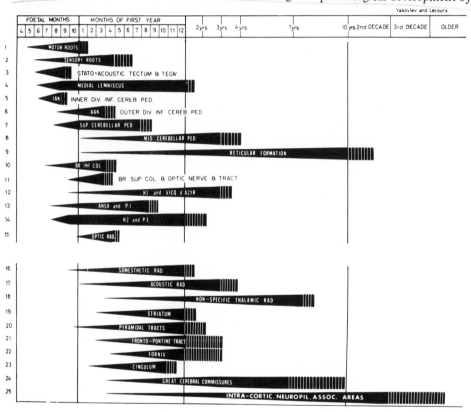

Figure 6. Cycles of myelination in the human nervous system. The length and width of each horizontal bar indicates progression in the intensity of staining and density of myelinated fibers. The vertical stripes at the end of each bar indicate the approximate age range of termination of myelination. From Yakovlev, P. I., and A. Lecours, The myelogenetic cycles of regional maturation of the brain. *In* Minkowski, A., ed., Regional Development of the Brain in Early Life. Oxford, Blackwell, 1967.

leaving these early stages of learning unencumbered by association of sounds with objects. The remarkable growth of vocabulary beyond the first year undoubtedly depends upon progressive maturation of the inferior parietal lobule and the mixing of auditory, visual, and somesthetic association area inputs that are mediated by this region. The cortical speech areas of the left hemisphere assume progressively disproportionate importance for the mediation of language function during the first decade of life (Basser, 1962; Piercy, 1964; Zangwill, 1964). This is the case for right- and left-handed individuals, although a significantly higher proportion of those individuals who make predominant use of the left hand will show representation of language function predominantly in the right hemisphere (Penfield and Roberts, 1959; Zangwill, 1964). If extensive damage is sustained by the left hemisphere during the first few years of life, later surgical removal of that hemisphere rarely produces language disability (Basser, 1962; Gardner et al., 1955; Krynauw, 1950; McFie, 1961; White, 1961). However, if the left hemisphere lesion is sustained after the first few years of life, the surgical removal of the left hemisphere is commonly associated with some disturbance of language function (Piercy, 1964). In addition, the use of dichotic listening tests has shown that spoken material presented to the right ear is reported more accurately than spoken material presented to the left ear as early as 4 years of age (Kimura, 1963). Previous studies in adults, utilizing the same tasks, had shown a definite superiority for the ear opposite the dominant hemisphere (Kimura, 1963). Extensive lesions involving the posterior temporal lobe on the left side show progressively more marked disturbance of language function the older the child at the time the lesion is sustained. However, at least until the age of about 10 to 12 years, extensive recovery is expected, usually within weeks or months, even after hemispherectomy. These several observations suggest that the left hemisphere gradually assumes disproportionate involvement in the mediation of language function. During the first decade, the nondominant hemisphere is capable of mediating normal language function (Obrador, 1964; Penfield and Roberts, 1959; Piercy, 1964; Roberts, 1958).

The plasticity of right and left hemisphere cortical speech areas, and the protracted maturation of geniculotemporal projections, auditory cortex, auditory association cortex, and inferior parietal lobule apparently, underlie the prolonged time period during which languages may be learned with considerable facility.

Reading and writing involve the learning of a set of visual forms and the association of these forms with the acoustic organization of the language. The selection of visual forms is completely arbitrary, as are the rules used for organizing these forms (Fries, 1962; Klapper, 1966). The visual forms need not be members of an alphabet. They may, for example, be pictorial representations of objects or ideas. Even if an alphabet is used, the question of whether it is written from right to left or from left to right is one of many organizational conventions that can be decided upon in any way that a group of users wishes. All these systems involve some degree of auditory-visual and visual-auditory association capability, mediated, in part, by the angular gyrus region of the dominant hemisphere. This region serves as a way-station for the transmission of information from visual association cortex to Wernicke's area. In addition, writing requires visual-somesthetic association capability that may be impaired by posterior parietal lesions, as well as intact connections linking the angular gyrus-Wernicke's area-Broca's area-hand area of the motor cortex and the association area just anterior to the hand area (Nielsen, 1962).

One of the important points that must be firmly in mind before attempting understanding of the neurology of language disorders in children is the crucial role of learning in language acquisition. A broad range of early sensory experience is necessary for the normal maturation of the physical structure of visual and auditory systems and the growth of sensory and perceptual capabilities that language learning requires (Fiske, 1961; Hernández-Peón, 1966; Horn, 1965; Melzack, 1965; Melzack and Burns, 1965; Riesen, 1961; Riesen, 1966; Worden, 1966). A broad experience in problem solving probably supports the development of logical capabilities related to the growth of grammatical competence. A broad social experience supports the development of social behaviors, including language (Bruner, 1959; Bruner, 1961; Casler, 1961; Gray, 1958; Harlow, 1959; Harlow, 1964; Hess, 1958; Hinde, 1962a; Hinde, 1962b; Newton and Levine, 1968; Scott, 1962; Scott, 1968; Spitz and Wolf, 1946). Early auditory experience supports the development of the phonological system. Precise determination of critical experiences essential to language development and the time periods during which these experiences must be made available has not yet been accomplished. Although no specific critical period has been defined for language learning, some general facts are at hand, suggesting that auditory experience during the early years of life is of great importance for normal speech development (Fry, 1966; Whetnall and Fry, 1964). Children who sustain a profound, bilateral deafness after the first year of life are far more likely to develop acceptable speech than their congenitally deaf counterparts (Mengel et al., 1967). It has also been demonstrated that children with bilateral impairment of hearing acuity that should not seriously interfere with speech development will, nonetheless, demonstrate very little speech capability if they have been unnecessarily deprived of normal early auditory experience (Whetnall and Fry, 1964). These observations, coupled with the observations on the general facility with which language learning normally proceeds during the first 5 years of life, strongly suggest that there is an extended, but quite real, optimal period for language learning. The fact that new languages can be learned throughout a lifetime attests to some residual capability for language learning at all times.

LANGUAGE DISORDERS IN CHILDHOOD: INTRODUCTION

Although there are a number of excellent general discussions of language disorders in children, there is, at the present time, no generally accepted terminology and classification system for these disorders (Brown, Darley, and Gomez, 1967; Darley, 1964; Hardy, 1965; Kastein and Fowler, 1954; Peacher, 1949; Rapin, 1959; Wood, 1964). The diagnostic classifications that are in use often place heavy emphasis upon behavioral observation, and although quite appropriate, such an approach often obscures the fact that the same behavioral alteration can result from a diversity of etiological mechanisms. The redundancy involved in many of the current classification systems is well known to all clinical workers in this field, and accounts, in part, for the fact that children with language disorders are often given different diagnostic labels by different examiners.

In addition to the difficulties presented by a lack of clarity in some of our concepts about the mechanisms of language disorders and the technical language that reflects our thoughts about these concepts, further difficulties arise when one specifically considers the neurological aspects of language disorders in children. The effects of focal brain lesions in children are often not the same as the effects of the same brain lesions in an adult. This makes it difficult to directly apply our more ample understanding of the adult patient in our clinical evaluation of children (Salam and Adams, 1966). The brain of an infant and young child is a rapidly changing system. It is changing as a result of genetically determined constraints as well as patterns of experience. As the structure of the nervous system changes so does the behavior of the child, and this changing behavioral repertoire can complicate the clinical evaluation of lesions of the nervous system. A departure from a stable behavioral baseline, as is more customary in an adult patient, presents a simpler problem for clinical interpretation. The patterns of brain injury observed in children are often different from those observed in adults. Conditions such as fetal anoxia (Saxon, 1961; Saxon, and Ponce, 1961; Windle, 1964), kernicterus (Carhart, 1967; Gerrard, 1952; Goodhill, 1950; Goodhill, 1956; Matkin and Carhart, 1966), and maternal viral infections during fetal development (Hardy, Monif, and Sever, 1966; Hardy, 1965; Monif, Hardy, and Sever, 1966) result in multiple lesions of both sides of the brain, whereas multiple, bilateral lesions are far less common in the case of vascular accidents, neoplasms, and traumatic injuries that account for so much of the spectrum of brain injury in adults. Finally, the clinical evaluation of certain brain lesions in the child must be undertaken largely in terms of the extent to which they interfere with learning rather than the extent to which they interfere with already well organized functions. Our understanding of structure-function interrelationships in this area is still at an early stage (Salam and Adams, 1966).

APHASIA

The term "aphasia" is generally used to indicate disturbance of speech. Many authors have pointed out that this term should properly be used only in the case of lesions that are sustained after some degree of speech competence has been acquired, with resultant impairment of or loss of this competence (Lenneberg, 1964; Strauss, 1954). However, current practice continues to favor use of this term to indicate many of the neurological conditions that significantly interfere with the acquisition of speech. Conditions that produce a loss of speech or impairment of speech are referred to as "acquired" aphasias. Conditions in which neonatal brain damage or genetic defects result in impairment of speech learning are referred to as "congenital" aphasias. The term "developmental" aphasia (or "specific developmental dysphasia") is often used in reference to congenitally aphasic children who have family histories of language disabilities (Ingram and Reid, 1956; Ingram, 1959; Ingram, 1960).

Acquired aphasia in children results from lesions in the same cortical areas that produce aphasia in adults (Guttmann, 1942). Frontal lesions result in motor disturbance of speech, often with an associated hemiplegia. Temporoparietal lesions disturb both speech comprehension and speech production. Lesions involving cortical speech areas do not produce the differential effects on speech production as a function of location that one observes in adult patients. Fluent aphasias are not observed in young children, and substitution of words that sound like the intended word, or have a meaning similar to that of the intended word, is less commonly observed (Alajouanine and Lhermitte, 1965; Benson, 1967; Benton, 1964; Benton, 1966; Geschwind, 1968; Karlin, 1954; Lenneberg, 1964; Lenneberg, 1967). The most striking clinical feature of the speech of a child with an acquired aphasia is the sharp reduction in the amount of speech that is voluntarily offered (Alajouanine and Lhermitte, 1965; Guttmann, 1942; Karlin, 1954). The reduction in speech may approach frank mutism. In adult patients, mutism rarely accompanies lesions of cortical speech areas except in the acute stage. In addition to the marked reduction in speech activity, many observers have commented on the reluctance of the aphasic child to communicate at all, noting that it is very difficult to motivate the child to exchange information, by speaking, writing, or using gesture (Alajouanine and Lhermitte, 1965; Karlin, 1954). When speech is produced, it is usually sparse and telegraphic in character. These characteristics obtain in the case of both frontal and temporal or temporoparietal lesions. However, as in the case of adult patients, frontal lesions often produce disturbances in articulation with accompanying hemiparesis, and temporal lesions often produce marked disturbance of speech comprehension. Large brain lesions sustained during the first few years of life, later treated by hemispherectomy, do not produce aphasia, independent of the side of the brain that is involved (Basser, 1962; Gardner et al., 1955; Krynauw, 1950; McFie, 1961; Piercy, 1964; White, 1961). Lateralization of language function apparently increases significantly during the first decade of life, and the tendency of left hemisphere lesions to disturb language function more than comparable right hemisphere lesions increases as a function of age. By the middle of the second decade, the clinical effects on language behavior of left versus right hemisphere lesions are usually close to that observed in the case of adults. As in adult patients, frontal lesions show a generally faster course of recovery than temporal lesions. Independent of the location of the cortical lesion, children recover language function far more rapidly, and usually far more completely, than adults (Alajouanine and Lhermitte, 1965; Guttmann, 1942; Kalrin, 1954; Lenneberg, 1964; Lenneberg, 1967). Significant recovery often occurs within weeks, or a few months in the case of children, whereas a longer period of months, or even years, might be required for an adult aphasic patient to realize significant recovery of language function (Schuell, Jenkins, and Jiménez-Pabón, 1964). Although there is universal agreement about the faster and more complete recovery of children with acquired aphasia, we should probably exercise caution in accepting the traditionally optimistic prognosis that is offered in the case of acquired aphasia in children. The most striking deficit is marked reduction in speech, and recovery of speech production capability is usually the major criterion used in evaluating recovery. There are many other dimensions of language usage, and some of these dimensions are still developing in children. The ability to comprehend long and complicated spoken messages; the ability to appreciate wit, humor, metaphor, sarcasm, rhetoric; the ability to utilize language as an instrument of thought and imagination, constitute dimensions of language that may be seriously affected by temporal and temporoparietal lesions in children (Alajouanine and Lhermitte, 1965; Bay, 1962).

Disturbances of reading and writing are to be expected in the majority of children with acquired aphasia. These disturbances are often more severe than disturbances of speech, and recovery may be slower and less complete than in disturbances of speech (Alajouanine and Lhermitte, 1965).

Congenital aphasia should be suspected if speech is delayed, and abnormal in character, with no family history of language disorder and no evidence of significant peripheral deafness, mental deficiency, or psychological disorder. One of the most striking clinical features of patients with congenital aphasia is the inconsistent and aberrant manner in which auditory input, particularly speech, is dealt with (Benton, 1964; Benton, 1966; Gordon and Taylor, 1964; Gordon, 1966; Myklebust, 1952; Myklebust, 1954; Reichstein and Rosenstein, 1964). Peripheral deafness is often suspected because of the extreme degree of inattention to auditory stimuli that may be demonstrated, particularly when the child is involved in visual or manual exploration. Evaluation of pure-tone hearing acuity often shows ability to hear at levels close to normal threshold, possibly with some impairment of acuity for high frequencies (Benton, 1964; Gordon and Taylor, 1964). Response to the same stimuli may be very inconsistent from one presentation to the next. Speech sounds apparently evoke very little interest or selective attention. It is, therefore, extremely difficult to teach the meanings of speech sounds. In addition, speech sounds do not elicit the imitative efforts required for normal speech learning. In extreme cases, there is no evidence whatever that speech, and possibly nonspeech sounds as well, conveys any meaning at all, and there is no development of speech. In other instances, speech may be understood if sentences are simple, spoken slowly, and efforts are made to avoid distractions while speech is being exchanged. In such instances, speech development is slow. Phonological development is impaired, although it has been observed that the patient's direct imitations of the examiner's speech can result in significant improvement in phonological structure. It may be difficult for any but the most familiar observers to understand the patient's speech. In addition to impaired phonological organization, speech is sparse, and grammatical structure is poorly differentiated (Ingram and Reid, 1956; Ingram, 1959; Ingram, 1960). Prepositions, conjunctions, and articles are often omitted, resulting in a "telegraphic" style of speech. A history compatible with brain damage in the neonatal period is frequently obtainable (Ingram, 1959). Distractability, short attention span, emotional lability, and hyperactivity may or may not accompany the language disturbance (Karlin, 1954).

A great deal of evidence favors the hypothesis that many children with congenital aphasia have suffered damage to the central auditory system (Allen, 1952; Benton, 1964; Benton, 1966; Bocca, 1958; Ewing, 1967; Gordon, 1966; Karlin, 1951; Landau, Goldstein, and Kleffner, 1960; Reichstein and Rosenstein, 1964; Worster-Drought and Allen, 1929; Worster-Drought and Allen, 1930). Bilateral lesions are postulated because of the plasticity of the young nervous system with respect to the development of language function and the fact that the auditory pathways are crossed (Sugar, 1952). In an adult, bilateral lesions of the geniculotemporal radiations and auditory cortex can impair the perception of all sounds (Kleist, 1962; Work and Haldane, 1966); and lesions of the geniculotemporal radiation on the left, combined with a callosal lesion interrupting the transmission of auditory information from the nondominant hemisphere, can result in inability to recognize any linguistic auditory stimulus (Geschwind, 1968; Nielsen, 1962). The latter set of lesions isolates Wernicke's area on the left from all auditory input. In the case of infants and very young children, however, it would presumably be sufficient to present undistorted speech to either hemisphere in order to allow normal development of speech production and speech perception. Although the production of bilateral lesions in the central auditory system requires a complicated and rare combination of lesions in the adult, a number of conditions that have long been suspected of playing a role in the etiology of congenital aphasia are now known to be capable of producing bilateral auditory system lesions. Prominent among these conditions are asphyxia neonatorum (Saxon, 1961; Saxon and Ponce, 1961; Windle, 1964), kernicterus (Carhart, 1967; Flower, Viehweg, and Ruzicka, 1966; Gerrard, 1952; Goodhill, 1950; Goodhill, 1956; Matkin and Carhart, 1966), and maternal viral infections that involve the fetus, particularly rubella (Hardy, Monif, and Sever, 1966; Hardy, 1968; Monif, Hardy, and Sever, 1966). The only reported case of congenital aphasia that has been subjected to postmortem examination showed atrophy of white and gray matter over large areas of both cerebral hemispheres, severely damaging the auditory radiations to the temporal lobes on both sides, with resultant retrograde degeneration of the medial geniculate nuclei (Landau, Goldstein, and Kleffner, 1960).

It is quite possible that differential involvement of different groups of nuclei of the central auditory system, and different portions of auditory cortex, auditory association cortex, and intracortical connections involving the auditory cortex, could account for the broad spectrum of auditory disorders that affect the development of language in children. Impairment of function of the efferent components of the auditory system might also contribute to the disturbances of auditory perception observed in these children. This might result from direct damage to efferent fiber tracts in the auditory system, or it might result as a secondary consequence of damage to the temporal cortex, or failure of normal functional development of the auditory cortex as a result of impaired function of lower stations of the auditory system.

There is a growing understanding of the physiology of the auditory system, including the efferent components of this system (Comis and Whitfield, 1968; Desmedt and Mecelse, 1958; Dewson, Nobel, and Pribram, 1966; Diamond and Neff, 1957; Galambos, 1964; Hernández-Peón, Jouvet, and Scherrer, 1957; Nobel and Dewson, 1966; Vardapetyan, 1967; Whitfield, 1967). There is, in addition, an enlarging capability for audiological evaluation of retrocochlear lesions, including lesions of the auditory cortex (Bender and Diamond, 1965; Bocca, 1958; Bocca and Calearo, 1963; Goodglass, 1967; Jerger, 1960; Jerger, 1964; Milner, 1962; Spinnler and Vignolo, 1966). New techniques for the audiological evaluation of infants and children are also being developed (Downs, 1967; Eisenberg et al., 1964; Eisenberg, Coursin, and Rupp, 1966; Frisina, 1963; Goldstein, 1967; Rapin and Graziani, 1967). Growth of knowledge in these areas should provide more rigorous evaluation of the hypothesis that most children with congenital aphasia have significant pathology involving the central auditory system bilaterally.

The prognosis for congenital aphasia is not nearly as favorable as is the case for developmental aphasia. The child's ability to acquire language capability is closely related to the nature and degree of his auditory impairment. The more severe degrees of auditory impairment preclude the development of speech, with resulting impairment of reading and writing. Special education plays a crucial role in the development of these children, for language skills must be taught with unusually heavy reliance on nonauditory sensory inputs.

Developmental aphasia (specific developmental dysphasia) is a type of congenital aphasia characterized by delayed, and sometimes aberrant, development of speech, reading, and writing in children with family histories of similar difficulties (Ingram, 1960). Genetic factors are thought to play a prominent etiologic role, and this disorder is considered by some to be the same basic disorder that is called "specific developmental dyslexia" in patients whose language disability involves reading and writing disproportionately (Ingram, 1960). All observers agree that a large number of children with developmental dyslexia have histories of delayed development of speech and poor articulation. It is also agreed that a large proportion of children with histories of delayed development of speech, poor articulation, and impaired speech comprehension later show difficulty in learning reading and writing skills (Gallagher, 1950; Ingram, 1959; Ingram, 1960; Ingram, 1963; Ingram, 1965). The possibility that a primary impairment of auditory language function underlies much of the spectrum of language disorders in children, including reading and writing disabilities, would seem to merit serious investigation.

Children with developmental aphasia may show delayed development of speech, usually accompanied by mild articulation difficulties, as their only clinical manifestation (Ingram, 1959; Ingram, 1960; Ingram, 1963; Morley et al., 1955; Morely, 1965). In such cases, the time of appearance of intelligible words, two-word phrases, and longer sentences may all be delayed by 1 or more years. When words do occur they are usually only intelligible to the parents and others close to the child. The fact that words are intelligible at all suggests that they are articulated in a consistent manner, but the fact that they are not intelligible to more casual observers tells us that adult speech models are not being replicated accurately. Some children will also show difficulties in their acquisition of grammatical structure, omitting prepositions, conjunctions, auxiliary verbs, and articles, with frequent errors in word order. As the vocabulary expands it can be appreciated that poor articulation is not the only cause of impaired production of intelligible speech. Syllables may be reversed, or omitted, and words similar in sound to the intended word might be substituted. It is commonplace to have parents raise questions about speech-comprehension ability, and it has been noted that many of these patients acquire the habit of frequently requesting that questions be repeated. A large number of children with early histories of these speech problems will later demonstrate the typical picture of specific developmental dyslexia (Cole and Walker, 1964; Gallagher, 1950; Ingram, 1960; Ingram, 1963). Developmental aphasia affects males more frequently than females. A higher incidence of incomplete or mixed patterns of preference with respect to the use of the hands, feet, eyes, and ears is thought to characterize this group by some observers, but observations on this matter remain controversial (Gordon and Taylor, 1964). The major milestones of general motor development are usually reached on schedule, and the neurological examination is usually negative. Pure-tone hearing acuity is characteristically within normal limits, although some inconsistency in responses may be noted.

The prognosis in this condition is generally quite good, the majority of children showing a fairly normal pattern of language development, with the delayed schedule of development constituting the major clinical manifestation of language disturbance (Ingram, 1960). It usually makes good sense to provide these children with supplemental language instruction. It is, of course, imperative that demands made on them in school do not exceed their available capabilities. This may require delaying the start of formal schooling. With appropriate management, improvement in all areas of language function over time is to be expected. The more severely affected individuals will show more marked residual impairment of language function, particularly reading. This is more likely to be the case for those children who show definite speech-comprehension deficits.

Reading Disability (Dyslexia)

The majority of reading disabilities in childhood are associated with inadequate or inappropriate instruction, emotional disturbances, lesser degrees of early brain damage (minimal cerebral dysfunction) (Clements, 1966a, 1966b; Eisenberg, 1959; Goldberg and Drash, 1968; Kawi and Pasamanick, 1958; Kawi and Pasamanick, 1959; Klapper, 1966), or the congenital form of reading disorder known as "specific" or "developmental" dyslexia (Eisenberg, 1959; Goldberg, 1968; Goldberg and Drash, 1968). Dyslexia will also often be present in association with aphasia (Ingram, 1960; Ingram, 1963), and, rarely, may result from focal, posterior brain lesions without associated aphasia (Ajax, 1964; Ajax, 1967; Bender, 1963; Ettlinger and Hurwitz, 1962; Russell and Espir, 1961).

Developmental dyslexia was first described at the end of the nineteenth century (Morgan, 1896), and since that time numerous studies have contributed to the definition of this entity (Money, 1962; Money, 1966; Shankweiler, 1964). Much of the literature has recently been reviewed by Critchley (1964). The child with developmental dyslexia has great difficulty attaching sound and meaning to written words. Oral reading is effortful and filled with errors. Words that have a similar appearance are often confused; letters are reversed, phonemes are mispronounced, phonemes or words may be omitted or inserted inappropriately. Vocalization often accompanies efforts at silent reading, and comprehension for oral or silent reading is markedly impaired. Disorders of writing are always present, consisting of poor structural formation of letters, and relationships between letters, rotation of letters, reversals of letters, omission and repetition of letters and words, and frequent misspellings. Difficulty with arithmetic and musical notation, drawing, right-left orientation, visual-motor coordination, and speech defects may or may not be present (Benton and Hemble, 1960; Benton, 1962; Critchley, 1964; Shankweiler, 1964). Left-handedness or ambidexterity; mild, generalized EEG abnormalities; and a positive family history of similar difficulties are common in this group. Males are affected about four times more frequently than females, and family studies suggest a monohybrid, autosomal dominant mode of inheritance (Drew, 1956; Hallgren, 1950; Pratt, 1967). The region of the angular gyrus has been often proposed as a possible site of lesion, but there has been no neuropathologic confirmation of this or any other lesion in this condition. The idea that maturation of the parietal lobe may be delayed in these patients seems to have attracted more favor than ideas concerning the possibility of more focal lesion (Critchley, 1964; Drew, 1956). Although inconsistent, the evidence concerning ambidexterity among dyslexics favors continued investigation of the possible role of altered patterns of cerebral dominance in this, as in most of the language disorders of childhood (Critchley, 1967; Eustis, 1947; Gooddy and Reinhold, 1961; McFie, 1952; Shankweiler, 1964; Spitzer, Rabkin, and Kramer, 1959; Zangwill, 1960; Zangwill, 1962). Perceptual studies provide further support in favor of such investigation, showing that dyslexic often fail to show normal directional effects in visual and auditory rivalry tasks (McFie, 1952; Shankweiler, 1964). The central defect would appear to be an impairment of auditory-visual, visual-auditory association function, with impairment of visual-spatial perceptual organization sometimes providing additional difficulty (Critchley, 1961; Critchley, 1964; Critchley, 1967; de Hirsch, 1957; de Hirsch and Jansky, 1968; Ingram, 1965; Kinsbourne and Warrington, 1963; Schenk, 1966). These patients may respond well to tutorial assistance, particularly if it is made available early and is so structured as to make clear the units of sound structure and visual structure used in language, and the relationships between the two (Klapper, 1966; Nicholls, 1960; Rawson, 1968).

Impairment of reading secondary to a focal brain lesion is quite rare in adults, and must surely be even rarer in children. Alexia without agraphia may be caused by a lesion in the dominant occipital lobe in combination with a lesion of the splenium of the corpus callosum (Cogan, 1965; Geschwind, 1962; Geschwind, 1967; Geschwind, 1968). The combination of lesions impairs visual association cortex input to Wernicke's area on the dominant hemisphere. Visual association cortex function is impaired on the dominant side, and comparable information from the nondominant side is prevented from crossing to the dominant Wernicke's area by the lesion in the posterior corpus callosum. The combination of lesions results from occlusion of the posterior cerebral artery (Cogan, 1965). Impairment of the visual recognition of words may also result from lesions of the geniculocalcarine projection, visual cortex, visual association cortex, and projections from visual association cortex to the region of the angular gyrus (Ajax, 1964; Ajax, 196?; Bender, 1963; Hécaen, 1967). Although a right homonymous hemianopsia is common in such instances, visual recognition defects are also found in association with occipital lesions on the right (Bender, 1963). Lesions that predominantly affect reading and writing together are usually located in the region of the angular and supramarginal gyri (Ajax, 1964; Brain, 1961; Geschwind, 1962; Nielsen, 1962).

Reading and writing are normally learned in reference to the initial auditory experience of a language. Reading and writing capability require, among other things, an accurate "mapping" of units of visual representation of the language onto units of auditory representation of the language. Such a formulation suggests two major ways in which reading might be impaired. There might be difficulty in the recognition of the visual organization of the language; or, there might be difficulty in developing an accurate system of appropriate visual-auditory associations (Ingram, 1970; Silver and Hagin, 1970). A number of studies show impairment of visual-auditory associations in commonly involved in the mechanism of dyslexia in children (Ingram, 1963; Schenk, 1966). Impairment of the initial development of speech would, of course, increase the probability of later difficulties with reading based on impairment of visual-auditory associations (Ingram, 1959; Ingram, 1960).

MINIMAL CEREBRAL DYSFUNCTION

During the past twenty years there has been increasing recognition of children with behavior disorders, attentional and perceptual deficits, and minor neurological deficits (Clements, 1966a, 1966b; Work and Haldane, 1966). The terms "minimal cerebral dysfunction" or "minimal brain damage" have been used as diagnostic labels for children who fit this description. This diagnosis is largely based on behavioral criteria. The characteristics most often cited as being descriptive of children with minimal cerebral dysfunction are hyperactivity; short attention span; impulsivity; emotional lability; perseveration; clumsiness; perceptual, cognitive and memory defects; impairments of reading, writing, spelling, and arithmetic; disorders of speech and hearing; and minor neurological signs and nonspecific EEG abnormalities (Clements and Peters, 1962; Clements, 1966a, 1966b; Cohn, 1964; Glaser and Clemmens, 1965; Gofman, 1965; Gubbay et al., 1965; Lucas, Rodin, and Simson, 1965; Paine, 1962; Paine, 1963; Paine, 1965; Pincus and Glaser, 1966; Stevens et al., 1967; Stevens, Sachdev, and Milstein, 1968). The minor neurological signs most frequently encountered are impairment of coordinated fine movements of the hands, general clumsiness, choreiform or athetoid movements, and strabismus (Clements, 1966b; Paine, 1962; Pincus and Glaser, 1966). These signs may be present in such a mild form that they can be easily overlooked in the course of a routine neurological examination. A history suggestive of possible injury to the nervous system in the perinatal period strengthens the diagnosis of minimal cerebral dysfunction. Etiological factors thought to be of significance are hemorrhage, use of toxic drugs, and viral infections during pregnancy; toxemia of pregnancy; prolonged and complicated labor; prematurity; subdural hematoma; cephalhematoma; anoxia; low birth weight; kernicterus; meningitis; encephalitis; arrested hydrocephalus; severe dehydration; lead intoxication; and head trauma (Kawi and Pasamanick, 1958; Kawi and Pasamanick, 1959; Knobloch and Pasamanick, 1959; Paine, 1965; Pincus and Glaser, 1966). It has been suggested that there is a continuum of severity in clinical patterns of early central nervous system damage. The most severe casualties result in abortions, stillbirths, and neonatal death. Less severe damage results in seizure disorders, cerebral palsy, mental retardation, and severe deficits of visual and auditory function. The mildest patterns of damage are associated with the deficits that have been reviewed above as being characteristic of the syndrome of minimal cerebral dysfunction (Kawi and Pasamanick, 1958, 1959; Paine, 1962, 1965).

Language disabilities most commonly cited in clinical descriptions of patients with minimal cerebral dysfunction are impairments of hearing and auditory perception, slow development of spoken language, articulation disorders, reading and writing disabilities (Clements, 1966b). Intelligence test scores often show scattered patterns of achievement, and some of the performance subtests commonly show very marked impairments

(Clements, 1966b; Pincus and Glaser, 1966). Delayed development of speech is commonly associated with left-handedness or ambidexterity without evidence for the diagnosis of focal brain damage (Ingram and Reid, 1956; Ingram, 1959, 1960, 1963, 1965; Morley et al., 1955; Morley, 1965; Pincus and Glaser, 1966). In such instances it is not at all clear whether early injury to the nervous system plays any role whatever. In the management of such cases, is it usually quite sufficient to reduce demands on the child with respect to language performance, including, at times, delaying the start of formal schooling. Even when language disorders are associated with other stigmata of minimal cerebral dysfunction, they are usually less marked than other deficits, and the prognosis is much more favorable than it is in conditions producing more isolated disturbances of language function. Many children diagnosed as having minimal cerebral dysfunction show general improvement in all areas over time, and the hyperkinesis that is so disturbing during the early years of life is rarely observed by the time these children reach adolescence (Paine, 1963). Hyperactivity, in association with perceptual deficits and mild language disorders, predisposes to patterns of early school failure. The destructive consequences of the psychological response to school failure can far exceed the destructive consequences of the primary functional deficits. Hyperkinesis is often successfully treated with amphetamines (Millichap and Fowler, 1967), but avoidance of psychological adjustment problems, particularly in the school setting, requires an understanding of this syndrome by parents and teachers, with suitable accommodation to the behavioral requirements of these children.

PSYCHOSES OF CHILDHOOD

Severe disturbances in behavior may be noted from very early infancy. A particularly well-defined constellation of early behavioral abnormalities consists of avoidance of physical and eye contact, obsessive efforts to maintain stereotopy in routines and physical arrangements, preference for physical objects instead of people, abnormal posture and motility patterns, and minimal use of meaningful speech in spite of other evidence for good general intelligence (Eisenberg, 1957; Kanner, 1944; Schain and Yannet, 1960). This syndrome has been given the name "early infantile autism." Descriptions of psychotic disorders in children usually include several of these features (Creak, 1963; Creak et al., 1964; Reiser, 1963), and at the present time there is no generally accepted classification of the psychotic disorders of childhood. Discussions about the possible differentiation of early infantile autism from other possible forms of psychotic disorder, such as schizophrenia, often refer to the absence of hallucinations and obvious thought disorder in psychotic children, which serves to obscure the relationship between schizophrenia in young adults and psychotic disorders in children (Rutter, 1965). The etiology of psychotic disorders in childhood is similarly obscure at this time. Some authors strongly favor disturbed patterns of parent-infant interrelationships as the most crucial causal factor, and other authors, noting the extremely early onset of symptoms in some patients, and the motor disturbances and obvious focal neurological signs and EEG abnormalities that frequently are revealed by diligent longitudinal study, favor frank brain damage as the most crucial etiological factor in most patients (Baer, 1961; Eaton and Menolascino, 1967; Menolascino, 1965; Reiser, 1963; Rutter, 1965; Schain and Yannet, 1960). There is no doubt whatever that many children described as autistic or psychotic do present abundant evidence for early brain damage, and the report of classical autistic behavioral patterns in children with neurolipidosis makes one additionally mindful of the possibility that structural brain lesions may be a sufficient cause of the autistic syndrome (Creak, 1963). It may well be the case that the behavioral syndrome we are discussing results from a variety of patterns of early brain damage, in much the same way that mutism so characteristically follows early acquired deafness as well as aphasia associated with temporoparietal or frontal lesions in children. For the present, we might accept early infantile autism as one psychotic disorder of childhood and acknowledge the fact that a great many of the children whose early behavior qualifies them for assignment into this diagnostic cateogry have definite evidence of early brain damage. This position does not foreclose any consideration of the pathogenicity of disturbed early relationships between infant and parents, nor does it diminish in any way our interest in the interpersonal context of the life of the autistic child.

The language behavior of the autistic child is quite characteristic. Usually, there is almost no spontaneous use of speech for purposes of interpersonal communication (Kanner, 1944; Rutter, 1965; Schain and Yannet, 1960). Frequently there has never been a demonstration of normal speech production capability, and this fact raises the possibility of deafness or aphasia. It is, however, almost always possible to demonstrate that the child can speak, and this fact, coupled with the observation that verbal commands are understood, rules out a profound hearing loss. A marked disinterest in sharing personal experience by any means helps to distinguish the autistic child from the aphasic child. This distinction is additionally reinforced by observing the autistic child's ability to repeat words, read, and write from oral and written models. Careful examination of these language capabilities often reveals a precocious pattern of language development characterized by large vocabularies containing many long words, with good spelling ability. The strikingly aberrant aspect of the language behavior of the autistic child is his pattern of language learning and language usage. Language is frequently learned without any appreciation of the behavioral context within which it is being elaborated, and impersonal sources of information, such as television, often function as major sources of new words. Learning to copy words from encyclopedias functions similarly. Repetition, by speech or writing, of words culled from such sources often shows marked evidence of perseveration, and is characteristically performed without obvious meaningful relationship to an interpersonal context. Words may be learned in the course of conversations in which the child's gross behavior suggests that he does not hear what is being said, or does not understand what is being said. Usually, neither supposition is correct, as later spontaneous usage of these words makes clear. Echolalia may be present, and this probably contributes to the confusion of pronouns in speech (Rutter, 1965). The presence of echolalia suggests the presence of a normally operative Wernicke's area and Broca's area, normally connected with each other, but inadequately influenced by brain mechanisms that guide language usage as a system for organizing and controlling behavior.

The articulation of autistic children is usually deficient. Several factors probably contribute to the inadequate development of articulation skills. The diminished usage of spoken language is probably the most significant single factor. This might also contribute to impairment of speech-perception capability. In addition, the motor disabilities that are often observed on examination of posture and locomotion may affect the motor control of speech also.

The sine qua non of early infantile autism is marked disturbance of the behavior exchanged between the infant and adults (Eisenberg, 1956, 1957; Kanner, 1944). The mother, particularly, trys to employ the range of supportive and nutritive behaviors that automatically appear, only to feel that the infant does not respond to, or even desire this attention. It would be surprising if some of this behavior did not begin to extinguish in the mother. It might be useful to consider that the brain lesion (or lesions) in autistic children serves to impair the growth of primary and other social bonds (Ambrose, 1963) and that, as a consequence, all behavior becomes "depersonalized." Functional deprivation of a marked degree can be superimposed upon the primary behavioral deficits as a result of extinction of adult supportive behavior. Some authors have suggested that limbic system lesions might be implicated in this syndrome (Pincus and Glaser, 1966; Schain and Yannet, 1960).

It is essential to realize that autistic children are almost always much brighter than they appear to be, and often have remarkable learning abilities (Goodwin and Goodwin, 1969). They do not usually have specific language disabilities in the traditional sense, but only appear to be so impaired because of their limited ability to employ language as a means of mediating social relationships. These children can often profit greatly from normal school settings once the essential nature of their disabilities is made clear to parents and teachers.

Child psychiatrists have called attention to a syndrome characterized by normal or near-normal development of communication and other social behaviors followed, at about 4 years of age, by severe regression in these areas of behavior. Emotional control becomes impaired, language usage is reduced, sometimes resulting in mutism, and profound disturbances in patterns of interpersonal relationships result. It has been proposed that the term "disintegrative psychosis" be provisionally used to refer to this form of childhood psychosis (Rutter et al., 1969).

PSYCHOMOTOR EPILEPSY

Seizures involving the limbic system often show behavioral automatisms, visceral disturbances, and personality, thought, and language disturbances. This complex seizure disorder is referred to by the terms "psychomotor epilepsy," "temporal lobe epilepsy," or "limbic epilepsy" and it accounts for about 25 percent of the seizure states in childhood (Glaser, 1967).

Although very few studies have been done on the language and speech disturbances associated with this type of epilepsy, studies which make observations on this question are in agreement that there is frequent alteration of language function both during and between active limbic seizures (Alajouanine and Sabouraud, 1960; Critchley, 1960a; Glaser, 1967; Hécaen and Piercy, 1956; Hécaen and Angelergues, 1960; Serafetinides and Falconer, 1963; Serafetinides, 1966). During seizure activity some patients will, while still conscious, and without apparent impairment of articulation or hearing, show difficulty with the ideational formulation of speech (ictal dysphasia). Others utter recognizable words or phrases after they have lost contact with the environment and are later found to be completely unable to recall these events (ictal speech automatisms). Ictal dysphasia is more commonly associated with left-sided EEG abnormalities and ictal speech automatisms are found in association with EEG abnormalities on either side with about equal frequency. Ictal speech automatisms have been produced by electrical stimulation in the region of the amygdala in unanesthetized patients, reproducing, in part, the behavior of a spontaneous seizure involving medial temporal structures (Driver, Falconer, and Serafetinides, 1964).

The release of automatic behavior, including speech, appears to result from excitation of the amygdala and adjacent medial temporal structures. The dysphasia accompanying limbic seizures, in all probability, results from abnormal electrical activity involving overlying temporal cortex, particularly posterior temporal cortex.

Evaluation during the inter-ictal period shows significant intellectual deficits, memory impairment, and persistent speech and language disorders in 25 to 50 percent of patients (Glaser, 1967). The speech and language disturbances characteristic of the inter-ictal state have not been studied in detail. The most striking characteristics of these children during the inter-ictal period is their disturbed general behavior. Many show excitability, irritability, and frankly aggressive behavior (Blumer, 1967; Glaser, 1967). Stubbornness, compulsiveness, depression and mood swings, sleep disturbances, and phobias are also common. The behavior of some of these patients can intermittently be frankly psychotic (Blumer, 1967; Glaser, 1967; Robertiello, 1953). Tumors of the limbic system produce a similar spectrum of behavior disorder (Malamud, 1967). It is quite clear that the disturbances in memory, and control of aggressive behavior, will aggravate the altered pattern of language development and use resulting from abnormalities in the function of temporal cortex, particularly the posterior auditory association cortex. School failure is common in this group.

This type of epilepsy is, unfortunately, notoriously difficult to manage with drugs. Only slightly more than half of these patients obtain even reasonably good seizure control with medications, and manipulation of medications is often required before the most effective program for a particular patient can be found. The rare patient with a focal lesion may realize significant reduction in the frequency of seizures following anterior temporal lobectomy.

Recently, a form of focal epilepsy has been described in which motor arrest of speech, somatosensory involvement of the tongue and mouth, excessive pooling of saliva, and movement of the face musculature occur with preservation of consciousness. Inter-ictal EEG studies often show midtemporal spike foci (Lombroso, 1967).

STUTTERING

The mechanisms underlying speech dysfluency characterized by repetitions and blocking continue to be a matter of controversy. Like many abnormalities of movement, stuttering is strongly influenced by emotional factors. Unlike most movement disorders, it is, under certain circumstances, completely reversible. Most stutterers are fluent when singing, or acting in a play (Bloodstein, 1941; Bloodstein, 1959). The possibility that stuttering is related to disturbed development of lateralization of language function has repeatedly been considered. Efforts to evaluate this question indirectly by observations on handedness have given conflicting results (Bloodstein, 1959). Some studies support the hypothesis that stutterers have a higher incidence of left-handedness or ambidexterity. However, other studies fail to support this hypothesis. The peak incidence of stuttering occurs between 3½ and 5 years of age, implicating the ideational and behavioral dimensions of language usage rather than simpler motor mechanisms for the regulation of speech. It should be kept in mind, however, that there must be functional differences between speech generated under circumstances in which dysfluency is to be expected and speech generated under circumstances in which dysfluency is not to be expected, and these differences must be mediated by neurological mechanisms that are different, at least in part. A comparable example is the relative sparing of stereotyped and emotive speech under conditions in which propositional speech is severely disturbed. This situation is commonly encountered among adult aphasic patients (Jackson, 1874, 1878, 1879; Smith, 1966). In general, a reduction in the propositional character of speech seems to favor fluency for patients who stutter (Bloodstein, 1941, 1959).

There have been a number of recent observations that provide additional motivation to search out possible neurological mechanisms in this disorder. Stuttering has been produced by electrical stimulation of the pulvinar in an unanesthetized human subject (Ojemann, Fedio, and Van Buren, 1968). In addition, stuttering is reported to have been markedly alleviated or completely eliminated following neurosurgical treatment of other conditions. Two patients are reported to have shown marked improvement in stuttering following anterior temporal lobectomy for the treatment of temporal lobe epilepsy (Blumer, 1967). Four other patients are also reported to have stopped stuttering following intracranial surgery. In this group surgery was performed for removal of a left frontal tumor and surgical treatment of aneurysms of the anterior cerebral, anterior communicating, and middle cerebral arteries (Jones, 1966). Three of the procedures involved the left side of the brain, and one procedure involved the right side of the brain. All the patients showed some degree of hemiparesis following surgery. Prior to surgery, carotid amytal tests showed that dysphasia, of similar degree, resulted from injection of either common carotid artery. Following surgery, dysphasia was far more marked following injection on the side opposite the lesion (Jones, 1966).

CHAPTER COMMENTARY

A summary of the differential diagnosis of language disorders in childhood is given in Table 1.

A bilateral impairment of hearing acuity resulting from cochlear or eighth-nerve lesions may delay speech acquisition and produce disturbances in articulation that can be correlated with the characteristics of the audiogram (Fry, 1966; Hirsh, 1966; McConnell and Ward, 1967; Whetnall and Fry, 1964). In some instances bilateral peripheral impairments of hearing acuity that are only moderate in degree result in sufficient

Table 1. Differential Diagnosis of Language Disorders in Childhood

1. Hearing loss
2. Oral-area sensory deficit
3. Aphasia
    a. Acquired
    b. Congenital
    c. Developmental
4. Dyslexia
    a. Acquired
    b. Developmental
5. Minimal cerebral dysfunction
6. Psychosis of childhood (including early infantile autism)
7. Nonpsychotic functional behavior disorders
8. Epilepsy
9. Mental retardation
10. Environmental deficits (sensory, emotional, and cultural deprivation; inadequate or incompetent instruction)
11. (Normal variation)

diminution of behavioral evidence of interest in sound to convince the mother that the child cannot hear, with a resultant sharp reduction in the amount of speech directed toward the child. This superimposed deprivation will, if allowed to continue, result in severe impairment of speech-perception and speech-production capabilities (Fry, 1966; Whetnall and Fry, 1964). Failure to provide appropriate amplification during the first few years of life can result in a similar picture of severe speech perception and speech comprehension deficits. These facts make clear the urgent nature of accurate diagnosis and management of impairments of hearing acuity during the early years of life. These facts also focus attention on the important issue of critical auditory experience during the early years of life as an essential determinant of normal speech and language development.

Clearer definition of the role of specific types of early experience, and specific periods of development during which these experiences have disproportionate behavioral implications, is also central to an understanding of the altered patterns of language development that accompany the deprivation syndromes.

Mental retardation may result from many different types of early central nervous system damage, and the etiologies in question overlap those that have already been implicated in the case of language disorders reviewed in the main body of this paper. The child with mental retardation will, by definition, show delayed and incomplete cognitive and perceptual development outside the language sphere. In addition, speech is usually late in developing, articulation is poor, grammatical competence develops slowly and incompletely, and language is not used as an effective mediator of experience (Carroll, 1967; Jordan, 1967; Lenneberg, Nichols, and Rosenberger, 1964; McCarthy, 1964). This group of children, heterogeneous with respect to both etiology and patterns of functional deficit, causes us to raise a myriad of questions concerning the relationships among language, thought, and intelligence (Jordan, 1967).

In order to achieve a modicum of clarity, a paper of this sort must construct the most useful diagnostic categories that current knowledge allows. The inexperienced clinician may, as a result, be tempted to fit every patient into one and only one diagnostic category. Children with disturbances of language function frequently defy such rigid diagnostic classification. It is often necessary to follow patients carefully over many months and often over many years before maximum clarification of diagnosis can be obtained. Even under such circumstances, it is often impossible to make a definitive diagnostic assignment. In such cases, a detailed statement of the findings obtained by history, physical examination, direct behavioral observation, laboratory procedures, and other specialized tests constitutes the best that can be done, and it is always preferable to a vague or simplistic diagnostic assignment.

This review of neurological aspects of language disorders in childhood brings into sharp relief a number of important research areas. The central role of early auditory experience for all aspects of language development has been repeatedly documented. And yet our knowledge of the ontogeny of auditory perception is very scant, and the armamentarium of audiological procedures that are useful in the diagnosis of lesions of the central auditory pathways, auditory cortex, and auditory association cortex in children is very small.

The extent to which inadequate lateralization of language function is a cause of language disorders or merely an accompaniment of language disorders, and the nature of the normal processes by which functions related to language become asymmetrically represented in the two halves of the brain, constitute questions of fundamental importance for the understanding of language disorders in children (Milner, 1962; Piercy 1964; Semmes, 1968; Zangwill, 1960, 1962, 1964).

An extensive review of research relevant to an understanding of language behavior and language disorders in children has recently been prepared by Chalfant and Scheffelin (1969).

REFERENCES

Ajax, E. T. 1964. Acquired dyslexia: A comparative study of two cases. Arch. Neurol. 11:66-72.
———1967. Dyslexia without agraphia. Arch. Neurol. (Chicago), 17:645-652.
Alajouanine, T., and F. Lhermitte. 1964. Aphasia and physiology of speech. In Rioch D. M., and E. A. Weinstein, eds., Disorders of Communication. Baltimore, Williams & Wilkins.
——— and F. Lhermitte. 1965. Acquired aphasia in children. Brain, 88:653-662.
——— and O. Sabouraud. 1960. Les perturbations paroxystiques de langage dans l'épilepsie. Encéphale, 49:95-133.
Allen, I. M. 1952. The history of congenital auditory imperception. New Zealand Med. J. 51:239-247.
Altman, J. 1967. Postnatal growth and differentiation of the mammalian brain, with implications for a morphological theory of memory. In Quarton, G. C., T Melnechuk, and F. O. Schmitt, eds. The Neurosciences. New York, Rockefeller University Press.

Ambrose, J. A. 1963. The concept of a critical period for the development of social responsiveness in early human infancy. *In* Foss, B. M., ed., Determinants of Infant Behavior, Vol. 2. New York, John Wiley & Sons.

Baer, P. E. 1961. Problems in the differential diagnosis of brain damage and childhood schizophrenia. Amer. J. Orthopsychiat., 31:728-737.

Barbizet, J. 1963. Defect of memorizing of hippocampal-mammillary origin: A review. J. Neurol. Neurosurg. Psychiat., 26:127-135.

Basser, L. S. 1962. Hemiplegia of early onset and the faculty of speech with special reference to the effects of hemispherectomy. Brain, 85:427-460.

Bay, E. 1962. Aphasia and non-verbal disorders of language. Brain, 85:411-426.

Bender, M. B. 1963. Disorders in visual perception. *In* Halpern, L., ed., Problems of Dynamic Neurology. New York, Grune & Stratton.

——— and S. P. Diamond. 1965. An analysis of auditory perceptual defects with observations on the localization of dysfunction. Brain, 88:675-686.

Benson, D. F. 1967. Fluency in aphasia. Correlation with radioactive scan localization. Cortex, 3:373-394.

Benton, A. L. 1962. Dyslexia in relation to form perception and directional sense. *In* Money, J., ed., Reading Disability. Baltimore, Johns Hopkins Press.

——— 1964. Developmental aphasia and brain damage. Cortex, 1:40-52.

——— 1966. Language disorders in children. Canad. Psychol., 7:298-312.

——— and J. D. Hemble. 1960. Right-left orientation and reading disability. Psychiat. Neurol., 139:49-60.

Bloodstein, O. 1941. Conditions under which stuttering is reduced or absent: A review of literature. J. Speech Hearing Dis., 6:187-203.

——— 1959. A Handbook on Stuttering for Professional Workers. Chicago, National Society for Crippled Children and Adults.

Blumer, D. P. 1967. The temporal lobes and paroxysmal behavior disorders. A study of patients with temporal lobectomy for epilepsy. Szondiana VII. Beiheft zur Schweizerischen Zeitschrift fur Psychologie und ihre Anwendungen, 51:273-285.

Bocca, E. 1958. Clinical aspects of cortical deafness. Laryngoscope, 68:301-309.

——— and C. Calearo. 1963. Central hearing processes. *In* Jerger, J., ed., Modern Developments in Audiology. New York, Academic Press.

Bonin, G. von. 1963. On the structure and function of the cortex. *In* De Bruyn, P. P. H., ed., The Evolution of the Human Brain. Chicago, University of Chicago Press.

Brain, R. 1961. Speech Disorders. London, Butterworth. pp. 69-91.

Bronson, G. 1965. The hierarchical organization of the central nervous system: Implications for learning processes and critical periods in early development. Behav. Sci., 10:7-25.

Brown, J. R., F. L. Darley, and M. R. Gomez. 1967. Disorders of communication. Pediat. Clin. N. Amer., 14:725-748.

Brown, R. 1965. Social Psychology, Chaps. 6, 7. New York, Free Press.

Bruner, J. S. 1959. The cognitive consequences of early sensory deprivation. Psychosom. Med., 21:89-95.

——— 1961. The cognitive consequences of early sensory deprivation. *In* Solomon, P., P. E. Kubzansky, P. H. Leiderman, J. H. Mendelson, R. Trumbull, and D. Wexler, eds., Sensory Deprivation. Cambridge, Mass., Harvard University Press.

Carhart, R. 1967. Lesions due to kernicterus. Acta Otolaryng. (Stockholm), Suppl. 221:5-41.

Carne, E. B. 1965 Artificial Intelligence Techniques, pp. 99-121. New York, Spartan Books.

Carroll, J. B. 1967. Psycholinguistics in the study of mental retardation. *In* Schiefelbusch, R. L., R. H. Copeland, and J. O. Smith, eds., Language and Mental Retardation. New York, Holt, Rinehart and Winston.

Casler, L. 1961. Maternal deprivation. Monogr. Soc. Res. Child Develop., 26:1-64.

Chalfant, J. C., and M. A. Scheffelin. 1969. Central Processing Dysfunctions in Children: A Review of Research. Washington, D. C., U. S. Department of Health, Education, and Welfare. U. S. Public Health Service.

Chase, R. A. 1967a. Abnormalities in motor control secondary to congenital sensory deficits: A case study. *In* J. S. Bosma, ed., Symposium on Oral Sensation and Perception. Springfield, Ill., Charles C Thomas.

——1967b. Verbal behavior: Some points of reference. *In* Research in Verbal Behavior and Some Neurophysiological Implications. Salzinger, K., and Suzanne Salzinger, eds., New York, Academic Press.

Ciemins, V. A. 1968. Aphasia with thalamic disorders. Neurology (Minneapolis),18:307.

Clements, S. D. 1966a. The child with minimal brain dysfunction. Lancet, 86:121-123.

——1966b. Minimal brain dysfunction in children. NINDB Monograph No. 3. Washington, D. C., U. S. Department of Health, Education, and Welfare, Public Health Service Publ. No. 1415.

—— and J. E. Peters. 1962. Minimal brain dysfunctions in the school-age child. Arch. Gen. Psychiat., 6:185-197.

Cogan, D. G. 1965. Alexia without agraphia, and the splenium. Arch. Ophthal. (Chicago), 73:2-3.

Cohn, R. 1964. The neurological study of children with learning disabilites. Except. Child., 31:179-185.

Cole, E. M., and L. Walker. 1964. Reading and speech problems as expressions of a specific language disability. *In* Rioch, D. M., and E. A. Weinstein, eds., Disorders of Communication. Baltimore, Williams & Wilkins.

Comis, S. D., and I. C. Whitfield. 1968. Influence of centrifugal pathways on unit activity in the cochlear nucleus. J. Neurophysiol., 31:62-68.

Creak, E. M. 1963. Childhood psychosis. A review of 100 cases. Brit. J. Psychiat., 109:84-89.

—— K. Cameron, Valerie Cowie, Sylvia Ini, R. Mackeith, G. Michell, G. O'Gorman, F. Orford, W. J. B. Rogers, A. Shapiro, F. Stone, G. Stroh, G. Vaughan, and S. Yudkin. 1964. Schizophrenic syndrome in childhood. Further progress report of a working party (April, 1964). Develop. Med. Child Neuro.., 6:530-535.

Critchley, M. 1960a. Troubles de la parole dans les cas d'épilepsie. Encéphale, 49:134-137.

——1960b. The evolution of man's capacity for language. *In* Tax, S., ed., The Evolution of Man; Mind, Culture and Society, Vol. 2 of Evolution After Darwin. Chicago, University of Chicago Press.

——1961. Doyne memorial lecture, 1961. Inborn reading disorders of central origin. Trans. Ophthal. Soc. U. K., 81:459-480.

——1964. Developmental Dyslexia. London, William Heinemann.

——1967. Some observations upon developmental dyslexia. *In* Williams, D., ed., Modern Trends in Neurology. New York, Appleton-Century-Crofts.

Crosby, E. C., T. Humphrey, E. W. Lauer. 1962. Correlative Anatomy of the Nervous System, pp. 282-284. New York, Macmillan.

Darley, F. L. 1964. Diagnosis and Appraisal of Communication Disorders. Englewood Cliffs, N. J., Prentice-Hall.

de Hirsch, Katrina. 1957. Tests designed to discover potential reading difficulties at the six-year-old level. Amer. J. Orthopsychiat., 27:566-576.

——— and J. J. Jansky. 1968. Early prediction of reading disability. In Keeney, A. H., and T. Keeney, eds., Dyslexia. Diagnosis and Treatment of Reading Disorders. St. Louis, C. V. Mosby.

Denny-Brown, D. 1963. The physiological basis of perception and speech. In Halpern, L., ed., Problems in Dynamic Neurology. New York, Grune & Stratton.

Desmedt, J. E., and K. Mechelse. 1958. Suppression of acoustic input by thalamic stimulation. Proc. Soc. Exp. Biol. Med., 99:772-775.

Deutsch, S. 1967. Models of the Nervous System, Chaps. 12, 13. New York, John Wiley & Sons.

Dewson, J. H., III, K. W. Nobel, and K. H. Pribram. 1966. Corticofugal influence at cochlear nucleus of the cat: Some effects of ablation of insular-temporal cortex. Brain Res., 2:151-159.

Diamond, I. T., and W. D. Neff. 1957. Ablation of temporal cortex and discrimination of auditory patterns. J. Neurophysiol., 20:300-315.

Downs, M. P. 1967. Testing hearing in infancy and early childhood. In McConnell, F., and P. H. Ward, eds., Deafness in Childhood. Nashville, Tenn., Vanderbilt University Press.

Drew, A. L. 1956. A neurological appraisal of familial congenital word-blindness. Brain, 79:440-460.

Driver, M. W., M. A. Falconer, and E. A. Serafetinides. 1964. Ictal speech automatism reproduced by activation procedures. Neurology (Minneapolis), 14:455-463.

Eaton, L., and F. J. Menolascino. 1967. Psychotic reactions of childhood: A follow-up study. Amer. J. Orthopsychiat., 37:521-529.

Eisenberg, L. 1956. The autistic child in adolescence. Amer. J. Psychiat., 112:607-612.

———1957. The course of childhood schizophrenia. Arch. Neurol. Psychiat., 78:69-83.

———1959. Office evaluation of specific reading disability in children. Pediatrics, 23:997-1003.

Eisenberg, R. B., D. B. Coursin, and N. R. Rupp. 1966. Habituation to an acoustic pattern as an index of differences among human neonates. J. Audit. Res., 6:239-248.

———E. J. Griffin, D. B. Coursin, and M. A. Hunter. 1964. Auditory behavior in the human neonate: A preliminary report. J. Speech Hearing Res., 7:245-269.

Ervin, S. M., and W. R. Miller. 1963. Language development. In Stevenson, H. W., ed., Child Psychology: The Sixty-second Yearbook of the National Society for the Study of Education, Part I. Chicago, University of Chicago Press.

Ettlinger, G., and L. Hurwitz. 1962. Dyslexia and its associated disturbances. Neurology (Minneapolis), 12:477-480.

Eustis, R. S. 1947. Specific reading disability. A familial syndrome associated with ambidexterity and speech defects and a frequent cause of problem behavior. New Eng. J. Med., 237:243-249.

Ewing, A. W. G. 1967. Aphasia in Children. New York, Hafner.

Fiske, D. W. 1961. Effects of monotonous and restricted stimulation. *In* Fiske, D. W., and S. R. Maddi, eds., Functions of Varied Experience. Homewood, Ill., Dorsey Press.

Flower, R. M., R. Viehweg, and W. R. Ruzicka. 1966. The communicative disorders of children with kernicteric athetosis: I. Auditory disorders. J. Speech Hearing Dis., 31:41-59.

Fries, C. C. 1962. Linguistics and Reading. Chap. 4. New York, Holt, Rinehart and Winston.

Frisina, D. R. 1963. Measurement of hearing in children. *In* Jerger, J., ed., Modern Developments in Audiology. New York, Academic Press.

Fry, D. B. 1966. The development of the phonological system in the normal and the deaf child. *In* Smith, F., and G. A. Miller, eds., The Genesis of Language: A Psycholinguistic Approach. Cambridge, Mass., The MIT Press.

Galambos, R. 1964. Physiology of central auditory mechanisms. *In* Fields, W. S., and B. R. Alford, eds., Neurological Aspects of Auditory and Vestibular Disorders. Springfield, Ill. Charles C Thomas.

Gallagher, J. R. 1950. Specific language disability. A cause of scholastic failure. New Eng. J. Med., 242:436-440.

Gardner, W. J., L. J. Karnosh, D. C. McClure, Jr., and A. K. Gardner. 1955. Residual function following hemispherectomy for tumour and for infantile hemiplegia. Brain, 78:487-502.

George, F. H. 1962. The Brain as a Computer. Elmsford, N. Y., Pergamon Press.

Gerrard, J. 1952. Kernicterus. Brain, 75:526-570.

Geschwind, N. 1962. The anatomy of the acquired disorders of reading. *In* Money, J., ed., Reading Disability. Baltimore, Johns Hopkins Press.

——1964. Non-aphasic disorders of speech. Int. J. Neurol., 4:207-214.

——1965. Disconnexion syndromes in animals and man. Brain, 88:237-294, 585-644.

——1967. Brain mechanisms suggested by studies of hemispheric connections. *In* Darley, F. L., ed., Brain Mechanisms Underlying Speech and Language. New York, Grune & Stratton.

—— 1968. Neurological foundations of language. *In* Myklebust, H. R., ed., Progress in Learning Disabilities. Vol. 1. New York, Grune & Stratton.

Glaser, G. H. 1967. Limbic epilepsy in childhood. J. Nerv. Ment. Dis., 144:391-397.

Glaser, K., and R. L. Clemmens. 1965. School failure. Pediatrics, 35:128-141.

Gofman, H. 1965. Etiologic factors in learning disorders of children. J. Neurol. Sci., 2:262-270.

Goldberg, H. K. 1968. Vision, perception, and related facts in dyslexia. *In* Keeney, A. H., and V. T. Keeney, eds., Dyslexia. Diagnosis and Treatment of Reading Disorders. St. Louis, C. V. Mosby.

—— and P. W. Drash. 1968. The disabled reader. J. Pediat. Ophthal., February 11-24.

Goldstein, R. 1967. Electrophysiologic evaluation of hearing. *In* McConnell, F., and P. H. Ward, eds., Deafness in Childhood. Nashville, Tenn., Vanderbilt University Press.

Gooddy, W., and M. Reinhold. 1961. Congenital dyslexia and asymmetry of cerebral function. Brain, 84:231-242.

Goodglass, H. 1967. Binaural digit presentation and early lateral brain damage. Cortex, 3:295-306.

Goodhill, V. 1950. Nuclear deafness and the nerve deaf child: The importance of the Rh factor. Trans. Amer. Acad. Ophthal. Otolaryng., 54:671-687.

——1956. Rh child: Deaf or "aphasic"? 1. Clinical pathologic aspects of kernicteric nuclear "deafness." J. Speech Hearing Dis., 21:407-410.

Goodwin, M. S., and T. C. Goodwin. 1969. In a dark mirror. Ment. Hyg., 53:550-563.

Gordon, N. 1966. The child who does not talk. Problems of diagnosis with special reference to children with severe auditory agnosia. Brit. J. Dis. Commun., 1:78-84.

—— and I. G. Taylor. 1964. The assessment of children with difficulties of communication. Brain, 87:121-140.

Gray, P. H. 1958. Theory and evidence of imprinting in human infants. J. Psychol., 46:155-166.

Green, J. D. 1964. The hippocampus. Physiol. Rev., 44:561-608.

Gubbay, S. S., E. Ellis, J. N. Walton, and S. D. M. Court. 1965. Clumsy children: A study of apraxic and agnosic defects in 21 children. Brain, 88:295-312.

Guttmann, E. 1942. Aphasia in children. Brain, 65:205-219.

Hallgren, B. 1950. Specific Dyslexia: A Clinical and Genetic Study. Copenhagen, Ejnar Munksgaard.

Hardy, J. B. 1968. Viruses and the fetus. Postgrad. Med., 43:156-167.

—— G. R. G. Monif, and J. L. Sever. 1966. Studies in congenital rubella, Baltimore 1964-65. II: Clinical and virologic. Bull. Johns Hopkins Hosp. 118:97-108.

Hardy, W. G. 1965. On language disorders in young children: A reorganization of thinking. J. Speech Hearing Dis., 30:3-16.

Harlow, H. F. 1959. Love in infant monkeys. Sci. Amer., 200:68-74.

—— 1964. Early social deprivation and later behavior in the monkey. In Abrams, A., H. H. Garner, and J. E. P. Toman, eds., Unfinished Tasks in the Behavioral Sicences. Baltimore, Williams & Wilkins.

Hécaen, H. 1967. Brain mechanisms suggested by studies of parietal lobes. In Darley, F. L., ed., Brain Mechanisms Underlying Speech and Language. New York, Grune & Stratton.

—— and R. Angelergues. 1960. Épilepsie et troubles du langage. Encéphale, 49:138-169.

—— and M. Piercy. 1956. Paroxysmal dysphasia and the problem of cerebral dominance. J. Neurol. Neurosurg. Psychiat., 19:194-102.

Hermann, K., J. W. Turner, F. J. Gillingham, and R. M. Gaze. 1966. The effects of destructive lesions and stimulation of the basal ganglia on speech mechanisms. Confin. Neurol., 27:197-207.

Hernández-Peón, R. 1966. Physiological mechanisms in attention. In Russell, R. W., ed., Frontiers in Physiological Psychology. New York, Academic Press.

—— M. Jouvet, and H. Scherrer. 1957. Auditory potentials at cochlear nucleus during acoustic habituation. Acta Neurol. Latinoamer., 3:144-156.

Hess, E. 1958. "Imprinting" in animals. Sci. Amer., 198:81-90.

Himwich, W. A. 1962. Biochemical and neurophysiological development of the brain in the neonatal period. Int. Rev. Neurobiol., 4:117-158.

Hinde, R. A. 1962a. Some aspects of the imprinting problem. In Imprinting and Early Learning, pp. 129-138. London, Symposia of the Zoological Society of London.

—— 1962b. Sensitive periods and the development of behaviour. In Barnett, S. A., ed., Lessons from Animal Behavior for the Clinician. London, National Spastics Society Study Group; and Heinemann Medical Books.

Hirsh, I. J. 1966. Teaching the deaf child to speak. In Smith, F., and G. A. Miller, eds., The Genesis of Language: A Psycholinguistic Approach. Cambridge, Mass., The MIT Press.

Horn, G. 1965. Physiological and psychological aspects of selective perception. In Lehrman, D. S., R. A. Hinde, and Evelyn Shaw, eds., Advances in the Study of Behavior. New York, Academic Press.

Ingram, T. T. S. 1959. Specific developmental disorders of speech in childhood. Brain, 82:450-467.

——1960. Pediatric aspects of specific developmental dysphasia, dyslexia and dysgraphia. Cereb. Palsy Bull., 2:254-277.

——1963. Delayed development of speech with special reference to dyslexia. Proc. Roy. Soc. Med., 56:199-203.

——1965. Specific learning difficulties in childhood. Public Health, 79:70-80.

——1970. The nature of dyslexia. In F. A. Young and D. B. Lindsley, eds., Early Experience and Visual Information Processing in Perceptual and Reading Disorders. Washington, D. C., National Academy of Sciences.

——and J. F. Reid. 1956. Developmental aphasia observed in a department of child psychiatry. Arch. Dis. Child.,31:161-172.

Jackson, J. H. 1874. On the nature of the duality of the brain. Med. Press Circ., 1:19, 41, 63. (Reprinted in Taylor, J., ed., Selected Writings of John Hughlings Jackson, Vol. 2. New York, Basic Books, 1958.)

——1878. On affections of speech from disease of the brain. Brain, 1:304-330. (Reprinted in Taylor, J., ed., Selected Writings of John Hughlings Jackson, Vol. 2. New York, Basic Books, 1958.)

——1879. On affections of speech from disease of the brain. Brain, 2:203-222. (Reprinted in Taylor, J., ed., Selected Writings of John Hughlings Jackson, Vol. 2. New York, Basic Books, 1958.)

Jerger, J. 1960. Observations on auditory behavior in lesions of the central auditory pathways. Arch. Otolaryngol. (Chicago), 71:797-806.

——1964. Auditory tests for disorders of the central auditory mechanism. In Fields, W. S., and B. R. Alford, eds., Neurological Aspects of Auditory and Vestibular Disorders. Springfield, Ill., Charles C Thomas.

Jones, R. K. 1966. Observations on stammering after localized cerebral injury. J. Neurol. Neurosurg. Psychiat., 29:192-195.

Jordan, T. E. 1967. Language and mental retardation: A review of the literature. In Schiefelbusch, R. L., R. H. Copeland, and J. O. Smith, eds., Language and Mental Retardation. New York, Holt, Rinehart and Winston.

Kanner, L. 1944. Early infantile autism. J. Pediat., 25:211-217.

Karlin, I. W. 1951. Congenital verbal-auditory agnosia (word deafness). Pediatrics, 7:60-68.

——1954. Aphasias in children. Amer. J. Dis. Child., 87:752-767.

Kastein, S., and E. P. Fowler, Jr. 1954. Differential diagnosis of communication disorders in children referred for hearing tests. Arch. Otolaryng. (Chicago), 60:468-477.

Kawi, A. A., and B. Pasamanick. 1958. Association of factors of pregnancy with reading disorders in childhood. J. Amer. Med. Assoc., 166:1420-1423.

——and B. Pasamanick. 1959. Prenatal and paranatal factors in the development of childhood reading disorders. Monogr. Soc. Res. Child Develop., 24:1-80.

Kimura, Doreen. 1963. Speech lateralization in young children as determined by an auditory test. J. Comp. Physiol. Psychol., 56:899-902.

Kinsbourne, M., and E. K. Warrington. 1963. The developmental Gerstmann syndrome. Arch. Neurol. (Chicago), 8:490-501.

Klapper, Z. S. 1966. Reading retardation: II. Psychoeducational aspects of reading disabilities. Pediatrics, 37:366-376.

Kleist, K. 1962. Sensory Aphasia and Amusia. Elmsford, N. Y., Pergamon Press.

Knobloch, H. and B. Pasamanick. 1959. Syndrome of minimal cerebral damage in infancy. JAMA, 170:1384-1387.

Koikegami, H. 1964. Amygdala and other related limbic structures; Experimental studies on the anatomy and function. Acta Med. Biol. (Niigata), 12:73-266.

Krynauw, R. A. 1950. Infantile hemiplegia treated by removing one cerebral hemisphere. J. Neurol. Neurosurg. Psychiat., 13:243-267.

Landau, W. M., R. Goldstein, and F. R. Kleffner. 1960. Congenital aphasia. A clinicopathologic study. Neurology (Minneapolis), 10:915-921.

Lenneberg, E. H. 1964. Language disorders in childhood. Harvard Educ. Rev., 34:152-177.

———1967. Biological Foundations of Language. New York, John Wiley & Sons.

———I. A. Nichols, and E. F. Rosenberger. 1964. Primitive stages of language development in mongolism. *In* Rioch, D. M., and E. A. Weinstein, eds., Disorders of Communication. Baltimore, Williams & Wilkins.

Lombroso, C. T. 1967. Sylvian seizures and midtemporal spike foci in children. Arch. Neurol. (Chicago), 17:52-59.

Lucas, A. R., E. A. Rodin, and C.B.Simson.1965. Neurological assessment of children with early school problems. Develop. Med. Child Neurol., 7:145-156.

Luria, A. R. 1961. The Role of Speech in the Regulation of Normal and Abnormal Behaviour. Elmsford, N. Y., Pergamon Press.

———1966. Higher Cortical Functions in Man. New York, Basic Books.

———1967a. The regulative function of speech in its development and dissolution. *In* Salzinger, K., and Suzanne Salzinger, eds., Research in Verbal Behavior and Some Neurophysiological Implications. New York, Academic Press.

———1967b. Problems and facts in neurolinguistics. Int. Soc. Sci. J., 19:36-51.

Malamud, N. 1967. Psychiatric disorder with intracranial tumors of limbic system. Arch. Neurol. (Chicago), 17:113-123.

Matkin, N. D., and R. Carhart. 1966. Auditory profiles associated with Rh incompatability. Arch. Otolaryngol. (Chicago), 84:502-513.

McCarthy, J. J. 1964. Research on the linguistic problems of the mentally retarded. Ment. Retard. Abstr., 1:3-27.

McConnell, F., and P. H. Ward. 1967. Deafness in Childhood. Nashville, Tenn.,Vanderbilt University Press.

McFie, J. 1952. Cerebral dominance in cases of reading disability. Neurol. Neurosurg. Psychiat., 15:194-199.

———1961. The effects of hemispherectomy on intellectual functioning in cases of infantile hemiplegia. Neurol. Neurosurg. Psychiat., 23:240-249.

Melzack, R. 1965 Effects of early experience on behavior: Experimental and conceptual considerations. *In* Hoch, P. H., and J. Zubin, Psychopathology of Perception. New York, Grune & Stratton.

——— and S. K. Burns. 1965. Neurophysiological effects of early sensory restriction. Exp. Neurol., 13:163-175.

Mendelson, J. H., L. Siger, P. E. Kubzansky, and P. Solomon. 1964. The language of signs and symbolic behavior of the deaf. *In* Rioch, D. M., and E. A. Weinstein, eds., Disorders of Communication. Baltimore, Williams & Wilkins.

Mengel, M. C., B. W. Konigsmark, C. I. Berlin, and V. A. McKusick. 1967. Recessive early-onset neural deafness. Acta Otolaryng. (Stockholm), 64:313-326.

Menolascino, F. J. 1965. Autistic reactions in early childhood: Differential diagnostic considerations. Child Psychol. Psychiat., 6:201-218.

Millichap, J. F., and G. W. Fowler. 1967. Treatment of "minimal brain dysfunction" syndromes. Pediat. Clin. N. Amer., 14:767-777.

Milner, Brenda. 1962. Laterality effects in audition. *In* Mountcastle, V. B., ed., Interhemispheric Relations and Cerebral Dominance. Baltimore, Johns Hopkins Press.

—— and H. L. Teuber. 1968. Alteration of perception and memory in man: Reflections on methods. *In* Weiskrantz, L., ed., Analysis of Behavioral Change. New York, Harper & Row.

Money, J., ed. 1962. Reading Disability. Progress and Research Needs in Dyslexia. Baltimore, Johns Hopkins Press.

—— ed. 1966. The Disabled Reader. Baltimore, Johns Hopkins Press.

Monif, G. R. G., J. B. Hardy, and J. L. Sever. 1966. Studies in congenital rubella, Baltimore 1964-65. I: Epidemiologic and virologic. Bull. Hopkins Hosp. 118:85-96.

Morgan, W. P. 1896. A case of congenital word blindness. Brit. Med. J., 2:1378.

Morley, M. E. 1965. The Development and Disorders of Speech in Childhood. Baltimore, Williams & Wilkins.

—— M. E., D. Court, H. Miller, and R. F. Garside. 1955. Delayed speech and developmental aphasia. Brit. Med. J., 2:463-467.

Myklebust, H. R. 1952. Aphasia in children. Except. Child., 19:9-14.

——1954. Auditory Disorders in Children. New York, Grune & Stratton.

——1960. The Psychology of Deafness: Sensory Deprivation, Learning, and Adjustments. New York, Grune & Stratton.

Neff, W. D. 1961. Neural mechanisms of auditory discrimination. *In* Rosenblith, W. A., ed., Sensory Communication. New York, John Wiley & Sons, and Cambridge, Mass., The MIT Press.

—— 1964. Temporal pattern discrimination in lower animals and its relation to language perception in man. *In* DeReuck, A. V. S., and M. O'Connor, eds., Disorders of Language. London, Churchill.

Newton, G., and S. Levine. 1968. Early Experience and Behavior. Springfield, Ill., Charles C Thomas.

Nicholls, J. V. V. 1960. Congenital dyslexia: A problem in etiology. Canad. Med. Ass. J., 82:575-579.

Nielsen, J. M. 1962. Agnosia, Apraxia, Aphasia. Their Value in Cerebral Localization. New York, Hafner.

Nobel, K. W., and J. H. Dewson, III. 1966. A corticofugal projection from insular and temporal cortex to the homolateral inferior colliculus in cat. J. Audit. Res.,6:67-75.

Obrador, S. 1964. Nervous integration after hemispherectomy in man. *In* Schaltenbrand, G., and C. N. Woolsey, eds., Cerebral Localization and Organization. Madison, University of Wisconsin Press.

Ojemann, G. A., P. Fedio, and J. M. Van Buren. 1968. Anomia from pulvinar and subcortical parietal stimulation. Brain, 91:99-106.

Paine, R. S. 1962. Minimal chronic brain syndromes in children. Develop. Med. Child Neurol., 4:21-27.

——1963. The contributions of neurology to the pathogenesis of hyperactivity in children. Clin. Proc. Child. Hosp. D. C., 19:235-247.

——1965. Organic neurological factors related to learning disorders. *In* Hellmuth, J., ed., Learning Disorders. Seattle, Special Child Publications of the Seattle Seguin School.

Peacher, W. G. 1949. Neurological factors in the etiology of delayed speech. J. Speech Hearing Dis., 14:147-161.

Penfield, W., and L. Roberts. 1959. Speech and Brain Mechanisms. Princeton, N. J., Princeton University Press.

Piercy, M. 1964. The effects of cerebral lesions on intellectual function: A review of current research trends. Brit. J. Psychiat., 110:310-352.

Pincus, J. H., and G. H. Glaser. 1966. The syndrome of "minimal brain damage" in childhood. New Eng. J. Med., 275:27-35.

Polyakov, G. I. 1961. Some results of research into the development of the neuronal structure of the cortical ends of the analyzers in man. J. Comp. Neurol., 117:197-212.

——1966. Modern data on the structural organization of the cerebral cortex. In Luria, A. R., ed., Higher Cortical Functions in Man. New York, Basic Books.

Pratt, R. T. C. 1967. The Genetics of Neurological Disorders, Chap. 12. New York, Oxford University Press.

Preston, M. S., Grace Yeni-Komshian, and R. E. Stark, 1967a. Voicing in initial stop-consonants produced by children in the pre-linguistic period from different language communities. Annual Report of the Neurocommunications Laboratory, Baltimore, The Johns Hopkins University School of Medicine.

——Grace Yeni-Komshian, and R. E. Stark. 1967b. A study of voicing in initial stops found in the pre-linguistic vocalizations of infants from different language environments. Status Report on Speech Research (SR-10). New York, Haskins Laboratories.

Rapin, Isabelle. 1959. The neurologist looks at the non-verbal child. Except. Chil., 26:48-52.

——and L. J. Graziani. 1967. Auditory-evoked responses in normal, brain-damaged, and deaf infants. Neurology (Minneapolis), 17:881-894.

Rawson, M. B. 1968. Developmental Language Disability. Adult Accomplishment of Dyslexic Boys. Baltimore, Johns Hopkins Press.

Reichstein, J., and J. Rosenstein. 1964. Differential diagnosis of auditory deficits—A review of the literature. Except. Child., 31:73-82.

Reiser, D. E. 1963. Psychosis of infancy and early childhood, as manifested by children with atypical development. New Eng. J. Med., 269:790-798, 844-850.

Richter, D. 1966. Aspects of Learning and Memory. New York, Basic Books.

Riesen, A. H. 1966. Sensory deprivation. In Stellar, E., and J. M. Sprague, eds., Progress in Physiological Psychology. New York, Academic Press.

Robertiello, R. C. 1953. Psychomotor epilepsy in children. Dis. Nerv. Syst., 14:337-339.

Roberts, H. L. 1958. Functional plasticity in cortical speech areas and integration of speech. Arch. Neurol. Psychiat., 79:275-283.

Russell, W. R., and Espir, M. L. E. 1961. Traumatic Aphasia. New York, Oxford University Press.

Rutter, M. 1965. The influence of organic and emotional factors on the origins, nature and outcome of childhood psychosis. Develop. Med. Child Neurol., 7:518-528.

——S. Lebovici, L. Eisenberg, A. V. Sneznevskij, R. Sadoun, Eileen Brooke, and Tsung-Yi Lin. 1969. A tri-axial classificiation of mental disorders in childhood. An international report. Child Psychol. Psychiat., 10:41-61.

Salam, M. Z., and R. D. Adams. 1966. New horizons in the neurology of childhood. Perspect. Biol. Med., 9:384-419.

Saxon, S. V. 1961. Differences in reactivity between asphyxial and normal rhesus monkeys. J. Genet. Psychol., 99:283-287.

—— and C. G. Ponce. 1961. Behavioral defects in monkeys asphyxiated during birth. Exp. Neurol., 4:460-469.

Schain, R. J., and H. Yannet. 1960. Infantile autism. An analysis of 50 cases and a consideration of certain relevant neurophysiologic concepts. J. Pediat., 57:560-567.

Schenk, V. W. D. 1966. Dyslexia and spatial disorientation. An examination of 77 dyslexic children. Psychiat. Neurol. Neurochir., 69:337-357.

Schuell, H. M., J. J. Jenkins, and E. Jiménez-Pabón. 1964. Aphasia in Adults. Diagnosis, Prognosis and Treatment. New York, Harper & Row.

Scott, J. P. 1962. Critical periods in behavioral development. Science, 138:949-958.

——1968. Early Experience and the Organization of Behavior. Belmont, Calif., Wadsworth.

Semmes, Josephine. 1968. Hemispheric specialization: A possible clue to mechanism. Neuropsychologia, 6:11-26.

Serafetinides, E. A. 1966. Speech findings in epilepsy and electro-cortical stimulation: An overview. Cortex, 2:463-473.

Shankweiler, D. 1964. Developmental dyslexia: A critique and review of recent evidence. Cortex, 1:53-62.

Sholl, D. A. 1967. The Organization of the Cerebral Cortex. New York, Hafner.

Silver, A. A., and R. A. Hagin. 1970. Visual perception in children with reading disabilities. In Young, F. A., and D. B. Lindsley, eds., Early Experience and Visual Information Processing in Perceptual and Reading Disorders. Washington, D. C., National Academy of Sciences.

Sloan, R. F. 1967. Neuronal histogenesis, maturation and organization related to speech development. J. Commun. Dis., 1:1-15.

Smith, A. 1966. Speech and other functions after left (dominant) hemispherectomy. J. Neurol. Neurosurg. Psychiat., 29:467-471.

Spinnler, H., and L. A. Vignolo. 1966. Impaired recognition of meaningful sounds in aphasia. Cortex, 2:337-348.

Spitz, R. A., and K. M. Wolf, 1946. Anaclitic depression; An inquiry into the genesis of psychiatric conditions in early childhood, II. Psychoanal. Stud. Child, 2:313-342.

Spitzer, R. L., R. Rabkin, and Y. Kramer, 1959. The relationship between "mixed dominance" and reading disabilities. J. Pediat., 54:76-80.

Stevens, D. A., J. A. Boydstun, R. A. Dykman, J. E. Peters, and D. W. Sinton. 1967. Presumed minimal brain dysfunction in children. Arch. Gen. Psychiat., 16:281-285.

Stevens, J. R., K. Sachdev, and V. Milstein. 1968. Behavior disorders of childhood and the electroencephalogram. Arch. Neurol. Psychiat. (Chicago), 18:160-177.

Stokoe, W. C., Jr. 1964. Language structure and the deaf child. Report on the Proceedings of the International Congress on Education of the Deaf. pp. 967-971. Washington, D. C., U. S. Government Printing Office.

Strauss, A. A. 1954. Aphasia in children. Amer. J. Phys. Med., 33:93-99.

Sugar, O. 1952. Congenital aphasia: An anatomical and physiological approach. J. Speech Hearing Dis., 17:301-304.

Taylor, W. K. 1964. Cortico-thalamic organization and memory. Proc. Roy. Soc. (London), 159:466-478.

Truex, R. A., and M. B. Carpenter. 1964. Strong and Elwyn's Human Neuroanatomy, pp. 409-410. Baltimore, Williams & Wilkins.

Uhr, L. 1966. Pattern Recognition. Theory, Experiment, Computer Simulations, and Dynamic Models of Form Perception and Discovery. New York, John Wiley & Sons.

Vardapetyan, G. A. 1967. Classificiation of single unit responses in the auditory cortex of cats. Neurosci. Trans., 1:1-11.

Whetnall, Edith, and D. B. Fry. 1964. The Deaf Child. London, William Heinemann.

White, H. H. 1961. Cerebral hemispherectomy in the treatment of infantile hemiplegia. Confin. Neurol., 21:1-50.

Whitfield, I. C. 1967. The Auditory Pathway. Baltimore, Williams & Wilkins.

Windle, W. F. 1964. Neurological deficits of asphyxia at birth of rhesus monkeys. Prevention and therapy. In Kellaway, P., and I. Petersen, eds., Neurological and Electroencephalographic Correlative Studies in Infancy. New York, Grune & Stratton.

Wood, N. E. 1964. Delayed Speech and Language Development. Englewood Cliffs, N. J., Prentice-Hall.

Worden, F. G. 1966. Attention and auditory electrophysiology. In Stellar, E., and J. M. Sprague, eds., Progress in Physiological Psychology. New York, Academic Press.

Work, H. H., and J. E. Haldane. 1966. Cerebral dysfunction in children. Amer. J. Dis. Child., 111:573-580.

Worster-Drought, C., and I. M. Allen. 1929. Congenital auditory imperception (congenital word-deafness): with report of a case. J. Neurol. Psychopathol., 9:193-208.

—— and I. M. Allen. 1930. Congenital auditory imperception (congenital word-deafness): and its relation to idioglossia and other speech defects. J. Neurol. Psychopathol., 10:193-236.

Yakovlev, P. I., and A. Lecours. 1967. The myelogenetic cycles of regional maturation of the brain. In Minkowski, A., ed., Regional Development of the Brain in Early Life. Oxford, Blackwell.

Zangwill, O. L. 1960. Cerebral Dominance and Its Relation to Psychological Function. Edinburgh, Oliver & Boyd.

——1962. Dyslexia in relation to cerebral dominance. In Money, J., ed., Reading Disability. Baltimore, Johns Hopkins Press.

——1964. The current status of cerebral dominance. In Rioch, D. M., and E. A. Weinstein, eds., Disorders of Communication. Baltimore, Williams & Wilkins.

5: Language disabilities of emotionally disturbed children

John S. Hicks

Emotionally involved children are often deeply caught up in the problems of adequate language development. Many times the type of emotional disorder can be recognized by a distinct language pattern or a distinct language disability. The child's problems of bizarre feelings, of developing appropriate affect, and the emotional conflict in their lives intrude upon their thoughts, speech patterns, and their desire to relate to others in terms of both verbal and nonverbal communication. Their discrepant language patterns often give the professional the only clues to the internal world of the mentally ill child. At the same time, language deficits can become the basis for emotional maladjustment as the handicapped child, such as the aphasic, attempts to interact with the people and objects in his or her environment. The relationships between emotional disorders and language disorders are complex. This chapter will attempt to define and to delineate the nature of these interrelationships as we now understand them and to present the evidence which is available on this topic in the literature.

It is important to note the crucial role of language and communication in the development of man from the periods of prehistory to the midtwentieth century. Man's language and ability to communicate meaningfully have both been a part of, and a cause of, the ever-growing complex nature of the many cultures which have survived through the thousands of years of recorded history. There is an interesting parallel between the growth of linguistic skills in one individual from childhood to maturity, and the growth of language in a culture as a nation develops from a small state to a complex power; or the growth of man's use of speech as a member of a nomadic tribe, to the sophisticated linguistic operations of the practicing psychoanalyst. The crucial point concerns the development of man as a member of a complex society—a society in which a child is

Acknowledgment of assistance in preparing this chapter is made to my wife, Eva; and to Hope Tama and Kathy Unger, graduate students of Hofstra University.

expected to learn and develop patterns of communication during early childhood which have been thousands of years in developing as a part of man's cultural heritage.

As many authors, such as Kessler (1966) and Graubard (1969), have pointed out, emotional disorders can be defined as the organism's inability to approximate culturally established patterns of behavior. The child's inability to function in the language area is taken as evidence that there are emotional problems present. Certain types of speech patterns, seemingly of and by themselves, confirm the child's diagnostic label, as Chess (1959, p. 134) points out: "Once a child has been described as showing echolalia, the diagnosis of schizophrenia has to all intents and purposes been made."

Thus, even in the area of defining emotional disturbance we see the significance of distorted speech and language. McCarthy (1954) made a similar conclusion that oral speech and language are important indicators of an individual's mental health. Chess (1944) noted that language disability may be an important factor in the development of personality distortions in childhood. To be mentally healthy is to be able and willing to communicate ideas, feelings, and experiences to other members of a culture. Rank (1932) noted that while speech at first may be an individual and creative act, the communicative function of language is superimposed upon this. Rank goes on to suggest that communication has developed because it was necessary in the development of family and community living. As man's culture developed so did the need for communication. As a child develops, so must the need for adequate communicative skills. An inability to develop in this sphere of activity labels a culture primitive, and a child, in many cases, disturbed.

While Miller (1964) and other anthropologists have indicated that linguistic codes do not differentiate between primitive and nonprimitive groups, they do argue that language types are socially rather than linguistically defined. Other writers, such as Deutsch (1965), have begun to delineate subcultural differences in language. Deutsch noted that in our American society both lower-class and minority-group status are associated with poorer language functioning. The problem of subcultural language patterns cannot be ignored. If emotional health is defined as the ability to pattern one's behavior, even in language, according to subcultural criteria, the problems of language conformity within a pluralistic culture somewhat disappear. However, as Szasz (1960) stated, the psychiatric and mental health professions have been guilty of supporting established language norms as representative of mental health. Definitional differentiation of mental health and illness in our pluralistic culture appears urgently needed.

Cultural parallels in linguistic development are mirrored even in the comparison of the speech of animals with that of people. Mowrer (1958) refers to the work done with talking birds as evidence of similarities in their form of speech and the beginning of speech in children. He notes that words are reproduced when they are first made to sound "good" in the context of affectionate care and attention. When words take on positive emotional meanings the stage is set for their reproduction and later on for their functioning as parts in the social process which we call speech. The child's production of babbling sounds, which are later turned into meaningful communication, parallels this development in the talking birds. On the broad scale of anthropological characteristics, children and adults seem to share the common developmental task of communicating with others. To be able to communicate in a meaningful way is a part of natural evolutionary growth. To communicate in the realm of feelings is a part of natural development—or mental health.

Two other ideas must be mentioned as part of this introduction: the several different aspects of speech and the sequency of growth. Benton (1966, p. 298) clearly defines some of the different aspects of language:

> . . . language consists of the use of symbols for the purposes of communication. On the expressive side, it is the utilization of conventional symbols to communicate one's perceptions, ideas, feelings or intentions to other persons or to oneself. This is the encoding aspect of language wherein the mental content evokes the symbol. On the receptive side, language is the utilization of symbols to apprehend the perception, ideas, feelings or intentions of other persons or oneself. This is the decoding aspect wherever the symbol evokes the mental content.

> . . . language is substitute behavior, which stands for or represents primary behavior processes. It has a referential function in that it links up external and internal events with speech behavior. The reference may be specific or general, precise or imprecise. This referential behavior serves the purposes of interpersonal and intrapersonal communication. While language is intrinsically related to symbolic thinking, it is important to realize that it is not synonymous with symbolic thinking. It is symbolic-communicative activity, i.e., that special mode of communication which employs conventional symbols. A disturbance in symbolic thinking will necessarily be reflected in language behavior but not all impairment in language behavior is referable to impairement in symbolic thinking.

Benton makes several critical points which must be kept in mind when discussing language disabilities in emotionally disturbed children. Language is symbolic, both in its expressive and receptive modes. The language seen or observed in disturbed children may be just that—symbolic of a certain type of disorder in emotional content. This disorder in emotional content can be either the inability to accept (receptive) or the inability to express (expressive) feelings. Benton also notes that language is substitute behavior, and that we can well remember when dealing with children with emotional disorders. The "feelings" involved in the emotional life of the child are not always translated into verbal or language behavior. The catatonic schizophrenic reminds us that feelings can remain locked inside the personality. Internal events in the lives of the disturbed child are not always made public through the process of verbalization; the neurotic types of adjustment to stress will attest to this. Finally, language is not synonymous with feeling. Distortions in language, such as aphasia, do not always represent distortions in feeling.

Shervanian (1967) outlines briefly the developmental stages in language and their concomitant emotional and personality growth needs. For the child to reach the stage of social speech where the healthy expression of feeling can be accomplished, there must be a convergence of the development of thought, speech, and interpersonal tools of communication. These three stages are (1) the development of thought from the primary processes and goal-directed thinking to the secondary processes of more logical, conceptual types of speech; (2) vocalization or speech changes from preintellectual babbling to meaningful sounds with the development of simple linguistic structures; and (3) development of communication from the expression of needs in crying to a meaningful verbal exchange based on a recognition of both oneself and others.

Speech and language problems in the emotionally involved child can be analyzed in terms of fixation at or regression to the primary processes, such as in the speech of the psychotic child. Language problems can sometimes be viewed as the emotional behavior of the intellectually deficient child, even though this analysis will not be attempted in this chapter. Finally, language problems associated with difficulties in interpersonal relations can clearly be recognized. The problems of emotional conflict during interpersonal communication will be discussed in the following section.

INTERPERSONAL NONVERBAL ASPECTS OF COMMUNICATION

Many types of emotional conflicts and distress are expressed directly through language. However, there is a broad area which must be kept in mind in which the emotional conflicts are expressed through nonverbal behavior. Language at times loses its communicative aspect and becomes a purely expressive activity. Often in this situation the speech will mirror an emotional feeling. At times speech serves as a process by which emotional feeling or conflict can be ventilated. In children emotional feelings will undergo a catharsis, at times directed toward a significant adult, but often more easily expressed toward an inanimate object, as in play therapy. Emotional conflicts can be repressed into alternative forms of action so that verbalization does not occur. The language of disturbed children includes aspects of expression which are nonverbal, just as the process of communication has its nonverbal aspects.

DeCarlo (1968) emphasized the importance of nonverbally oriented interaction between a significant adult and a young child in terms of the effects these interactions have on the development of language. Des Lauriers and Carlson in 1969 noted:

> It is in the reciprocity of this direct physical, preverbal, and affective communication between the child and his mother that the foundations are laid for the development in the child of a truly human form of life expression. In some ways this could be called a silent language, where words are not needed, nor images, nor symbols; it is a communication expressed in the direct physical presence of one to another. . . . This then is a language of body, of physical space, of time, but mostly of affective and sensory arousal and stimulation.[1]

More subtle, but nonetheless as important, are the effects of nonverbal communication on the natural growth and progression of language. Indeed, nonverbal physical interaction predates the development of speech and communication. Eisenberg and

---

[1] Reprinted with permission of Des Lauriers, A. M., and C. F. Carlson, Your Child Is Asleep, (Homewood, Ill., Dorsey Press , p. 362.)

Kanner (1956) noted the hesitancy of parents of autistic children to interact physically with the young infant, and considered this a critical factor in the emotional response lag of the autistic child. The parents felt no need for nonverbal communication with the young infant, and the stage was set for permanent fixation at a nonverbal level of communication. Wolf and Ruttenberg (1967) reported that autistic children appear to try to communicate through nonverbal means. Verbal communication appears to demand a degree of sophistication in ego functioning that the autistic child does not possess; consequently, the autistic child uses nonverbal and more primitive communication techniques.

In general, severely ill children and psychiatric patients do not express a normal need for verbal communication. Weiland and Legg (1964) and de Hirsch (1967) point out that shared or social experiences seem to have far less significance for psychotic children and that speech and language is less often used as a means of interpersonal contact. Without the need for interpersonal communication little verbalization is reinforced. Another aspect of this problem is the child's desire to maintain distance from other people as a form of protection or defense. Barbara (1959) in the American Handbook of Psychiatry noted that there were patients, whom he called "resigned" stutterers, who see to it that they maintain emotional distance from others, rarely becoming emotionally involved with anyone. Along with the desire to stay apart from other people is a panic reaction to speech—because it represents communication with others.

Ruesch (1959) also reported this tendency for the very ill child to express his conflicts in nonverbal terms through body movement and other forms of expression. He suggests that the therapies which have developed for the psychoses focus on a nonverbal approach to the patient, as opposed to the traditional verbal therapies of psychoanalysis. Ruesch noted that verbal communication is nearly impossible when nonverbal perception and expressions do not function. He correctly points to the fact that the psychoanalysts have worked out in minute detail the relationships of verbal content of speech to the therapeutic process. However, Ruesch asserts that it has been the psychiatrists who have worked with psychotic patients and children—Sullivan, Fromm-Reichman, Redl and Wineman, and Szurek—who have made us aware of the importance of nonverbal communication.

Therapists have long accepted the need for the expression of feeling in children through the medium of nonverbal language. The literature is replete with examples of therapeutic approaches which use play, art, music, the dance, and other forms of physical expression. Dibs: In Search of Self by Virginia Axline is only one of many excellent books which detail the nonverbal communication of feelings between a child and a therapist. DeCarlo (1968, p. 362) noted that "expressiveness locked in without words will need to flow forth in art, crafts, music and dance." For the release of these locked-in feelings it is often necessary for the adult to have what Spiegel (1959, p. 915) called empathic communication:

> Empathic communication occurs through the reading of subliminal signs of another person's behavior, emotions, etc. . . . . Empathic communication is not verbal, does not depend on a statement of the feeling-state, but may accompany language, for instance, through the ring of the voice.

Body language includes the sense of the basic physical presence of another person, the sense of the impact of another person, his quality of movement. It includes gestures, the body attitudes, that the person does not intend but which reveal him, and also those which he does intend and by means of which he communicates.

Certain characteristic patterns of nonverbal communication and language appear to be substituted for normal speech in the psychotic illnesses in children. In describing the physical response characteristics of 12 schizophrenic children, Goldfarb and co-workers (1956) noted that if spoken language was present, it was not reinforced by gestures of face and body as is usually seen in the normal child. They reported the characteristic wooden features of almost pathogenic dilation and the absence of facial expression in the children. De Hirsch (1967) noted that often there seems to be a complete absence of verbal communicative intent. Spiegel (1959) observes that in schizophrenia there are strikingly characteristic patterns of physical posture, stance, movement, muscle tension, and facial expression which give a wide range of information about the patient's inner state of emotion and communication. Body language in the schizophrenic is often linked to his communicative needs and verbal language is less often directed toward expressing social and communicative needs.

Similar evidence appears to present itself in the case of the autistic child. Accompanying autism and/or echolalic speech, there is a highly developed nonverbal pattern of communication. Pronovost and co-workers (1966) noted that autistic children were not responding to verbal reflections but were responding to physical contact and gesture language. If gestures were deleted, the children no longer responded appropriately. They concluded that the verbal language of these children seemed limited to the level of concrete nouns, similar to that of a 2- or 3-year-old, with an absence of abstract and collective nouns. Ruttenberg and Gordon (1967) also report that conversation among autistic children is basically nonverbal, and that vocalization for the autistic child often serves an autoerotic function rather than an interpersonal function of communication. Fay (1969) suggests that the autistic child indeed does try, though unsuccessfully, to maintain contact with the verbal world through his echolalic speech.

A useful analysis of the nonverbal communication patterns of the autistic child is presented by Ruttenberg and Gordon (1967). They outline 10 nonverbal levels of speech in the autistic child. The levels represent a sequential growth pattern in the use of nonverbal language for communication. The following are parts of the Behavior-Rating Instrument for Autistic Children reported originally by Ruttenberg et al. (1966) and reprinted here from Ruttenberg and Gordon (1967, pp. 317-319):

Nature and Degree of Relationship to an Adult as a Person

Level 1. Imperviousness, or obliviousness to people. There is almost continuous lack of response; the child behaves as if no one is present; he looks right through a person or ignores the person as a whole. However, he may use part of the person—the person's hand, for example—as a tool or instrument. Persistent attempts to become involved with the child, or even physical proximity to him, may trigger off diffuse rage or panic.

Level 2. Withdrawal or intermittent imperviousness. When someone comes close, the child withdraws into imperviousness, stops visual following. This implies that he has noted the other person and then responds via withdrawal into imperviousness.

Level 3. Resistiveness. This is a continued but less extreme way of warding off a relationship. The child turns away, averts his gaze, or looks just past the person's face rather than through the person. In certain instances he may shift his gaze to maintain a tangential position as the adult moves his gaze toward the child.

Visual following is the clinically observable behavior which may be used to differentiate the above three levels. In Level 1 the child constantly looks through the adult; in 2 he intermittently looks through the adult; and in 3 he looks away from or past the adult.

Level 4. The child will attend to a familiar person at a distance of approximately six feet or more. Usually the child's gaze is limited to the face or, more specifically, the eyes of the person. However, he will withdraw from an approaching adult.

Level 5. Brief, sporadic, but recurrent attending to one familiar adult at close range. Typically this is in conjunction with gratification of primitive needs, such as food, relief of tension or pain, and sleep.

Level 6. Regularly recurring response to one person as a whole. For the first time the child establishes and maintains eye-to-eye contact, his gaze having an exploring, searching quality. He explores the adult's face visually and manually. He tries to maneuver the entire adult physically, in contrast to his behavior at previous levels when only part of the body was manipulated.

At Level 6 the physical response to adults is more sustained than at Level 5, and is observed in a greater variety of modes and situations, such as clinging, pulling, hitting, stalking, cuddling, looking, and need-related vocalizing and gesturing. There are also beginning signs of possessiveness and jealousy.

Level 7. A consistent searching out and attending to one person for comfort, approval, help, and play. An active relationship is established through reciprocal games and teasing, but things are done on the child's own terms.

Level 8. The child is beginning to anticipate approval and disapproval and can control his behavior accordingly. In contrast to Level 7, he no longer relates only on his own terms but is regularly responsive to requests and suggestions from a familiar person.

Level 9. Sharing of experiences. The child seeks mutuality and direction; he expresses pride in achievement and acquisition to the adult. This is not merely a quest for help; it is a giving as well as a taking. He attempts to direct the adult's attention to what he is doing and what he has acquired, and somehow tries to involve the adult in his activity.

Level 10. Identification and empathy. The child may respond to another with a similar affective state. He also can do something to please or help another without obvious direct gain for himself. This implies a high order of awareness of another person as a human being.

Specific deficits in the nonverbal communication of emotionally involved children is an area which to a great degree has not been charted. That emotional disorders often interfere with the verbal communication of disturbed children and that emotional conflict is often expressed through bodily functions, movements, and empathic responses is readily accepted. The role of nonverbal communication in the lives of normal children as compared with the role of nonverbal communication among disturbed children needs to be researched. Clinical experience suggests that these areas may be fruitful in understanding and dealing with severely disturbed children. At this point let us turn our attention to language and communication deficits associated with the neurotic disorders.

LANGUAGE DEFICITS ASSOCIATED WITH NEUROTIC DISORDERS

There is ample evidence concerning types of language disabilities found in neurotic disorders. It almost appears to be a natural result that an internalized state of anxiety interferes with communicative language. Expressive and receptive languages are both extremely susceptible to the effect of anxiety. Many of the processes which produce language are also processes which function in neurotic disorders. Myklebust (1957) noted that internalization was an essential process for the normal development of language. He also suggests that the process of identification must be intact for adequate growth in language, and that an infant's first babbling can be understood as the first signs of identification taking place. Mowrer (1950) points out that intrapsychic satisfaction in the young infant is related to the child's desire to play with and perfect the sounds he has associated with the pleasurable sensations evoked by his mother, his first love object.

As early as 1932 the American Speech and Hearing Association noted that some speech defects occur partially as a result of frustration and discouragement in interpersonal relations. Feelings of insecurity related to social relationships are expressed in speech. Emotional disorders which produce anxiety, feelings of insecurity, or deficient self-concepts are found to be basic components in many types of distorted interpersonal verbal communications. As a handicapped personality, with weakened defenses and heightened vulnerability, approaches other people in private or social interchange, the usual result is a reticence in communication, or perhaps at times the inappropriate, irrelevant, or insensitive use of language. Barbara (1959, p. 953) in the *American Handbook of Psychiatry* describes one form of neurotic speech disorder, stuttering, and explains its functioning in the following manner:

> So-called symptoms of neurosis are not essentially constituents, but they develop as an outgrowth of the neurotic character structure and can be understood only on that basis. Stuttering is to be considered as an expression of anxiety, which results when the protective structure of the organism in a neurotic process becomes threatened and disorganized.

Stuttering, which is but an outward expression of anxiety in conflict, is secondary to an unhealthy personality development and is manifested specifically and implicitly in speaking where lines of normal verbalization and communication are disturbed ... The syndrome of stuttering must then be considered as a problem involving both interpersonal and interpsychic aspects of inner conflict.

Thus the stutterer is to a large degree a person with a primary emotional conflict which is being expressed through language. The neurotic conflict which is the base of some stuttering is not accepted as explanatory of all types and cases of stuttering. Stuttering does not represent a large portion of neurotic reactions in children or a large percentage of all the emotional disorders found in children. Emotionally involved children, as a group, do not use stuttering as the sole resolution of their neurotic interpersonal or interpsychic conflicts. Phobias, compulsions, and anxiety states are other common resolutions of neurotic disorders in children, yet very little information is available about the speech and language patterns of these manifestations of neurotic adjustment. Perhaps it is the nonverbal or "action" character of phobias, anxiety states, and compulsions which accounts for their having impact on the child's communicative speech.

There is a series of studies which suggests that stuttering is a result of conflict in the parent—child relationship, specifically the mother—child relationship. Despert (1946) noted in her study of 50 stuttering children that there was a common element of anxiety which appeared to be the result of pressure from a neurotic, compulsive mother at critical periods of language development. She also found the mothers to be overprotective. These findings were supported by Kinstler (1961) and Moncur (1963), whose works suggest covert or overt rejection by mothers and parental domination. Discordant interpersonal relationships between the mother and child appear to be able to produce one basic language disorder in young children—stuttering.

Some evidence appears in the literature concerning the use of mutism as a neurotic solution to conflict in the lives of children. As early as 1943, Rose indicated that one of the characteristics of withdrawn, silent, or mute children was that as an attempt to cope with basic fear, they let speech stand for the feared object and solved the conflict by remaining mute. Barbara (1957) noted that a common element in disturbed speakers was the intense emotional reaction precipitated by the fear of speaking situations where the personality is the focus of attention by others, leaving it vulnerable in the case of neurotic organization. Thus they may appear to be quiet or withdrawn due to a desire to stay out of the center of attention in a group. In general Barnard et al. (1961) and Zimbardo et al. (1963) report the same type of findings. In the first study anxiety was found to impede verbal behavior but not to impede basic cognitive understanding of words that express emotion. In the second study the speech of the anxious child was shown to be less comprehensible and to include more intrusions of inappropriate affect than speech of the nonanxious child. They also indicated that the anxious children's speech is more readily affected under stressful conditions. Subjected to stress the anxious child's speech deteriorates even further.

Aronson et al. (1965) also studied the relationship between situational conflicts and voice disorders and found that the voice disorders represented primary gains for a majority of the subjects studied. These subjects were classified into four classes: muteness, continually whispered speech, intermittently phonated whispered speech, and continually phonated speech. One of the striking characteristics of that population was their inability to deal with feelings of anger in a mature manner. Their lifelong patterns of neurotic adjustment appeared to turn their inability to handle anger into mutism, or near mutism. These findings may be understood better in light of the fact that in several other studies (Taffel, 1955; Davids and Eriksen, 1955) it was found that subjects with higher levels of anxiety conditioned quicker and developed more chained verbal associations. Highly anxious children, consequently, may be seen as vulnerable to conditioning processes associated with their language development. Because of their built-in internalization tendencies, they usually internalize enough guilt to lead to a reduced verbal output, or in extreme cases to mutism.

Thus, in general, neurotic adjustment in children can be seen as having one of three effects on their speech patterns and communications. The processes of internalizing anxiety and guilt, so common in neurotic disorders, appear to be central in the speech pattern which develops. First, the neurotic conflict can be resolved through the use of nonverbal or physical expression, as in the cases of compulsions, phobias, or conversions into somatic disorders, each with its own disordered body or action language. Second, the neurotic conflict can be expressed through disordered speech, such as stuttering. Finally, the anxiety may produce withdrawal from verbal exchanges, reduced verbal output, or mutism. Which of the three patterns develops depends on a large variety of situational variables.

INNER LANGUAGE—THE WORLD OF THE PSYCHOTIC

The American Psychiatric Association's Diagnostic and Statistical Manual: Mental Disorders (1965) defines psychoses as having three distinct parts: (1) "a varying degree of personality disintegration"; (2) "a failure to test and evaluate, correctly, external reality"; (3) "an inability to relate themselves to other people and to their own work." The language disabilities found in psychotic disorders mirror these three psychological disabilities. In children these psychological disabilities can perhaps be better described as the following: (1) distortions of language, including mutism, which represent the disintegrated inner world of the psychotic child, with all of the distortions of feelings and ideas which accompany this personality disintegration or disharmony; (2) distorted language patterns which the child uses in trying to describe, identify, and explore the world of reality outside himself—the reality which is shared by others in his environment but is so different from his point of view; and (3) the distorted verbal systems he uses in his attempt to make contact, to communicate, to relate to others either verbally or nonverbally. This section will be an attempt to analyze the speech patterns of the various types of psychotic disorders in children through these three functions of language. Hopefully, patterns will develop which may give more clues to the nature of the pathology as the linguistic modes of the psychotic child are considered.

A slight digression must be permitted at this point, for in reality the past 30 years has seen the recognition of several distinct types of psychotic reactions in childhood. Along with this delineation has come disagreement and professional differences of opinion concerning the types of psychotic disorders in childhood. It is not the intent of this section to argue these several points, but for the sake of a frame of reference the points of view of Jane Kessler (1966) will be followed. Kessler describes and delineates four distinct types of psychotic disorders in children: infantile autism, symbiosis, infantile psychosis, and childhood schizophrenia. These four types of psychotic reactions in childhood can be conceptualized easier if one considers the two factors of age and introversion-extroversion as dimensions. In that case the four types of psychotic reactions fall into the pattern shown in Table 1.

Table 1. Psychotic Reactions in Childhood

Introversion-extroversion dimension	Age dimension			
	Birth	Infancy	Early childhood	Latency
High degree of introversion		Infantile autism	Infantile psychosis	
High degree of extroversion		Symbiosis	Childhood schizophrenia	

The clinician or educator must ask the relevant question, are there also four distinct language disability patterns which coincide with the several types of psychotic disorders in childhood? The following discussion is an attempt to review the evidence in each case.

Infantile Autism

In the case of infantile autism, the evidence clearly indicates that the distinct diagnostic category has been accepted, and a distinct language pattern can be seen developing. The works of Kanner (1946), Rimland (1964), Bettelheim (1967), and Des Lauriers and Carlson (1969) have become classic works on the subject and are widely known as having introduced the pathology of childhood autism to both the professional and the public educator.

Infantile autism presents an almost perfect example of the effects of a psychosis on language in the three areas of functioning, i.e., personality disintegration, reality testing, and interpersonal communication. The severity of the disorder is such that all three aspects of the psychotic disorder are observable, and representative language deficits in each area can be noted. Wolf and Ruttenberg (1967) suggest that infantile autism is a disorder which pervades the entire range of ego functioning and consequently thought, speech, and communication are all impaired to a degree. This severe disorder involves the total functioning of the child and consequently presents a comprehensive picture of language deficits in emotional disorder.

In infantile autism the child appears to live in an inner, mental world which is for all intents and purposes devoid of emotion and feeling. There is a unique type of disharmony between the parts of the personality in that the id, ego, and superego seem to be only partially functioning in each case. Instincts for survival are apparent yet do not appear to include aggression; reality needs of the ego are often disregarded in that the child lives in the psychotic, withdrawn, nonhuman environment of objects and his own mind. The superego demands seem almost irrelevant to the inner controls and stimulation which is present. Consequently the inner, subjective world of the autistic child is unique in its use of linguistic material. This inner world appears extremely distorted and nonemotional. Kanner (1946) points to the autistic "privacy" of these children's thoughts, that the metaphorical language they use is not communicative but is undoubtedly creative in a self-sufficient and self-contained way. Verbal responses when given suggest that memory and understanding are present (Ruttenberg and Gordon, 1967) but resemble the responses of lucid catatonics. Pronovost (1961) also points out the evident existence of an internal comprehension of nonaffective parts of linguistic communication.

Distorted perceptions of reality are also observable. Constant and repeated evidence indicates that autistic children rigidly select the aspects of reality that they want to respond to, or that they are capable of responding to (Rimland, 1964). Pronovost (1961) points to their highly developed awareness of reality and relationships within their environment—especially among objects. Characteristics of their speech suggest, however, that their understanding of reality is only partial. This can be seen in their mute or echolalic speech patterns. While they are attracted to objects, they seldom use the names of them. Often, the child may not utter any sounds, or only produce phonetic sounds (Shervanian, 1967). The autistic child is often thought of as depersonalizing or making inanimate many living things. There appears to be no desire or ability to relate to the reality of the emotional aspects of life. Feelings and emotions appear to be locked up inside the child (Des Lauriers and Carlson, 1969; Bettleheim, 1967). Consequently, speech, when used, is flat, emotionless, and void of feeling (Goldfarb et al., 1956). The reality of other people's existence is even negated, as is, seemingly, his own existence through the use of pronoun reversals and echolalic, parrot-like speech patterns. The autistic child has neither strong contact with nor emotional investment in the real world—the shared world of other people. His speech mirrors this defect.

Finally, the autistic child sees little need for interpersonal contact. Communication between the autistic child and other people is almost nonexistent. This appears to be true in their receptive language. Speech is not utilized as extensively as nonverbal cues in understanding others in his environment. Hingtgen and Coulter (1967) found that the comprehension of autistic children dropped sharply as gestures and visual cues were reduced or stopped by the person trying to communicate with them. Ruttenberg and Gordon (1967) and Despert (1938) found much the same thing—autistic children do not use verbalization for communication. Their communication is usually autoerotic in nature and devoid of communicative intent. Often gestures from others must be used if the autistic child is to understand the intent of another's communication. Verbalization, when it does occur, usually represents a type of energy release through the vocal mechanisms, devoid of intent, except in the same sense that many creative acts are basically self-sufficient and self-fulfilling.

Pronovost et al. (1966) describe the vocalizations of autistic children as being unique. They note a high degree of monotonal sounds as well as a high pitch to the voice of many autistic children in their study. They also perceive a wide variety of intensity levels in autistic children's speech as well as hoarseness, harshness, and hypernasality. At times the verbal autistic child was echolalic, and at times combined speech with musical phrases.

Kanner (1946) noted that several of the autistic children he studied used speech effectively on occasions, such as uttering whole sentences in emergency situations. Kanner notes that some autistic children use words as magical protection against unpleasant occurrences. He also cited instances where the seemingly irrelevant phrases could be traced back to earlier conversations, wherein the phrases assumed definite meanings even though the associations were still "peculiar." Finally, he suggests that a type of metaphorical substitution may be common among autistic children. In this type of situation, an autistic child being asked to subtract 4 cents from 10 cents did not reply directly, but said instead "I'll draw a hexagon." Obviously, the inner language and thought systems were intact, if not superior, but the forms of interpersonal communication used were irregular, in this case metaphorical.

Symbiosis

Symbiotic psychosis is at once the easiest and most difficult to describe linguistically. The concept of symbiotic psychosis as a separate psychotic disorder was introduced by Margaret Mahler in 1952. She describes it as a borderline psychosis, that is, on the border between psychosis and neurosis. It is accompanied by behavior patterns which include the child's clinging to the mother, panic upon separation from the mother, having a "symbiotic" tie to the mother, and being oversensitive or crying readily. Symbiotic children cannot tolerate frustration and never achieve "individuation" or independence. The psychosis develops between the ages of 2½ and 5. Extreme anxiety reactions, a growing discrepancy between the rate of maturation of the ego and physiological processes, and catatonic-like temper tantrums are all a part of Mahler's (1952) description of the disorder.

In terms of language or communication, the symbiotic child appears to have the most severe malfunction in the distortion of efforts to communicate with other people—that is, with the mother. These language distortions are both verbal and nonverbal. They are described as "cry-babies," as reacting in verbal panic to separation, and as reacting in almost catatonic temper tantrums of explosive speech. Their nonverbal or physical communication is just as striking. Mahler (1952) describes a conflict between a craving for body contact with the mother and a shrinking from it, as well as diffuse anxiety reactions which reflect seemingly real organic distress. This organic distress is real to the child, and it is often supported by physiological signs—the children are unhealthy. This particular point exemplifies the "personality disintegration" in symbiosis. As the young child experiences this psychotic disorder the decompensation process is translated directly into physiological distress.

The "newness" of the diagnostic category, as well as its borderline status, seem to have worked against extensive research on language deficits in this area. The symbiotic child expresses his feelings of anxiety both through language and body states, much like the neurotic child does in phobias and compulsions. The point which argues for its inclusion among the psychotic disorders is the disintegration or decompensation of ego defenses which are so complete as to leave the organism in a psychotic and undefended state. This type of vulnerability does not lead to withdrawal into the mute world of the schizophrenic but to a seemingly primitive level of linguistic organization which consists of undifferentiated verbal panic under stress. Perhaps the future will provide further research efforts into the linguistic patterns of the symbiotic child.

Infantile Psychosis

The third category of infantile psychosis shares with symbiosis its nonestablished position in professional literature. It is defined as being apart from the other three types of psychotic reactions, yet sharing certain symptoms with each of the others. It is considered more serious than symbiosis, yet more general than autism or schizophrenia as a type of psychosis. Reiser (1963) describes infantile psychosis as an impairment of contact with reality, an absence of meaningful verbal communication, a withdrawal from social interaction, an unevenness between mental and emotional functioning, as well as a disparity among motor, verbal, social, and adaptive behavior.

The verbal and nonverbal aspects of childhood psychosis were described by Brown (1960). Among the verbal aspects were an odd quality to the voice, echolalia, pronoun reversals, no facial gestures or communicative expressions, and often an uncertain understanding of the speech of others. Nonverbal aspects of their communication included preoccupation or apparent attention to internal speech, bizarre movements, primitive use of objects and persons not usually for communication, avoidance of interpersonal contact, and an inhibition of motor activity.

Other writers have attempted to describe the speech of the psychotic child. Shervanian (1967) notes that psychotic children range from a lack of speech for communication to an inconsistent use of speech for communication. He notes that the major determinants of speech, thought, and communication disorders in psychotic children are related to the ego defenses erected against anxiety-producing stimuli from within or outside the organism. Lenneberg (1964) also notes the wide variability in speech patterns of psychotic children. He indicates that there may be long periods of muteness accompanied by purposeful behavior requiring an internal language. Lenneberg also notes that increased verbalization is one alternative, as opposed to mutism. Both appear to be variations of a common and constant theme—speech and language has its roots in abnormal motivational and emotional states; its use is limited and often interferes with interpersonal communication more than it facilitates it.

Language analysis by Weiland and Legg (1964) suggests that psychotic children develop a pattern of increased variability in the use of nouns, pronouns, and prepositions. They indicate that psychotic distortions of reality and of interpersonal relationships produce this increase in rates of usage of these parts of speech. Benton (1966) notes a lack of a need to communicate with others in psychotic disorders, which often produces a kind of incomprehensible word salad full of word substitutions, syntactic distortions, and neologisms. Other authors, such as Despert (1938) and Bradley and Bowen (1941), indicate that this garbled speech may be indicative of impaired thought processes. Spiegel (1959) notes that two forms of communication are really impaired—communication with others or interpersonal communication, and relatedness to himself—his intrapsychic communication.

The linguistic pattern of infantile psychosis, as compared with the three other psychotic reactions in childhood, does not yet appear to have been fully delineated. This author felt that some of the confusion resulted from the diagnostic category itself. Several authors used the terms infantile or childhood psychosis, but it did not seem to mean the same disorder as that described by Kessler (1966) as one of four distinct types of childhood psychoses.

Childhood Schizophrenia

In childhood schizophrenia a similar comparison can be made, utilizing the three aspects of psychotic behavior—personality disintegration, distorted perceptions of reality, and confused interpersonal relationships. De Hirsch (1967) points out that schizophrenic behavior is expressed through personality disintegration. She notes that the disorder is pervasive; it involves ego boundaries and the totality of personality organization. Receptive language in schizophrenic children indicates responsiveness to both external stimuli and internal stimuli, which at times may create auditory hallucinations. Spiegel (1959) notes that schizophrenia presents a montage of disturbed communication, seriously damaged in intrapsychic, perceptual, and interpersonal modes. Spiegel notes that disassociation, autism, symbolism of imagery and myth, discursive logic, and nonverbal language which includes body movement are all signs of the disordered inner mental state. Regression of thought patterns producing a greater use of nouns reflects a concreteness of thought in schizophrenic processes (Ellsworth, 1952). Ellsworth also points to a lessened use of verbs, which he interprets as a sign of emotional instability among schizophrenic children. De Hirsch (1967) notes the primitiveness of the personality organization among schizophrenics as being evidenced by their higher auditory threshold, their memory for meaningless material, and their ability to incorporate sophisticated linguistic rules. Obviously, the evidence suggests an inner turmoil, a discordance about the interfunctioning of personality within the schizophrenic's speech patterns.

Their perception of reality and their relationship to the outer world are also affected, and produce distinct language deficits. De Hirsch (1967) notes that schizophrenic language often does not serve as referents—words lose their symbolic status; they become concrete entities of and by themselves and as such may acquire magical status. She further notes that communication is subject to primary process distortions; instead of speech being at the service of the ego, it is tied to early instinctual processes. Words do not serve reality and have no conventional objective significance. Ellsworth (1952) attributes their use of more pronouns to their egocentricity and their projection of ideas onto others in their environment.

Many authors have cited the uncommon associations which are present in schizophrenic language. Sommer et al. (1960) note that their study found the use of less

Table 2. Language Patterns in Psychoses During Childhood

Type of psychosis	Verbal speech patterns	Nonverbal communication patterns	Thought patterns
Infantile autism	1. noncommunicative energy release 2. parrot-like speech 3. echolalia, pronoun reversals 4. flat, devoid of feeling with no emotional content 5. emergency use of speech only	1. no body language for communication 2. movement is autoerotic in nature 3. depersonalized life, contact with inanimate objects preferred	1. a creative inner language 2. lack of meaningful association with reality or past experiences 3. little use of abstract or collective nouns, lack of generalization 4. high degree of rote memory
Symbiosis	1. cry-babies 2. verbal panic 3. explosive speech 4. high degree of interpersonal content or emotional content in speech	1. temper tantrums 2. catatonic rage 3. ambivalence—both craving for physical contact and shrinking from interpersonal contact	1. basically normal, with tendencies toward projected deindividuation or symbiotic thought agreement with mother

Infantile psychosis	1. no meaningful verbal communication 2. odd quality to voice 3. many word salads, and neologisms 4. increased variability of the use of nouns, prepositions, and pronouns	1. inhibited motor activity 2. bizarre movements 3. lack of facial gestures to accompany speech	1. attention to internal thought and language as opposed to speech as a communicative act
Childhood schizophrenia	1. wide variation of meaningfulness of speech from realistic speech to auditory hallucinations 2. complex patterns of verbal responses 3. speech is full of emotional content 4. often includes symbolic use of words and images	1. great variety of facial expressions depending on type of reaction 2. catatonic reactions 3. often wooden faces, staring unseeing eyes 4. possible acting out, aggressive, violent physical acting out of conflict	1. regressed thought—primitive thinking 2. highly developed logical thought with many associative chains 3. symbolism, myths, metaphorical use of language 4. magical thinking often present

popular associations by schizophrenic patients, and that the schizophrenic is less likely to give the same associations from one occasion to another. However, they concluded that the schizophrenic was aware of his own uncommon choices and uncommon associations. Bleuler (1955) and Arieti (1955) have also commented on these uncommon associations and uncommon responses. Sommer et al. (1960) explain these uncommon associations as the end of association chains, or associations linked to a series of associations. This is commonly called the knight's move, and refers to associational chains in which the middle associations are missing, or not related verbally.

In relation to the schizophrenic's inability to maintain interpersonal communication, here again we see a wide variety of patterns emerging. Communicative intent appears often to be absent, irrelevant, yet at other times is quite evident and functional. Schizophrenia is often differentiated from autism through the differences in interpersonal relations, the schizophrenic displaying distortions in ability to communicate while the autistic withdraws completely from interpersonal communication. The schizophrenic child may be aggressive, acting out, panic stricken, or mute and withdrawn. Goldfarb et al. (1956) point out a greater variety and wider range of speech deviations in schizophrenics. They note an unpredictable variety of distortions and completely idiosyncratic patterns of communicative signals. The voice and characteristics of the utterances are not utilized to convey meaning and emotions. Their speech patterns are often flat and unexpressive; the word is given magical powers and becomes a concrete weapon.

Spiegel (1959) notes that among adolescent and adult schizophrenic patients there are distinct speech patterns similar to the different types of schizophrenia. Catatonics are mute, verbal communication is given up, and the remaining communication is empathic and in body language while intrapsychic activity remains. In the paranoid type, schizophrenics communicate quite well, using symbolism and logic, although the imagery and meaning are distorted. Hebephrenic schizophrenia is noted for its silliness of speech, use of language fragments, and verbal "noise," which appears to protect them from other people. Simple schizophrenia is associated with a reduced and constricted communicative language. It appears more uniform to the observer and does involve verbal speech as well as gestures used to express a feeling state, appearing like children who are to be seen but not heard.

Table 2 attempts to summarize the language patterns which are suggested by the literature on childhood psychosis. Each type of childhood psychosis is described in terms of its verbal and nonverbal speech patterns as well as the characteristic thought patterns.

Language in infantile autism is almost disregarded as a vehicle for the expression of the disorder. In symbiosis language is overwhelmingly used as the vehicle for the expression of conflict through the panic reactions of the child. In infantile psychosis the picture is not clear. In the schizophrenic it seems that language is often used as the vehicle for the expression of the emotional disorder. Frequently it will mirror a distorted inner reality as well as a distorted grasp on the world of others. The study of the language deficits suggests focal points about the nature of the disorder. The muteness of the autistic child characterizes it as an interpersonal deficit, the panic of the symbiotic child characterizes it as a distortion of feelings evoked by interpersonal relationships, and the variety of verbal patterns in schizophrenia appears to reflect the disabilities in many spheres—in the intrapsychic world as well as the communicative act.

SUMMARY

This chapter described several important theories, as well as evidence which suggests distinct patterns of language disabilities among emotionally disordered children. It has been suggested that the ability to communicate is central to the definition of emotional health in our culture. Often the professional must be aware of the sophisticated bodily expressive or nonverbal aspects through which an emotional disorder is channeled in children. The evidence for distinct patterns of language deficit associated with the various forms of neurotic and psychotic disorders has been outlined.

While a serious effort was made to include most of the pertinent literature, an exhaustive study is a life's work. There is a tremendous complexity in the relationship between emotional disorders in children and their communicative patterns. Much of the research evidence concerning the conditioning of verbal responses was not included simply because it did not appear central to the discussion. Students interested in the effect of conditioning on speech rates are referred to the following studies: Hartman (1955), Isaacs et al. (1960), Lovaas et al. (1966), Schell et al. (1967), Hewett (1965), and Hagen et al. (1968). The works of Ullman and Krasner (1965) as well as Krasner and Ullman (1968) include important articles concerning the techniques of conditioning verbal speech. Most of the work that pertained to the description of verbal behavior has been included. Information about modifying verbal behavior in disturbed children has not been included.

REFERENCES

American Psychiatric Association. 1965. Diagnostic and Statistical Manual: Mental Disorders. Washington, D. C., American Psychiatric Association.

American Speech and Hearing Association, Committee on the Mid-Century White House Conference. 1952. Speech disorders and speech correction. J. Speech Hearing Dis., 17:129-137.

Arieti, S. 1955. Interpretation of Schizophrenia. New York, Robert Brunner.

Aronson, A. E., H. W. Peterson, and E. M. Litin. 1965. Psychiatric symptomatology in functional dysphonia and aphonia. J. Speech Hearing Dis., 32:115-127.

Axline, V. 1964. Dibs: In Search of Self. Boston, Houghton Mifflin.

Barbara, D. A. 1957. Neurosis in speaking. Psychoanal. Rev., 44:41-50.

———1959. Stuttering. In Arieti, S., ed., American Handbook of Psychiatry, Vol. 1. New York, Basic Books.

Barnard, J. W., P. G. Zimbardo, and S. Sarason. 1961. Anxiety and verbal behavior in children. Child Develop., 32:379-392.

Benton, A. L. 1966. Language disorders in children. Canad. Psycho., 7a(4):298-312.

Bettelheim, B. 1967. The Empty Fortress. New York, Free Press.

Bleuler, E. 1955. Dementia Praecox or the Group of Schizophrenias. New York, International Universities Press.

Bradley, C., and M. Bowen. 1941. Behavior characteristics of schizophrenic children. Psychiat. Quart., 15:296-315.

Brown, J. L. 1960. Prognosis from presenting symptoms of preschool children with atypical development. Amer. J. Orthopsychiat., 30:382-391.

Chess, S. 1944. Developmental language disability as a factor in personality distortions in childhood. Amer. J. Orthopsychiat., 14:483-490.

Davids, A., and C. W. Eriksen. 1955. The relationship of manifest anxiety of association productivity and intellectual attainment. J. Consult. Psychol., 19:219-222.

—— 1959. An Introduction to Child Psychiatry. New York, Grune & Stratton.

DeCarlo, M. 1968. The nonverbal child. Child. Educ., 44:358-362.

De Hirsch, K. 1967. Differential diagnosis between aphasic and schizophrenic language in children. J. Speech Hearing Dis., 32:3-10.

Des Lauriers, A. M. 1962. The Experience of Reality in Childhood Schizophrenia. New York, International Universities Press.

—— and C. F. Carlson. 1969. Your Child Is Asleep. Homewood, Ill., Dorsey Press.

Despert, J. L. 1938. Schizophrenia in children. Psychiat. Quart., 12:366-371.

—— 1946. Psychosomatic study of fifty stuttering children. Amer. J. Orthopsychiat., 16:100-113.

Deutsch, M. 1965. The role of social class in language development and cognition. Amer. J. Orthopsychiat., 35:78-88.

Eisenberg, L., and L. Kanner. 1956. Early infantile autism, 1943-55. Amer. Orthopsychiat., 26:556-566.

Ellsworth, R. B. 1952. The regression of schizophrenic language. J. Consul. Psychol., 15:387-391.

Fay, W. H. 1969. On the basis of autistic echolalia. J. Commun. Dis., 2:38-47.

Fromm-Reichman, F. 1950. Principles of Intensive Psychotherapy. Chicago, University of Chicago Press.

Goldfarb, W., P. Braunstein, and I. Lorge. 1956. A study of speech patterns in a group of schizophrenic children. Amer. J. Orthopsychiat., 26:544-555.

Graubard, P., ed. 1969. Children Against Schools. Chicago, Follett Educational Corporation.

Hagen, J. W., B. G. Winsberg, and P. Wolff. 1968. Cognitive and linguistic deficits in psychotic children. Child Develop., 39:1103-1117.

Hartman, C. H. 1955. Verbal behavior of schizophrenic and normal subjects as a function of types of social reinforcement. Dissertation Abstr., 15:1652-1653.

Hewett, F. M. 1965. Teaching speech to an autistic child through operant conditioning. Amer. J. Orthopsychiat., 35:926-936.

Hingtgen, J. M., and S. K. Coulter. 1967. Auditory control of operant behavior in mute autistic children. J. Percept. Motor Skills, 25:561-565.

Isaacs, W., J. Thomas, and I. Goldiamond. 1960. Application of operant conditioning to reinstate verbal behavior in psychotics. J. Speech Hearing Dis., 25:8-12.

Kanner, L. 1946. Irrelevant and metaphorical language in early infantile autism. Amer. J. Psychiat., 103:242-246.

Kessler, J. W. 1966. Psychopathology of Childhood. Englewood Cliffs, N. J., Prentice-Hall.

Kinstler, D. B. 1961. Covert and overt maternal rejection in stuttering. J. Speech Hearing Dis., 26:145-155.

Krasner, L. 1958. Studies of the conditioning verbal behavior. Psychol. Bull., 55:148-168.

—— and L. Ullman. 1968. Research in Behavior Modification. New York, Holt, Rinehart and Winston.

Lenneberg, E. 1964. Language disorders in childhood. Harvard Educ. Rev., 34:160-163, 173-175.

Levy, D. M. 1943. Maternal Overprotection. New York, Columbia University Press.

Lovaas, I. O., J. B. Berberich, B. F. Perloff, and B. Schaeffer. 1966. Acquisition of imitative speech in schizophrenic children. Science, 151:705-708.

Mahler, M. S. 1952. On Childhood Psychosis and Schizophrenia: Autistic and Symbiotic Infantile Psychoses. New York, International Universities Press.

McCarthy, D. 1954. Language disorders and parent-child relationships. J. Speech Hearing Dis., 19:514-523.

Miller, W. R. 1964. The acquisition of formal features of language. Amer. J. Orthopsychiat., 34:862-867.

Moncur, J. P. 1963. Parental domination in stuttering. J. Speech Hearing Dis., 28:155-165.

Mowrer, O. H. 1950. Learning Theory and Personality Dynamics. New York, Ronald Press.

——1958. Hearing and speaking: An analysis of language learning. J. Speech Hearing Dis., 23:143-151.

Myklebust, H. R. 1957. Babbling and echolalia in language theory. J. Speech Hearing Dis., 22:356-360.

Pronovost, W. 1961. The speech behavior and language comprehension of autistic children. J. Chronic Dis., 13:228-233.

——P. Wakstein, and J. Wakstein. 1966. A longitudinal study of the speech behavior and language comprehension of fourteen children diagnosed atypical or autistic. Except. Child., 33:19-26.

Rank, O. 1932. Art and Artist. New York, Knopf.

Redl, F., and D. Wineman. 1952. Controls from Within. New York, Free Press.

Reiser, D. E. 1963. Psychosis of infancy and early childhood, as manifested by children with atypical development. New Eng. J. Med., 269:790-798, 844-850.

Rimland, B. 1964. Infantile Autism. New York, Appleton-Century-Crofts.

Rose, J. A. 1943. Dynamics and treatment of speech disorders. Amer. J. Orthopsychiat., 13:284-289.

Rosen, J. N. 1953. Direct Analysis. New York, Grune & Stratton.

Ruesch, J. 1959. General theory of communication in psychiatry. In Arieti, S., ed., American Handbook of Psychiatry, Vol. 1, New York, Basic Books.

Ruttenberg, B. A., and E. G. Gordon. 1967. Evaluating the communication of the autistic child. J. Speech Hearing Dis., 32:314-324.

——M. L. Dratman, J. Fraknoi, and C. Wenar. 1966. An instrument for evaluating autistic children. J. Amer. Acad. Child Psychiat., 5:453-478.

Schell, R. E., J. Stark, and J. J. Giddan. 1967. Development of language behavior in an autistic child. J. Speech Hearing Dis., 32:51-64.

Shervanian, C. C. 1967. Speech, thought, and communication disorders in childhood psychoses: Theoretical implications. J. Speech Hearing Dis., 32:303-313.

Sommer, R., R. Dewar, and H. Osmond. 1960. Is there a schizophrenic language? Arch. Gen. Psychiat. (Chicago), 3:665-673.

Spiegel, R. 1959. Specific problems of communication in psychiatric conditions. *In* Arieti, S., ed., American Handbook of Psychiatry, Vol. 1. New York, Basic Books.

Sullivan, H. S. 1953. The Interpersonal Theory of Psychiatry. New York, W. W. Norton.

Szasz, T. 1960. The Myth of Mental Illness. Amer. Psychol., 15:113-118.

Szurek, S. A. 1956. Childhood schizophrenia: Psychotic episodes and psychotic mal-development. Amer. J. Orthopsychiat., 26:519-543.

Taffel, C. 1955. Anxiety and the conditioning of verbal behavior. J. Abnorm. Social Psychol., 51:496-501.

Ullman, L., and L. Krasner. 1965. Case Studies in Behavior Modification. New York, Holt, Rinehart and Winston.

Weiland, I. H., and D. R. Legg. 1964. Formal speech characteristics as a diagnostic aid in childhood psychosis. Amer. J. Orthopsychiat., 34:91-94.

Wolf, E. G., and B. A. Ruttenberg. 1967. Communication therapy for the autistic child. J. Speech Hearing Dis., 32:331-335.

Zimbardo, P. G., J. W. Barnard, and L. Berkowitz. 1963. The role of anxiety and defensiveness in children's verbal behaviors. J. Personality, 31:79-96.

—— G. F. Mahl, and J. W. Barnard. 1963. The measurement of speech disturbance in anxious children. J. Speech Hearing Dis., 28:362-370.

6: Language disabilities
of hearing-impaired children

Donald Moores

Of all the subareas of education perhaps none has generated more heat and less light than that of the hearing-impaired. Almost from the time of the establishment of the first school for the deaf in Paris more than 200 years ago, the field has been riven by debilitating controversies which have drained the energies of its most gifted educators, individuals who consequently have approached problems within the framework of overly simplistic either—or, black—white polarizations. It has been noted in a report entitled Education of the Deaf in the United States (1965) that in the opinion of many, for 100 years, emotion has been accepted as a substitute for research in education of the deaf. The incontrovertible evidence that children pour out of programs for the hearing-impaired in an endless stream unable to read at the fifth-grade level, unable to write a simple sentence, unable to speechread anything but the most common expressions, and unable to speak in a manner understandable to any but their immediate family stands as mute testimony to an inability, or unwillingness, to come to grips with the generic problem of children with severe auditory deficits—language.

Part of the frustration may be accounted for by the extremely difficult nature of the task. The ease with which a child acquires language varies inversely with the severity of his hearing loss. Not to hear the human voice is not to hear spoken language. While other children are able to utilize an intact auditory modality to build up automatic integrative mechanisms leading to early mastery of the sound, shape, and sense of their language, the severely hearing-impaired child is unique in that his language acquisition is heavily dependent on vision.

The child with normal hearing can be said to be linguistically proficient in every sense of the word. He has a knowledge of the basic rules of his language. He can produce a potentially infinite number of novel yet appropriate utterances. Because of his unconscious mastery over the grammatical structure of his language, he can combine and recombine its elements indefinitely. He can produce and understand utterances to which he has never been exposed. He then enters the formal educational situation with an

159

already fully developed instrument for learning—language and communication ability—an ability which he has acquired with no conscious effort on the part of his parents or himself.

A profoundly deaf 5-year-old, one with no functional response to speech, on the other hand, presents an entirely different picture. He cannot be expected to acquire language naturally. Without training he would lack linguistic competence completely; he might even be unaware that such things as words exist. For this child, language is not a facilitating device for the acquisition of knowledge. Rather it is an obstacle that stands between the child and learning, an obstacle that must be overcome slowly, painfully, and, usually, imperfectly. Input and output must be filtered through a distorted system and the child, although of potentially normal intelligence, finds his range of experience constrained by communication limitations. Much of the curriculum in a program for hearing-impaired children is designed to provide them, through formal instruction, a modicum of the linguistic proficiency which hearing children bring to the educational process. The process by which most deaf children presently learn a language is a necessarily different, more laborious, and conscious procedure. The norm of language acquisition varies both qualitatively and quantitatively from that of the hearing. The hearing child employs his early knowledge of the phonological structure of his language as a vehicle to choose from a wealth of language forms pervading much of his environment leading to unconscious mastery of morphology. The profoundly deaf child must for the most part bypass phonology in his quest for morphological competence. Language, such as it is perceived by the deaf child through primarily visual means, must be received through speech reading, informal or formal gestures, and/or graphemic presentation as well as through the auditory channel. Proficiency in speech reading (lipreading), the interpretation of words or meaning of a speaker by watching the movement of his lips, is really a form of closure by which an individual decodes a message based on fragmentary bits of information transmitted through a noisy distorted channel. It is dependent on past experience with the redundancies and predictability of language based on previous linguistic experience and, therefore, is of limited utility by itself in the development of grammatical proficiency.

There is little doubt, at least to the author, that all children have innate propensities toward the learning of language and that the child is an active agent in the learning process, not some passive organism to be shaped completely by contingencies of reinforcement. However, for people dealing with children with profound hearing losses, it is of little benefit to learn that the environment merely triggers the language acquisition process. Unfortunately, for these children the trigger has not yet been found.

DEFINITION OF TERMS

Hearing-Impaired

It should be emphasized that the term hearing-impaired is not limited to an individual with a profound hearing loss. It covers the entire range of hearing loss and encompasses not only the deaf child but also the one with a mild impairment who may have adequately developed morphologic-syntactic structures and whose only difficulty may lie in imperfect discrimination and production of a small number of phonemes. The number of children involved decreases from the mild to moderate to severe to profound levels.

Much of the confusion found among professionals dealing with children with hearing losses may be traced to an unfortunate inability to reach consensus on terminology. For some the term hearing-impaired occurs in free variation with hard-of-hearing. For others it also includes deaf children. In addition, one man's hard-of-hearing is another man's deaf.

In the final analysis, any definition must be a functional one and can be accepted only within broad limits. It is no more defensible to classify a child as deaf or hard-of-hearing solely on the basis of an audiogram than it is to judge a child trainable or educable mentally retarded purely on the basis of performance on a Stanford-Binet intelligence scale. Other factors such as age of onset of the hearing loss, configuration of the loss, age of instigation of training, age of fitting and appropriateness of fit of the hearing aid, and family climate all can be important considerations. As Hirsh (1963, p. 73) has stated: ". . . a child with a 90 decibel loss, high IQ, a history of amplified home training, and a good attitude toward the sounds, things and people around him is more likely to be our successful student than a child of lesser loss, like 70 decibel, with less favorable IQ, no home training, and an introverted aspect that may likely be related to his acoustic isolation."

Within this framework, terms such as limited hearing, acoustically handicapped, and hearing-impaired include both of the more frequently used terms, hard-of-hearing and deaf. The distinction is usually made between those for whom the auditory channel is affected but functional and those for whom the sense of hearing is nonfunctional. It has been suggested (Hirsh, 1963) that the deaf child is one who, without special training, is not aware of normal spoken conversation. The line between the deaf and hard-of-hearing for convenience sake is usually drawn around a 75-decibel loss. However no satisfactory definition, other than a behavioral one, has been developed. The difficulties lie, first, in trying to dichotomize levels of hearing loss when, in actuality, they exist on a continuum and, second, in attempting to generalize from an audiogram alone when so many other factors may also influence the behavior of an acoustically handicapped child. A misleading and inaccurate practice which has added to the confusion is the tendency to report an individual's loss on the basis of an *unaided* audiogram. This practice has been criticized (Pollock, 1964) on the grounds that substantial differences frequently exist between aided and unaided hearing. With proper early fitting and training many children can move across the invisible line from deaf to hard-of-hearing. There is an increasing movement toward early diagnosis of hearing loss and fitting of hearing-impaired children with aids for all ranges of impairment. In some preschool programs for the hearing-impaired today, for example, every child is equipped with an individual hearing aid. It is much more reasonable, then, to refer to an individual's hearing loss under his normal listening condition. For a majority of young hearing-impaired children the normal condition includes a hearing aid.

Severe Loss

In the United States approximately 50,000 children with severe hearing losses are receiving special educational services. The figure is consistent with estimates placing the incidence of deafness in the school-age population from between 7 per 10,000 to 10 per 10,000 (Carhart, 1969). The numbers are affected by cyclical epidemics such as the rubella epidemic which swept the United States from east to west from 1963 to 1965 and left in its wake twice the numbers of deaf children which would normally be expected for that period.

The characteristics of children served by classes for the severely impaired appear to be changing. In the past, large numbers of children were adventitiously deaf; one study of successful graduates of Gallaudet College, the world's only college for the deaf, reported that 64 percent of its sample became deaf after the age of 3 (Quigley et al., 1969). Vernon (1969) has reported on the effects of advances in medicine on the area of the hearing-impaired. Twenty years ago a typical hearing-impaired child with an etiology of cerebral-spinal meningitis would have lost his hearing around the age of 4 or later. For younger children the prognosis for successful recovery would have been greatly reduced. The additional sequelae for a child affected after the age of 4 usually would be minimal, perhaps involving no more than a somewhat affected sense of balance. He would also have some base of linguistic competency on which to build.

Given improved medical treatment, a typical hearing-impaired child with an etiology of meningitis in a program today would have lost his hearing preverbally, i.e., sometime before the age of 3. Older children, treated with antimicrobiotics, may reasonably be expected to recover with no lasting aftereffects. The younger child, who previously might have died, is the one now being saved and finds himself in a program for the hearing-impaired. The educational prognosis for this child, in contrast to the postverbal meningitic one, is quite limited because of his lack of a language base and because the sequelae for the preverbal child more frequently involve other severe handicaps in addition to hearing impairment. Vernon (1969) argues that growing numbers of children in programs for the hearing-impaired reflect etiological factors related to multiple handicapping conditions. Children with etiologies of maternal rubella and preverbal meningitis, for example, have tended to achieve academically at levels lower than other hearing-impaired children.

Hard-of-Hearing

Estimation of the number of school-age hard-of-hearing children in the United States, those children whose hearing is mildly or moderately affected, is almost impossible. No accurate data exist. In contrast to many Western European countries, there are very few programs specifically designed for the hard-of-hearing child. A conservative incidence estimate of 1 percent of the school-age population (Carhart, 1969) would place the number at approximately 500,000 children, of whom only a minority are receiving special attention. Research on this type of child and his special problems is almost nonexistent, and the research contained in this chapter has primarily been conducted with deaf children. It is quite possible that the increasing emphasis on individualization of instruction which is leading to expanding programs in learning disabilities, remedial reading, and speech pathology will unearth large numbers of children achieving far below their potential largely because of a moderate hearing loss.

STUDIES OF EXPRESSIVE LANGUAGE

Because of the difficulty inherent in comprehension of the speech of most severely hearing-impaired children, the majority of studies concerned with assessing their language proficiency have concentrated on written compositions in expressive language and on performance on standardized reading tests in the receptive sphere. Comparisons of the written language of the deaf and hearing suggest that the deaf are significantly inferior in all aspects of language development and facility, illustrating the importance of an intact auditory channel in language development and emphasizing the limitations imposed on output by inefficient input.

Heider and Heider (1940) compared the written language of children at three residential schools from 11 to 17 years of age to that of hearing students at two public schools from age 8 to 14. A traditional grammatical analysis of 1,118 compositions describing a short motion picture shown to the subjects indicated that the deaf children exhibited simple, rigid, and immature patterns of written behavior. The investigators stated that the differences between the deaf and hearing were of such a nature as to prevent their description in completely quantitative terms.

Walter (1955) studied the written sentence construction of 102 children from the ages of 6 years 0 months to 12 years 11 months at a school for the deaf in Australia and noted a lack of flexibility and an absence of sentence complexity. Walter (1959), in a later study of three Australian and four English schools for the deaf, analyzed written work of a total of 58 children from 9 years 11 months to 12 years 11 months. She noted similar patterns of language development and usage, although the level of sentence complexity and forms of sentence structure were somewhat more complex than in the original study.

Thompson (1936) analyzed 16,000 written compositions by 800 students attending 10 schools for the deaf in the United States and found an average of 104 mistakes per 1,000 words. Birch and Stuckless (1963), in an investigation of the written language of deaf children employing basically the same techniques, reported a total of 5,044 grammatical errors from a corpus of 50,050 words, or slightly more than 100 errors per 1,000 words, a result in close agreement with the findings of Thompson.

Myklebust (1964) adapted the classifications used by Thompson to develop a syntax score to measure written language based on categories including word order, additions, substitutions, omissions, punctuation, and carrier phrases. He compared deaf and hearing children from the ages of 7 to 17 and found significant differences at every level in favor of the hearing. He reported that the mean score of the 17-year-old deaf children tested, 86.2, approximated the score of 86.8 achieved by the average 7-year-old hearing child.

Myklebust noted that in the hearing children significant differences appeared between the 7- and 9-, and the 9- and 11-year age groups but not at the older age levels. From this he concluded that the structure of written language is rapidly developed based upon previously developed maturity in spoken language. It would be interesting to investigate whether the reported maturity of hearing children in written language syntax would be evident at an even younger age than 11 if errors of punctuation were not included in the syntax score.

Wells (1942), using written samples of deaf and hearing subjects and performance on a completion test, attempted to trace differences in growth of abstract language forms. He concluded that the deaf function in abstract language on a level similar to that of younger hearing children; they displayed comprehension equal to that of the hearing for concrete words but were retarded from 4 to 5 years in understanding abstract terms. Conjunctions and adverbs were commonly omitted, resulting in the type of expression observed in the verbal utterances of young children and characterized by Brown and Fraser (1964) as "telegraphic." It should be noted, however, that the telegraphic nature of the utterances of young hearing children differs from the writing of deaf children. Although in both cases messages are cut down and words omitted, the patterns of word combinations used and the types of omissions vary between the two groups.

Simmons (1959) used a type-token ratio (TTR) to determine the relative flexibility or rigidity of deaf and hearing subjects in word usage. Five written compositions and one spoken composition, elicited by picture sequences, of 54 students at the Central Institute for the Deaf and 112 hearing students attending public schools in the St. Louis area were studied. The type-token ratio, a measure of vocabulary diversity, is computed by dividing the number of different words (types) in a language sample by the total number of words (tokens). As a result of her analysis Simmons emphasized the redundancy found in the language of deaf children. Commenting on the rigidity and stereotypy of expression employed by the deaf as contrasted to the richness of the language of hearing children, she used the following example to illustrate how even relatively grammatically correct sentences are frequently stilted and repetitive (Simmons, 1959, p. 35).

> A girl threw a ball to a boy. The boy bat a ball. The boy bat the ball to the window and the window was broken. The mother heard the boy broke the window. The mother saw a broke the window. She went to see the ball game.

Simmons commented that deaf children would repeatedly refer to the child in a picture as a *boy*, where the hearing children would call him the *kid, boy, urchin, friend, young man, youngster, him, Tom*, and so forth. She also reported a lower TTR for Class II words due to a tendency for repetition of four verbs—*have, be, go*, and *feel*. A glance at the example presented above also illustrates the relatively low TTR found in the use of determiners. Although, like the deaf, hearing children frequently used *a, an*, and *the*, other definite articles such as *these, that*, and *those*, and possessives were also employed by the hearing.

Tervoort and Verbeck (1967) investigated the ingroup communication of students ranging from 7 to 17 over a 6-year period in four schools for the deaf: two in the United

States, one in Belgium, and one in the Netherlands. They filmed the conversations of students informally interacting in pairs and reported that among themselves the children conversed in a relaxed fluent manner, using their hands regularly sometimes with and sometimes without speech. Their communication with normally hearing individuals, on the other hand, frequently showed hesitance, awkwardness, and embarrassment. Tervoort attempted to study the relationship between what he perceived as two separate systems and concluded that the private, or esoteric, system is predominant for younger children and is the main reason for the stereotyped mistakes which characterize the children's attempts to use the language of the adult society, termed the exoteric system. The exoteric system influences the esoteric even at an early age to the extent that normal vocabulary and structure penetrate into private communication.

Tervoort reported a consistent growth in grammatically correct usage through the elementary years with continued improvement in the American students through adolescence in contrast to the students in the Benelux schools. American students showed the influence of the exoteric system by their more efficient use of word order, auxiliary verbs, conjunctions, and other function words, especially prepositions. Only 2 percent of the utterances of the American children consisted of imitative gesture sentences as compared to 10 percent of the European total.

At all ages the most common mode of expression was the use of signs, with fingerspelling increasing with age. Speech, when used, was most frequently combined with signs and spelling. At first the results seem contradictory. The subjects continue to use esoteric means (signs and spelling) but use them increasingly within the context of an exoteric grammatical (English or Dutch) structure. Tervoort resolves the paradox to his own satisfaction by treating speech and language as functionally separate. In support of his thesis he claimed the data showed no consistent relationships between speech and language; i.e., some children showed good articulation and poor grammatical skills and some had poor articulation but adequate grammatical abilities. All possible combinations existed.

Two explanations for the superiority of the American students in language, but not necessarily in speech, have been advanced. First is the suggestion that the influence of a structured approach to teaching language is evident in the sentences of the American students and appears to be more beneficial in terms of grammaticality than the "natural language" approach employed in the European schools. Another possible factor, which raises the question of the effect of manual communication on the development of speech and language skills, is the availability of an arbitrary system to the American students. Tervoort has presented his findings as a challenge to exclusively oral methods of instruction (Tervoort and Verbeck, 1967, p. 148):

> ... the sign language of the American adult deaf is a source from above, strongly influencing the interchange of the deaf teenager, on campus too, and on the contrary the fact that no such source from above is available for their mates across the ocean with whom they are matched. Once the esotericity of at least part of the subjects' private communication is established as a fact (whether this is a fact that should have been prevented, should be corrected,

or even denied, is not the issue here), it is evident that normal need for communication finds a better outlet in an adult arbitrary system, than in uncontrolled and half-grown symbolic behavior not fed from above. In educational terms: it seems clear that the choice has to be: either well controlled, monitored signing tending towards an adult level, semantically and syntactically, or no signing whatsoever; but no signing that is uncontrolled and left to find its own ways.

Johnson (1948) reported on the ability of 253 children in the Acoustic (hard-of-hearing), Oral, and Manual departments of the Illinois School for the Deaf to understand various methods of communication. All children were given tests of reading, speech-hearing ability, speechreading ability, hearing plus speechreading, fingerspelling only, and signs plus fingerspelling. The results suggested that the Acoustic group functioned most effectively. For the three groups as a whole only fingerspelling, with a mean score of 74 percent, and reading, with a mean of 72 percent, were reasonably successful. Johnson recommended that fingerspelling be added to the instructional method with the Oral group and that it be emphasized even more, in relation to signs, with the Manual group. Montgomery (1966) studied 59 prelingually deaf Scottish students and reported that a mere 7 percent could produce fairly fluent intelligible speech and 25 percent could follow a normal conversation reasonably well by speechreading. Even though officially no form of manual communication was allowed in the classroom, Montgomery found that 71 percent of the students could communicate fluently by means of the finger alphabet.

STUDIES OF RECEPTIVE LANGUAGE

Results of investigations on performance on standardized tests of reading achievement suggest that deaf children are also retarded in the ability to decode linguistic signs. Wrightstone et al. (1963) tested 5,307 deaf students in the United States and Canada between the ages of 10 years 6 months and 16 years 6 months on the Metropolitan Achievement Test, Elementary Level, in reading and found that less than 10 percent read on a fourth-grade level. They estimated that 54 percent of all eligible children with performance IQs of 75 or above were tested. In emphasizing the linguistic deficiencies of the deaf, Furth (1966) notes that in comparison with hearing norms, the data published by Wrightstone and co-workers indicated that the mean reading score of the deaf rose between the ages of 11 and 16 from a grade equivalent of 2.6 to 3.4, that is, less than 1 year of improvement in 5 years of schooling.

Myklebust (1964), using the Columbia Vocabulary Test as a measuring instrument, compared the reading vocabulary of deaf and hearing children at four age levels. The average score of 11.32 for the deaf students at age 15 was inferior not only to the score of his hearing contemporary, but also to the average score of 21.37 made by the 9-year-old hearing group. Another point of interest is the large increase in mean scores achieved by the hearing subjects at each successive age level. The improvement in the scores for the deaf, on the other hand, appears to taper off between the ages of 13 and 15, presenting a situation in which the hearing children are consistently consolidating and increasing their relative superiority in reading vocabulary.

Goetzinger and Rousey (1959), in a study of 101 students at a residential school for the deaf, concluded that deaf children of average mentality tend to plateau between the ages of 14 and 21 at grade 5 in vocabulary and paragraph meaning as measured by the Stanford Achievement Test. Magner (1964) reported that the 11 members of the graduating class of the Clarke School, a private residential school for the deaf, achieved reading scores at the sixth-grade level on the Stanford Achievement Test.

Pugh (1946) established reading norms for the deaf at different age levels on the Iowa Silent Reading Test on the basis of the performance of students at 54 day and residential schools for the deaf. In her standardization no group scored above a seventh-grade level on any of the subtests. Her finding that improvement in reading achievement scores was slight from the seventh to thirteenth year of schooling, and that during this period the gap between the hearing and deaf is widened, is in agreement with the previously mentioned studies of Goetzinger and Rousey, Myklebust, and Wrightstone et al.

An amount of justifiable criticism has been leveled at the use of reading achievement test scores as a measure of linguistic proficiency for deaf students. Cooper and Rosenstein (1966) have made the point that a person may be illiterate and unable to respond to the demands of a reading test, which measures skills commonly acquired in the educational process, and still possess a high degree of linguistic competence. This is usually the case with normally hearing children who typically enter school without the skills necessary for reading proficiency but who may be assumed to possess relatively sophisticated morphological and syntactical abilities.

The difficulty of interpreting a reading achievement score is compounded in the case of a deaf child. The tests have been standardized on hearing subjects and assume the presence of a base of linguistic competence. The normally hearing child already has at his disposal predictive integrations by which he is capable of handling automatically the structure of his language. Even by the age of 6 he has mastered the basic foundations of morphology. For him, performance on a standardized reading test is less an indication of linguistic proficiency, which has been established prior to the initiation of instruction in reading, than it is a measure of skills necessary for the reading process. The deaf child does not have a comparable linguistic competence built up as a function of the redundancy, frequency, and contiguity of auditory input variables. He has not internalized the structure of his language. Thus, given a relatively low score in reading achievement for a deaf child, it is difficult to ascertain the extent to which the basic weakness may be attributed to inadequate language facility or to poor development of skills basic to reading proficiency. With deaf subjects, mastery of the structure of language cannot be an assumed base.

Performance scores of deaf children on standardized tests of reading, despite their relative inferiority to scores for the hearing, may give a spuriously inflated estimate of the language capabilities of deaf subjects. Standardized reading tests require a multiple choice response; the student is instructed to select the most appropriate of four or five alternatives. The range of choices typically falls within one of the five general grammatical classes (i.e., nouns, verbs, adjectives, adverbs, or function words) and thus limits the selection procedure to a grammatically correct subset. Such a procedure, by failing to account for grammatical insufficiencies, might tend to artificially raise estimates of reading ability in many deaf children. In relation to this, Fusfeld (1955) found a discrepancy between apparent command of language as measured by the Stanford Achievement Test and written compositions of 18- and 19-year-old deaf students entering the Preparatory Class at Gallaudet College, reporting median achievement scores of grade 6 for vocabulary and grade 8 for paragraph meaning, both well above the levels reported in other studies. In spite of the relatively high reading achievement scores of this group, however, Fusfeld stated (1955, p. 70) that the written compositions submitted by the students represented a "tangled web type of expression in which words occur in profusion but do not align themselves in orderly array."

Moores (1970a) investigated the sensitivity of Cloze procedures in differentiating between deaf and hearing students matched on reading achievement scores. The experimental group consisted of 37 students with an average age of 16 years 9 months and mean grade reading achievement of 4.77 in the Metropolitan Achievement Test. They were matched with 37 fourth- and fifth-grade hearing students with an average age of 9 years 10 months and a mean grade reading achievement of 4.84. Three passages of 250 words were chosen from fourth-, sixth-, and eighth-grade textbooks and every fifth word deleted. Subjects were instructed to fill in the blanks with the most appropriate words. Responses were scored for each passage for (1) verbatim reproduction—replacing the exact word deleted from the text, (2) form-class reproduction—supplying a word of the same grammatical class as the original word; and (3) verbatim given form-class reproduction—the percentage of correct verbatim responses given correct form-class responses.

Results showed the hearing group to be superior on all measures. The inferiority of the deaf on verbatim scores supported the argument that standardized reading scores overestimate general language ability of the deaf. The form-class scores suggest that at least part of the inferiority may be explained by inadequately developed grammatical structures. By scoring subjects on the basis of verbatim given form-class scores, it was possible to compare the vocabulary level of the groups while holding grammatical proficiency constant. The lower performance of the deaf group on this measure indicated that, in addition to poorly developed grammatical skills, the deaf are further handicapped by redundant stereotyped modes of expression and limited vocabulary.

Schmitt (1969) used a transformational-generative model of language to explore the abilities of 8-, 11-, 14-, and 17-year-old deaf children to comprehend and produce sentences varying on the dimensions of transformations (kernel, negative, passive, passive-negative) and tense (past, present, progressive, future) and to contrast them with 8- and 11-year-old hearing students. Both groups of hearing children were superior to the deaf subjects at all ages. Qualitative analysis of the data led Schmitt to postulate that the deaf children were using incorrect underlying rules to process sentences and that three rules could account for most errors. He designated these: (1) the $NP_2 = NP_1$ rule, which permits reversal of noun phrase 1 and noun phrase 2 in transitive verb, reversible sentences; (2) the passive-active rule, which specifies the ignoring of passive transformation markers and permits the processing of passive sentences as actives; and (3) the no-negative rule, which specifies the ignoring of negative markers and permits the processing of negative sentences as positives.

METHODOLOGY

The Methods Controversy

The methods controversy, which has been raging for over 200 years, perhaps has accounted for more confusion than any other question concerned with the hearing-impaired. The issues have been distorted beyond recognition and it is not surprising that these are misunderstood by professionals on the periphery. It is inaccurate to speak of an oral-manual controversy, because no present-day educators of the hearing-impaired advocate a "pure" or "rigid" manual position. All educators of the hearing-impaired in the United States are oralists and all are concerned with developing the child's ability to speak and understand the spoken word to the highest degree possible. The difference is between oral-alone educators, who argue that all children must be educated by purely oral methods, and the oral-plus educators who argue that at least some children would progress more satisfactorily with simultaneous or combined oral-manual presentation. At present, although variations exist, four basic methods of instruction may be identified in the United States: the oral method, the auditory method, the Rochester method, and the simultaneous method.

1. *Oral method.* In this method, also called the oral-aural method, the child receives input through speechreading (lipreading) and amplification of sound and he expresses himself through speech. Gestures and signs are prohibited. In its purest form reading and writing are discouraged in the early years as a potential inhibitor to the development of oral skills.

2. *Auditory method.* This method, as opposed to the oral method, is basically unisensory. It concentrates on developing listening skills in the child who is expected to rely primarily on his hearing. Reading and writing are usually discouraged in the child, as is a dependence on speechreading. Although developed for children with moderate losses, some attempts have been made to use it with profoundly impaired children.

3. *Rochester method.* This is a combination of the oral method plus fingerspelling and is usually restricted to children with profound losses. The child receives information through speechreading, amplification, and fingerspelling, and he expresses himself through speech and fingerspelling. Reading and writing are usually given great emphasis. When practiced correctly, the teacher spells in the manual alphabet every letter of every word in coordination with speech. A proficient teacher can present at the rate of approximately 100 words per minute.

4. *Simultaneous method.* This is a combination of the oral method plus signs and fingerspelling. The child receives input through speechreading, amplification, signs, and fingerspelling. He expresses himself in speech, signs, and fingerspelling. Signs are differentiated from fingerspelling in that they represent complete words or ideas. A proficient teacher will sign in coordination with the spoken word, using spelling to illustrate elements of language for which no signs exist, e.g., some function words, such as *of* and *the* and indications of some verb tenses. This method is also limited to use with children with profound losses.

Recent Trends

Until quite recently, the oral method has been unquestionably predominant. Its ascendency may be traced as far back as the International Congress on Deafness in Milan in 1888, in which a resolution was passed stating the use of manual communication of any kind would restrict or prevent the growth of speech and language skills in deaf children.

Almost without exception programs for the deaf have followed a completely oral approach. This includes even the "manual" schools in which simultaneous methods of instruction typically have not been introduced into the classroom below the age of 12. In view of this, it might be argued that the history of failure of education of the deaf is a history of failure of the completely oral method, that it is more appropriate for children with moderate to severe losses than for those with severe to profound losses. A spate of articles (Karlin, 1969; Bruce, 1970; Miller, 1970) appearing in the Volta Review, a journal dedicated to the advancement of oral methods, has strongly reacted to such an interpretation.

Although one of the goals of education of the hearing-impaired is to produce children proficient in speech and speechreading, the possibility must be faced that rigid adherence to learning language by means of speech and speechreading, even with the best of auditory training, might be self-defeating for some children. A straight oral approach is committed to teaching language through speech and speechreading, although research indicates (Lowell, 1957-58; Lowell, 1959; Wright, 1917) that a primary requisite for speechreading is grammatical ability. Deaf people, after years of training in speechreading, cannot speechread as well as hard-of-hearing people (Costello, 1957), because they lack the ability to utilize context and anticipate, integrate, and interpret in consistent grammatical patterns those sounds, words, and phrases which are difficult to distinguish from the lips. Many distinct sounds either look like other sounds (e.g., [p], [b], [m]), or present very limited clues (e.g., [k], [g], [h]). The less residual hearing the individual possesses, the more difficult decoding becomes. The task of a speechreader, then, is a complex one: to understand utterances he must differentiate between sounds that look similar on the speaker's lips and at the same time perform closure, i.e., fill in on parts of the message which are not readily available to the eyes. A. G. Bell, a leading exponent for the development of oral skills in hearing-impaired children, was aware of these difficulties and was quoted (Deland, 1923) as stating:

> Spoken language I would have used by the pupil from the commencement of his education to the end of it; but spoken language I would not have as a means of communication with the pupil in the earliest stages of education, because it is not clear to the eye, and requires a knowledge of language to unravel the ambiguities. In that case, I would have the teacher use written language and I do not think that the manual language (fingerspelling) differs from written language except in this, that it is better and more expeditious.

The auditory method, in its unisensory form, may be traced to the success of people such as Wedenberg (1954) in Sweden and Whetnall and Fry (1964) in Great Britain with severely hard-of-hearing children. The auditory method in the United States and Canada has been used mostly with children of preschool ages (Stewart et al., 1964; Griffiths, 1967; Ling, 1964; McCroskey, 1968) and some attempts have been made to extend it to even the most severely hearing-impaired child (Stewart et al., 1964; Griffiths, 1967; McCroskey, 1968).

The work of Gaeth, who has been studying the effects of unimodal and bimodal sensory presentation since 1957, is of great relevance to consideration of the oral (bimodal) and auditory (unimodal) methods. The results of his investigations (1963, 1966) with deaf, hard-of-hearing, and normally hearing students suggest that bimodal presentation is never better than the better of two unimodal presentations and that in bimodal presentation attention is directed to the modality which is most meaningful. The results contradict the finding of Numbers and Hudgins (1948) that bimodal presentation (look and listen) was superior to visual (look) or auditory (listen) alone. It is possible that Numbers and Hudgins, in comparing groups, overlooked individual differences and interaction effects. Within any group of students with varying degrees of hearing impairment some may be oriented toward vision and some toward audition, a factor not readily apparent using group statistics.

Gaeth (1966) reported that hard-of-hearing subjects, defined as having a loss less than 60 decibels in the better ear, although somewhat inferior, functioned much as normal subjects in that they attended to the modality, either visual or auditory, which was most meaningful. There was some indication that the performance of the hard-of-hearing group in the bimodal situation was affected by a confusion as to which modality was more meaningful. Deaf students, defined as those with a loss greater than 60 decibels in the better ear, attended to the visual modality.

As opposed to possible interference between simultaneous bimodal presentation, Broadbent and Gregory (1961) and Gaeth (1966) report no inhibition in the use of two stimuli presented simultaneously to the same modality. If so, this could lend support to the simultaneous use of speech and fingerspelling, or speech signs, and fingerspelling for children with severe losses.

Whetnall and Fry were especially effective in promoting the educational separation of deaf and hard-of-hearing children and in providing services for more hard-of-hearing children within the regular public school situation in Great Britain. The benefits for the hard-of-hearing child were immediate. Separate treatment of the deaf child has served so far to point up the extent of his failure. In a survey of children born in 1947 who were in schools for the deaf in Great Britain in 1962-1963 they reported (1964) that only 11.6 percent of the students could carry on a reasonably clear conversation in speech and speechreading.

The question of methodology was deemed serious enough to appoint a committee to investigate the possible use of signs and fingerspelling in Great Britain. The result, commonly referred to as the Lewis Report (The Education of Deaf Children, 1968), concluded that more study was needed. An interesting sidelight to the Lewis Report was the enthusiastic reaction of educators sent to observe programs in the Soviet Union, which had rejected as unsatisfactory traditional oral methods in favor of neo-oralism, a combination of speech and fingerspelling similar to the Rochester method in the United States. The observers reported (1968, pp. 44-45):

The children of four, five, and six years old whom we saw in class certainly understood their teacher well, and mostly spoke freely and often with good voice, although they were regarded as being profoundly deaf and were unselected groups. We could not judge the intelligibility of the speech, but our interpreter (who had never previously seen a deaf child) said that she could understand some of them. The children were also very lively and spontaneous, and did not appear to be oppressed by the methods used, which might strike someone accustomed to English methods as unsuitable for young children.

It appeared to us, from what we were shown, that the Russians are more successful than we are in the development of language, vocabulary and speech in deaf children once they enter the educational system. This seemed to us a strong point in favor of their method (use of fingerspelling from the very start as an instrument for the development of language, communication and speech), the investigation of which was the main object of our visit.

Their enthusiasm matched that of Morkovin's (1960) observations after visiting the Soviet Union. The Russians claim that by starting fingerspelling in the home and nursery at age 2 the child is able to develop a vocabulary of several thousand words by 6 years of age. They also report that, rather than inhibiting oral development, the use of fingerspelling enhanced speech and speechreading skills. Although the claims have been received skeptically in the United States, they have created a renewed interest in the Rochester method and anecdotal substantiation is provided by the case of Howard Hofsteator (1959), a deaf individual whose parents provided him an early language environment through fingerspelling all conversations. They would read to him from books by placing their hands close to the printed page, spelling the stories, enabling him to read at a very early age. Several preschool programs using the Rochester method have recently been developed and their numbers appear to be increasing.

A reservation concerning the use of the method with young children should be noted. Possibly the presentation of connected English by means of rapidly changing hand configurations would place too great a burden on the perceptual and cognitive abilities of a child. His ability to form letters manually may also be limited. No such difficulty was encountered by Hofsteator but perhaps he was an exceptional case. It might be more beneficial to develop pivot-type grammars by means of selected signs, later placing an emphasis on spelling congruent with the introduction of the printed word after the age of 3.

The possible use of the simultaneous method with very young children is also gaining support throughout the country, support which may be traced to a number of factors. Among these are (1) the evidence that deaf children with deaf parents achieve more than those with hearing parents, (2) the growing tendency to accept the language of signs as a legitimate mode of communication, (3) dissatisfaction with results of traditional methods with the profoundly deaf, and (4) the increasing militancy of deaf adults who are only beginning to make an impact on the field, the majority of whom, despite their own rigid oral training, strongly support the use of the simultaneous method. *The Deaf American*, a journal produced by deaf professionals, has been particularly active on this question. It is interesting that the first public school program, in 1968, to use the simultaneous method with young deaf children, Santa Ana, California, was also the only program for the hearing-impaired in the United States at the time to be directed by a deaf person.

Research and Opinion on Methodology

In view of the frequent bitterness involved in the methods controversy, it is somewhat surprising to find that except for the citations previously made hard data is almost nonexistent. Most of the available literature consists of position papers in favor of one or another of the various methodologies. A situation worthy of note is the fact that while most educators of the hearing-impaired have preferred straight oral methods, many psychologists, psychiatrists, and "outside" educators who, for one reason or another, have become interested in the problems of limited hearing argue for some form of early manual communication (Moores, 1970b).

In a paper presented to the International Conference on Oral Education of the Deaf, Lenneberg (1967) stressed that the primary goal of education must be language, not its subsidiary skills. Lenneberg went on to criticize educators of the deaf for not distinguishing between speech and language. Stressing that the key is to get as many examples of English into the child as possible, he developed the argument that the establishment of language is not inseparably bound to phonics and, echoing Bell's earlier cited position (Deland, 1923), urged that graphics (reading and writing) be introduced in addition to oral methods at the earliest possible time. Lenneberg included fingerspelling and signs within his definition of graphics. Lenneberg's theoretical position is consistent with Tervoort's and Verbeck's (1967) finding that manual communication had no deleterious effects on speech. It should be emphasized that both Lenneberg and Tervoort recognized the primary importance of oral communication in our society. They advocate balanced, as opposed to rigid manual or rigid oral, communication. Their position, of course, is in direct opposition to the Congress of Milan.

In his study of the relationship of manual and oral skills, Montgomery (1966) came to the same conclusion based on the findings that (1) no negative correlations existed between any measures of oral skills and manual communication ratings, and (2) positive significant correlations were recorded between the manual communication rating and the Donaldson Lipreading Test. In his discussion, Montgomery stated (1966, p. 562): "There thus appears to be no statistical support for the currently popular opinion that manual communication is detrimental to or incompatible with the development of speech and lipreading."

Kohl (1967), more widely known for his work in education of the culturally disadvantaged, produced a highly controversial study on language and education of the deaf. Equating the position of the deaf to a large extent to that of the disadvantaged, Kohl noted that, although not one school officially taught sign language, it was the means of communication used by most deaf children with each other, no matter what the educational policies of the particular school. Kohl argued that teachers of the deaf should master sign language and utilize it in the schools, with oral language used as the child's second language occupying more of the curriculum as he grows older. Kohl's suggestions drew a storm of protest. It was dismissed by Quigley (1969, p. 18) as representative of " . . . support for the use of manual communication by individuals with only a superficial knowledge of the problems of education of deaf children, who apparently believe that the use of manual communication will correct most of the inadequacies of the educational system." According to a follow-up report on Kohl's study (Lederer, 1968), reaction was violent to an extreme. The editor of the Volta Review "attempted to discredit Kohl as patently unqualified to write or speak on the subject" (Lederer, 1968, p. 8) and was quoted by Lederer (1968, p. 9) as threatening that "another Kohl type report with federal funds might lead to an investigation by some powerful people who sit in committees." The superintendent of an exclusively oral school in New York was quoted (Lederer, 1968, p. 10) as dismissing Kohl's work as an "expanded master's thesis" and as agreeing only to answer specific questions put to him by a bona fide specialist on the deaf.

In a less emotional vein, Quigley (1969) attempted to assess the effects of the Rochester method (oral plus fingerspelling) on achievement and communication in two studies. The first involved a comparison over 5 years of three residential schools receiving instruction at the high school level in the Rochester method matched with three control schools in contiguous states. The experimental group was superior on fingerspelling and no differences were found in speechreading or speech intelligibility. The experimental group scored higher on all subtests of the Stanford Achievement test with an overall battery median of grade 5.88 compared to 5.04 for the contrast schools. In various analyses of written language, one statistically significant difference, grammatical correctness ratio, in favor of the experimental group, was found. Applications of Moores' (1967) Cloze procedures revealed the experimental groups to be superior in form class (grammatical functioning) with no differences in verbatim and verbatim given form class performance.

Quigley reported that in two of the three experimental schools studied, the Rochester method was not introduced until age 12. The school which used the method with children beginning at a younger age was the one which enjoyed the greatest advantage relative to its control (1969, p. 77). Quigley's second study involved a comparison of two preschool programs for the hearing-impaired, one using the Rochester method and one a traditional oral method. After 4 years of instruction, as shown in Table 1, Quigley reported that the students taught through the Rochester method were superior in fingerspelling, one of two measures of speechreading, in five of seven measures of reading, and in three of five measures of written language. The control group received superior scores on grammatical correctness ratio, which was attributed to a function of their limited language production (1969, p. 89). Quigley drew the following implications from the two studies:

1. The use of fingerspelling in combination with speech as practiced in the Rochester method can lead to improved achievement in deaf students particulary on those variables where meaningful language is involved.

2. When good oral techniques are used in conjunction with fingerspelling, there need be no detrimental effects on the acquisition of oral skills.

Table 1. Achievement of Hearing-Impaired Children Receiving Preschool Instruction in the Rochester and Oral Methods

	Students taught by Rochester method (N = 16)		Students taught by oral method (N = 16)			Level of significance
	Mean score	S. D.	Mean score	S. D.	t	
Age	7.81	0.40	7.85	0.68	0.34	—
Fingerspelling	33.71	21.60	2.34	3.74	8.32	0.001
Speechreading						
Craig Word	44.85	16.73	39.79	14.81	1.06	—
Craig Sentence	37.73	12.02	23.21	9.78	3.42	0.01
Reading						
SAT Paragraph	2.28	0.53	2.10	0.68	1.49	—
SAT Word Meaning	2.31	0.50	2.02	0.61	2.81	0.01
SAT Combined Reading	2.27	0.49	2.04	0.57	2.19	0.05
Metro. Word Knowledge	2.09	0.59	1.83	0.57	2.69	0.02
Metro. Reading	1.96	0.54	1.70	0.62	3.35	0.05
Gates Vocabulary	2.21	0.81	1.68	0.64	2.55	0.02
Gates Comprehension	2.00	0.61	1.74	0.59	1.57	—
Written language						
Total Words Written	61.53	29.24	37.47	18.54	2.46	0.02
Sentence Length	5.79	1.60	4.49	1.44	3.45	0.01
Strings Analysis	3.59	1.16	4.07	1.36	1.52	—
Subordination Ratio	3.23	6.41	2.22	7.61	2.94	0.01
Grammatical Correctness Ratio	79.53	19.70	89.33	21.82	2.42	0.05

3. Fingerspelling is likely to produce greater benefits when used with younger rather than older children. It was used successfully in the experimental study with children as young as 3½ years of age.

4. Fingerspelling is a useful tool for instructing deaf children, but it is not a panacea.

Deaf Children with Deaf Parents

The influence of the work of people such as Tervoort, Lenneberg, Montgomery, and Kohl in recent years has resulted in a renewed interest in the use of combined methods in the education of at least some hearing-impaired children. Because of the relatively small number of programs using any form of manual communication with young children, some investigators have turned to the study of deaf children who have received manual communication in the home, those with deaf parents.

Stevenson (1964) examined the protocols of all 134 children of deaf parents enrolled at the California School for the Deaf at Berkeley between 1914 and 1961 and matched them to deaf children of hearing parents. He reported that 38 percent of those with deaf parents went to college compared to 9 percent of those with hearing parents and that of the 134 paired comparisons those students with deaf parents were better students and had attained a higher educational level in 90 percent of the cases.

Stuckless and Birch (1966), in a matched pair design, compared 38 deaf students of deaf parents to 38 deaf students of hearing parents from five residential schools for the deaf. The deaf parents had used the language of signs with their children as babies. Pairs were matched on age, sex, age of entrance to school, extent of hearing impairment, and intelligence test scores. No differences between the groups were found on speech intelligibility or teachers' ratings of psychosocial adjustment. Children with deaf parents were superior on measures of speechreading, reading, and written language.

In an unplanned ramification of a study of the effects of institutionalization, Quigley and Frisina (1961) studied 16 deaf students of deaf parents from a population of 120 deaf day students. They reported that the group with deaf parents were higher in fingerspelling and vocabulary with no differences in educational achievement and speechreading. The group with hearing parents had better speech.

Meadow (1967) compared 59 children of deaf parents to a carefully matched paired group of children with hearing parents. She reported that children with deaf parents ranked higher in self-image tests and in academic achievement showed an average superiority to their matched pairs of 1.25 years in arithmetic, 2.1 years in reading, and 1.28 years in overall achievement. The gap in overall achievement increased with age, reaching 2.2 years in senior high school. Ratings by teachers and counselors favored children with deaf parents on (1) maturity, responsibility, independence; (2) sociability and popularity; (3) appropriate sex-role behavior; and (4) appropriate response to situations. In communicative functioning the group with deaf parents was rated superior in written language, use of fingerspelling, use of signs, absence of communicative frustration, and willingness to communicate with strangers. No differences were reported for speech or lipreading ability.

In a commentary on the child's reaction to deafness, Meadow (1967, p. 306) claimed that children with hearing parents viewed their deprivation in terms of an inability to *speak* rather than an inability to *hear*. Children of hearing parents tend to ask questions regarding their deafness at a later age than children of deaf parents.

The results reported by Stevenson, Quigley and Frisina, Stuckless and Birch, and Meadow, interesting in themselves, should be evaluated in relation to the richer environment to which children of hearing parents theoretically should be exposed. The socioeconomic status of children with hearing parents is superior; e.g., Meadow had to equate deaf fathers who were skilled craftsmen with professional, managerial, clerical, and sales workers among the hearing fathers. The language and speech limitations of deaf adults have been documented extensively. In addition, deaf children of hearing parents are far more likely to receive preschool training and individual tutoring. Meadow reported that 60 percent of the children with deaf parents received no preschool training as compared with only 18 percent of those with hearing parents. Half of the group with hearing parents not only attended preschool but had additional experience either at home or at a speech clinic. Almost 90 percent of the hearing families interviewed in the study had had some involvement with the Tracy Correspondence Course, but none of the deaf families had sent for it. Given the higher socioeconomic levels, more adequate linguistic and speech skills, and higher academic attainments to be found in the hearing families in addition to preschool educational and speech training for children with hearing parents, the educational, social, and communicative superiority of those with deaf parents takes on added significance. One can only speculate on the attainments of deaf children with hearing parents if, in addition to other advantages, they had benefited by early systematic communication with their parents.

PRESCHOOL PROGRAMS

Consistent with developments in other areas, educators of the hearing-impaired have been turning with more and more emphasis to the development of programs for children below the age of 5. The main reasons for such a movement may be traced to the increased awareness of the importance of the first 5 years of life, to dissatisfaction with results obtained with older children, and to growing awareness and appreciation of the tremendous potential of very young children which has been documented by modern research in psycholinguistics, perception, and cognition. Of perhaps more importance than purely methodological considerations which have already been discussed extensively are what might be referred to as the two different philosophies of education which are developing in preschool programs for the hearing-impaired.

The first philosophy has its roots in the pioneering work of educators of the hearing-impaired in Western Europe, with much of the leadership coming from Great Britain. This may be labeled the home-centered socialization philosophy. Attention is focused on activities around the home and "natural-language" environment is emphasized. Parent guidance is a major aspect of such a program and physical placement contiguous to hearing peers is usually an essential component. Stress is placed on the spontaneous development of language skills and of speech skills. Descriptions of such programs may be found in the writings of Pollock (1964), Reed (1963), Griffiths (1967), and Knox and McConnell (1968).

The second major philosophical approach, which may be labeled child-centered cognitive-academic, is exerting influence on many new programs. The impetus has grown out of the failure of traditional socially oriented preschool and nursery programs to serve disadvantaged children in the United States and, to a lesser extent, Israel. Beginning in 1966, a number of research investigations have suggested that the only successful programs for the disadvantaged have been those which contain a highly structured component with specific academic-cognitive training. The work of investigators such as Bereiter and Engelmann (1966), Di Lorenzo (1969), and Karnes and co-authors (1968) has had the greatest impact.

As the work of these researchers has become more widely known among educators of the hearing-impaired, a change in the orientation of many systems toward increased attention to the development of cognitive-academic skills has been witnessed. Generalizing from the few programs of such a type presently in existence, the focus may be expected to shift from the parent to the child and skills such as reading readiness and number concepts would be begun as early as 2 years of age. Moores (1970c) has described a public school program for the hearing-impaired developed on these principles.

Related Research

The paucity of educational research with the hearing-impaired is especially marked in regard to the effectiveness of various intervention programs for the very young hearing-impaired child. Most of the literature cited as research or "proof" for the benefits of one approach or another may more properly be classified as program description. The typical article or paper involves a program being described, defended, and praised by a person who has developed it or who in some way is closely related to it. With the exception of an occasional tape or audiogram, no data are presented. Position papers and descriptive works can serve an important function, but too often they have been treated as evidence.

In the few attempts at assessment, measured benefits have been negligible. Comparisons of children receiving traditional preschool training with children having no preschool training suggest a wash-out effect (Phillips, 1963; Craig, 1964). By 9 years of age there appear to be no differences between experimental and control groups. The results are consistent with those reported for traditionally based preschool programs for the disadvantaged. One of two conclusions may be reached. The first is that such a preschool experience is of no benefit to the children. The second holds that it was effective but the benefits were dissipated by the failure of the schools to take advantage of them in the primary-grade years.

McCroskey (1968) compared children who participated in a home-centered program with auditory emphasis to children who received no training and found few differences between the groups. What differences existed tended to favor the control group, those with no previous training. The investigator postulated that the experimental group consisted of a "basically inferior product" which had been brought to a position of quality with the control group. However this must remain conjecture.

The only study which directly compared preschool hearing-impaired children receiving instruction under two different methodologies has been discussed. Quigley 1969) reported that children being taught by the Rochester method (oral plus ingerspelling) were superior to those taught by the oral-only method.

The lack of research studies is not surprising considering that the difficulties of valuation of any type of educational intervention are multiplied when dealing with the preschool hearing-impaired. Underlying the hostility and suspicion endemic to the field is he tremendous complexity of the task only hinted at by some of the following questions. How does one measure the speech, language, and communication ability of 3-, 4-, and 5-year-old children with severe hearing impairments? Are there any valid measures of parent attitude? Are differential program effects transitory? Do or can children in one program who are behind at age 4 in one area close the gap by age 8? Is it possible to develop measurement techniques which will be fair to children in programs which have different goals and therefore different concepts of success?

The University of Minnesota Research and Development Center has attempted to meet the problem (Moores, 1970d) by adapting Cronbach's (1957) Characteristics by Treatment Interaction Model to an assessment of 12 programs for the hearing-impaired in he United States. Cronbach has argued that group comparisons are of limited value because they frequently hide individual effects and because they are geared toward finding the one "best" approach for a particular educational problem such as "basal" vs. "linguistic" instruction, oral-aural vs. aural-only instruction of the hearing-impaired, segregated vs. integrated classes for the retarded, and so on. Looking only for group differences obscures the fact that one treatment may be preferable for some children and another treatment for other children.

Such a situation apparently does exist in the field of reading. Comparisons of linguistic and basal approaches suggest there is no one best method. In a cooperative study involving 27 individual projects, Bond and Dykstra (1967) reported no consistent differences between groups. No one approach was successful for all children. Within each treatment some children failed to read, but the characteristics of the failures varied as a function of treatment. The finding is supported by Hurley's (1968) report that learning disabilities or reading failures in Champaign, Illinois, and its sister city, Urbana, had different characteristics, presumably because the two school systems had different approaches to the teaching of reading. Theoretically, then, judicious matching of treatment to subject would reduce the number of failures produced by imposition of one method of instruction on all students regardless of individual differences.

The longitudinal study being conducted by the University of Minnesota, then, is not designed to unearth the "best method or philosophy per se." It is primarily concerned with individual differences and only secondarily with group effects. It is possible that one approach and one method will prove beneficial to all children but the investigation is predicated on Gallagher's (1967) "unthinkable thought" that all methods of teaching the hearing-impaired, when applied to all children, are to some extent failures. Hopefully the most fruitful part of the search will unearth indicators of the best method for a particular child at a particular stage of development.

CONCLUSIONS

On balance, the author, whose world view generally leads him to equate the past with failure, the present with change, and the future with success, looks to the future of education of the hearing-impaired with cautious optimism. The advances of recent years in the field have come in medicine, primarily in the near elimination of postlingual hearing loss in children, and in technology in the form of improved hearing aids and sophisticated audio-visual hardware. Education, the final component of the triad, alone has failed to make any substantial new contribution in the ongoing struggle against severe hearing impairment. Educators of the hearing-impaired, long given to inbreeding traditionally have been isolated from the main body of education and therefore have not benefited adequately from improvements in general education.

It is to be expected that advances in medicine and technology will continue However, there is little reason to believe that elimination of severe hearing losses, in the form of complete breakthroughs in medicine, or the development of hearing aids capable of presenting normal, undistorted speech to even the profoundly deaf child will precede man's colonization of Mars. The burden is now on educators to begin to contribute their share. In this context the signs are encouraging. The growing research by scientists on the effects of severe hearing loss on cognitive, linguistic, perceptual, and social functioning has surfaced many of the problems attending education of hearing-impaired children Educators of the hearing-impaired are now branching out into "pure" disciplines, such as psycholinguistics and cognition, and "applied" disciplines, such as reading and special learning disabilities.

Although the tiresome oral-manual controversy has taken on different dimensions other issues exist which could create new lines of division. Educators will have to exercise great care before solidifying positions on questions such as unimodal vs. bimodal presentation and social vs. cognitive preschool programs. However, for years lip service has been paid to the concept of individual needs and individualization of instruction. If the ideal or the pursuit of the ideal becomes a reality in the near future, such either-or dichotomies will become meaningless and we will actually fit the method to the child rather than vice versa.

REFERENCES

Bereiter, C., and S. Engelmann. 1966. Teaching Disadvantaged Children in the Preschool Englewood Cliffs, N. J., Prentice-Hall.

Birch, J., and E. Stuckless. 1963. Programmed Instruction as a Device for the Correction of Written Language in Deaf Adolescents. Washington, D. C., U. S. Office of Education Project Report 1769.

Bond, G., and R. Dykstra. 1967. The cooperative research program in first grade reading instruction. Reading Res. Quart., 2:180-209.

Broadbent, D., and M. Gregory. 1961. On the recall of stimuli presented alternately to two sense organs. J. Exp. Psychol., 13:103-109.

Brown, R., and C. Fraser. 1964. The acquisition of syntax. *In* Bellugi, U., and R. Brown, eds., The Acquisition of Language. Monogr. Soc. Res. Child Develop., 29(1):43-79.

Bruce, W. 1970. Assignment of the seventies. Volta Rev., 72:78-80.

Carhart, R. 1969. Human Communication and Its Disorders. Bethesda, Md., National Institutes of Health.

Cooper, R., and J. Rosenstein. 1966. Language acquisition of deaf children. Volta Rev., 68:58-67.

Costello, M. 1957. A study of speech reading as a developing language process in deaf and in hard of hearing children. Doctoral dissertation, Evanston, Ill., Northwestern University.

Craig, W. 1964. Effects of preschool training on the development of reading and lipreading skills of deaf children. Amer. Ann. Deaf, 109:280-296.

Cronbach, L. 1957. The two disciplines of scientific psychology. Amer. Psychol., 12:671-684.

Deland, F. 1923. An ever-continuing memorial. Volta Rev., 25:34-39.

Di Lorenzo, L. 1969. Prekindergarten Programs for the Disadvantaged. Albany, New York State Office of Research and Evaluation, December 1969.

Education of the Deaf in the United States. 1965. The Report of the Advisory Committee on Education of the Deaf. Washington, D. C., United States Government Printing Office.

Furth, H. 1966. Research with the deaf: Implications for language and cognition. Volta Rev., 68:34-56.

Fusfeld, I. 1955. The academic program of schools for the deaf. Volta Rev., 57:63-70.

Gaeth, J. 1963. Verbal and Nonverbal Learning in Children Including Those with Hearing Losses. Washington, D. C., United States Office of Education Project 1001.

————1966. Verbal and Nonverbal Learning in Children Including Those with Hearing Losses: Part II. Washington, D. C., United States Office of Education Project 2207.

Gallagher, J. 1967. New directions in special education. Except. Child., 33:441-447.

Goetzinger, C., and E. Rousey. 1959. Educational achievement of deaf children. Amer. Ann. Deaf, 104:221-224.

Griffiths, C. 1967. Conquering Childhood Deafness. New York, Exposition Press.

Heider, F., and G. Heider. 1940. A comparison of sentence structure of deaf and hearing children. Psychol. Monogr., 52(1):52-103.

Hirsh, I. 1963. Communication for the deaf. Proc. 41st Convention of American Instructors of the Deaf, pp. 164-183. Washington, D. C.

Hofsteator, H. 1959. An Experiment in Preschool Education: An Autobiographical Case Study. Washington, D. C., Gallaudet College.

Hurley, O. 1968. Perceptual integration and reading problems. Except. Child., 35:207-215.

Johnson, E. 1948. The ability of pupils in a school for the deaf to understand various methods of communication. Amer. Ann. Deaf, 98:194-213.

Karlin, S. 1969. Et tu oralist? Volta Rev., 71:478e-478g.

Karnes, M., A. Hogens, and J. Teska. 1968. An evaluation of two preschool programs for disadvantaged children: A traditional and a highly structured experimental preschool. Except. Child., 34:667-676.

Knox, L., and F. McConnell. 1968. Helping parents to help deaf infants. Children, 15:183-187.

Kohl, H. 1967. Language and Education of the Deaf. New York, Center for Urban Education.

Lederer, J. 1968. A Follow-up Report on: Language and Education of the Deaf. New York, Center for Urban Education.

Lenneberg, E. 1967. Prerequisites for language acquisition. Proc. Int. Conf. on Oral Education of the Deaf, New York, 1967, pp. 1302-1362.

Ling, D. 1964. An auditory approach to the education of deaf children. Audecibel 4:96-101.

Lowell, E. 1957-1958. John Tracy Clinic Research Papers III, V, VI, and VII. Los Angeles, John Tracy Clinic.

————1959. Research in speech readings: Some relationships to language development and implications for the classroom teacher. Proc., 34th Convention of American Instructors of the Deaf, 1959, pp. 68-73.

Magner, M. 1964. Reading: Goals and achievement at Clarke School for the Deaf. Volta Rev., 66:464-468.

McCroskey, R. 1968. Final progress report of four-year home training program. Paper read at A. G. Bell National Convention, San Francisco, July 1968.

Meadow, K. 1967. The effect of early manual communication and family climate on the deaf child's development. Doctoral Dissertation, Berkeley, University of California.

Miller, J. 1970, Oralism. Volta Rev., 72:211-217.

Montgomery, G. 1966. The relationship of oral skills to manual communication in profoundly deaf adolescents. Amer. Ann. Deaf, 111:557-565.

Moores, D. 1967. Applications of "Cloze" procedures to the assessment of psycholinguistic abilities of the deaf. Doctoral Dissertation, Urbana, University of Illinois.

————1969. Communication, psycholinguistics and deafness. Proc. Mid-Atlantic Institute on Deafness. Frederick, Md. Council of Organizations Serving the Deaf, October 1969, pp. 4-15.

————1970a. An investigation of the psycholinguistic functioning of deaf adolescents. Except. Child., 36:645-652.

————1970b. Psycholinguistics and deafness. Amer. Ann. Deaf, 115:37-48.

————1970c. The St. Paul, Minnesota Model Preschool Program for the Hearing Impaired. Paper read at Minnesota Speech and Hearing Association Annual Meeting, St. Paul, April 1970.

————1970d. Evaluation of preschool programs. An interaction analysis model. Proc. Conference of Executives of American Instructors of the Deaf Annual Convention. St. Augustine, Fl., April 1970.

Morkovin, B. 1960. Experiment in teaching deaf preschool children in the Soviet Union. Volta Rev., 62:260-268.

Myklebust, H. 1964. The Psychology of Deafness. New York, Grune & Stratton.

Numbers, M., and C. Hudgins. 1948. Speech perception in present day education for deaf children. Volta Rev., 50:449-456.

Phillips, W. 1963. Influence of preschool training on achievement in language arts, arithmetic concepts, and socialization of young deaf children. Doctoral dissertation, New York, Teachers College, Columbia University.

Pollock, D. 1964. Acoupedics: A uni-sensory approach to auditory training. Volta Rev., 66:400-409.

Pugh, G. 1946. Summaries from the appraisal of the silent reading abilities of acoustically handicapped children. Amer. Ann. Deaf, 91:331-349.

Quigley, S. 1969. The Influence of Fingerspelling on the Development of Language, Communication, and Educational Achievement in Deaf Children. Urbana, Ill., University of Illinois.

——— and R. Frisina. 1961. Institutionalization and Psycho-Educational Development in Deaf Children. Washington, D. C., Council for Exceptional Children.

——— W. Jenne, and S. Phillips. 1969. Deaf Students in Colleges and Universities. Washington, D. C., Alexander Graham Bell Association.

Reed, M. Preprimary education. 1963. Proc. 41st Convention of American Instructors of the Deaf. Washington, D. C., June 1963, pp. 543-550.

Schmitt, P. 1969. Deaf children's comprehension and production of sentence transformations and verb tenses. Doctoral dissertation, Urbana, University of Illinois.

Simmons, A. 1959. A comparison of the written and spoken language from deaf and hearing children at five age levels. Doctoral dissertation, Washington University of St. Louis.

Stevenson, E. 1964. A study of the educational achievement of deaf children of deaf parents. Calif. News, 80:143.

Stewart, J., D. Pollock, and M. Downs. 1964. A unisensory approach for the limited hearing child. ASHA, 6:151-154.

Stuckless, E., and J. Birch. 1966. The influence of early manual communication on the linguistic development of deaf children. Amer. Ann. Deaf, 111:452-460, 499-504.

Survey of children born in 1947 who were in schools for the deaf in 1962-63. 1964. The health of the school child, 1962-63. Report of the Chief Medical Office of the Department of Education and Sciences. London, Her Majesty's Stationery Office.

Tervoort, B., and A. Verbeck. 1967. Analysis of communicative structure patterns in deaf children. Groningen, The Netherlands: V. R. A. Project RD-467-64-45 (Z. W. O. Onderzoek, N. R.: 583-15).

The education of deaf children: The possible place of fingerspelling and signing. 1968. London, Department of Education and Science, Her Majesty's Stationery Office.

Thompson, W. 1936. An analysis of errors in written composition by deaf children. Amer. Ann. Deaf, 81:95-99.

Vernon, M. 1969. Multiple handicapped deaf children: Medical, educational and psychological considerations. Washington, D. C., Council for Exceptional Children Research Monograph.

Walter, J. 1955. A study of the written sentence construction of profoundly deaf children. Amer. Ann. Deaf, 100:235-252.

———1959. Some further observations on the written sentence construction of profoundly deaf children. Amer. Ann. Deaf, 104:282-285.

Wedenberg, E. 1954. Auditory training for severely hard of hearing preschool children. Acta Otolaryng. (Stockholm), Suppl. 110.

Wells, C. 1942. The Development of Abstract Language Concepts in Normal and in Deaf Children. Chicago, University of Chicago Libraries.

Whetnall, E., and D. Fry. 1964. The Deaf Child. Springfield, Ill., Charles C Thomas.

Wright, J. 1917. Familiarity with language the prime factor. Volta Rev., 19:222-223.

Wrightstone, J., M. Aronow, and S. Moskowitz. 1963. Developing reading test norms for deaf children. Amer. Ann. Deaf, 108:311-316.

7: Language problems of disadvantaged children

Roger W. Shuy

THE EMERGING CONCERN FOR LANGUAGE PROBLEMS OF THE DISADVANTAGED

During the decade of the 1960s American linguistic scholarship witnessed an important rebirth of interest in the systematic study of language as a social phenomenon. The importance of language in social interaction had been noted earlier by social psychologists such as George Herbert Mead, by sociologists such as C. Wright Mills and Joyce Hertzler, and by many antropological linguists and dialectologists. It was not until the 1960s, perhaps because of a national awakening to the problems of the poor, the minorities, and the uneducated, that the impact of this earlier work began to take hold. This now obvious and necessary interaction between language and society was also deterred by the natural desire for autonomy which emerging disciplines seem to demand. It was important, in the early days especially, for linguists to clearly separate that which was their territory from that which belonged to other fields. But now that linguistics has devoted most of its energies to linguistic theory for a decade or so, the cycle is once again beginning to move toward relational matters.

The growing interest in language problems of disadvantaged[1] children owes its origins to a number of factors. Educators and psychologists were attracted to the language

[1] The terms "disadvantaged," "lower class," and "working class" are used frequently in this paper. With reference to these terms it should be made clear that only a small subset of the total possible language difference observed between groups places speakers at an educational disadvantage. In addition, any group designations such as the above should be regarded as only gross approximations of classifications that are useful in research on language and society at this time. As this chapter points out, the study of this area is changing and developing rapidly and its current classification must be taken as preliminary and by no means does every individual who falls within such designations maintain all or any of the generalized group characteristics. By "disadvantaged" in this chapter I refer to those of monolingual experience as distinguished from native speakers of Spanish, French, or other languages.

185

problems of disadvantaged children earlier than linguists, social scientists, or speech specialists. The early work of psychologists in this area quite naturally followed the framework of experimental psychology, including pre- and post-testing, experimental and control groups, and other research techniques which are perfectly appropriate when the experimental variables are pure. In the case of the language of disadvantaged children however, the variables had not yet been isolated and most of the early work of the 1960 treated the speech of disadvantaged children as a deviation from a nondisadvantaged norm rather than as a culturally patterned difference. One surely cannot blame psychologists for approaching the language problems of disadvantaged children from the research assumptions with which they were most familiar, but it has become increasingly clear that the psychologists' preference for comparative and correlational research methodologies tends to overlook the need for a preceding ethnological and linguistic description.

Educators, as might be expected, were also early to assess the importance of a child's language. It is only natural that problems would be noticed first in the frustrations of teaching. As is often the case when there is a sudden national awakening to a social or pedagogical problem, the development of theory, materials, and the training of personnel relating to the general area of social dialects was dictated by expediency more than by any careful, well-developed plan. As absurd as it may seem to produce classroom materials before establishing a theoretical base for their development, that is exactly what happened in this field. To complicate matters even more, sensitive teachers, realizing that their training had not been adequate for their needs, began asking for that training, preferably in condensed and intensive packages. And healthy as this situation appeared to be, it only triggered still another problem—that of finding adequately prepared professionals to provide this training.

In all fairness to both psychologists and educators, however, it must be admitted that researchers in these fields were among the first to tackle the problems which had been almost completely ignored by linguists and social scientists. To be sure, they charged into areas without adequate interdisciplinary breadth and descriptive depth, but this does not diminish the fact that they noted the problems and put forth solutions while other fields were still tending to internal matters.

The field of speech, like psychology and education, has held to the assumption that the normal or the correct are definable primarily in light of Standard English language production. The common measures of speech behavior in this field, the Goldman-Fristoe Articulation Test, the Peabody Picture Vocabulary Test, and the Illinois Test of Psycholinguistic Ability, are all based on Standard English. Although speech clinicians are continuously engaged in descriptive research in a diagnostic mode, little or no significant research on the form and function of various social dialects is being undertaken by speech specialists. There is a growing awareness, however, that extant training programs for speech clinicians do not prepare these specialists adequately in the differences between socially induced language variation and actual pathologies. The literature now abounds with horror stories of black children who were given speech therapy when their speech was quite acceptable in the black community.

Social scientists have only scarcely begun to realize the potential usefulness of language data to their fields. American sociology, like American linguistics, has been so busy formalizing its field (with considerable justification) that it has tended to move away from its earlier focus on the ethnology of social problems toward sophisticated techniques of quantitiative analysis and large-scale social structure. Of this tendency of sociologists to overlook language as a resource, Fishman (1968, p. 8) observes:

> A concern with language has been contraindicated on yet another score; namely, language is often considered to be omnipresent and therefore of no significance in differentiating social behavior. The latter view is undoubtedly related to the monoglot and urbanized nature of the societies best known to the founding fathers of American and European sociology. In addition, American sociology has long been primarily non-comparative and American sociologists themselves, overwhelmingly monolingual.

It was only recently that sociologists have become at all interested in this area, largely as a result of their increased interest in small group dynamics, social change in the community, communications networks, and the problems of developing nations. At this time, however, very few sociologists are making contributions to this area.

Linguists, as has been mentioned already, have turned the major share of their recent attention to concerns other than problems involving language and society.

Anthropologists and linguists share many of the same research assumptions and the history of these fields in relationship to the language problems of the disadvantaged are so intertwined that it is more profitable to view them together. American anthropologists such as Boas, Kroeber, and Herskovitz viewed cultures descriptively rather than against some norm from which deviation takes place. Concepts such as "primitive language," "underdeveloped speech," or "substandard grammar" were denounced, in the anthropological tradition, as pure ethnocentrism. Linguists adopted this tradition, rejecting the language norms of a familiar society as measures of those of an unfamiliar one. Thus, when linguists examine the speech of disadvantaged children they tend not to view it as deviant but simply as different. Likewise, anthropologists and linguists assume that different surface forms of behavior do not interfere with the development of conceptualization.[2] Consequently, when nonlinguists such as Carl Bereiter and Sigfried Engelmann (1966) observe that certain black children suffer cognitive deficits because of their inability to produce Standard English, linguists are quick to be suspicious of these claims.

Anthropologists and linguists also assume the adequacy of all behavior and language systems as communication systems for members of the social groups which use them.

---

[2] Walt Wolfram observes that one should be careful to distinguish between "interference in conceptual development" and the Whorfian hypothesis. The latter maintains that language categories predetermine conceptualizations of the external world, although no value judgment is to be made concerning them. In contrast, by "interference in conceptual development" is meant that a value judgment is placed on the adequacy of conceptualization. See Wolfram, 1971.

Thus, when nonlinguists label disadvantaged children as verbally destitute or linguistically deficient, linguists seriously question their labels. Linguists tend to account for the same child-language behavior as a sign of the child's unfamiliarity with the particular language production context in which the label was originally attached or as an indication that the language elicitor or monitor is interfering in some way with the normal language flow.

Anthropologists and linguists further agree that behavior and language are systematic and ordered. Linguists therefore reject the interpretations of many educators and speech therapists that specific social dialects are irregular and faulty. The classic quotation for linguists to attack on this score is from speech pathologist Charles Hurst, who coined the term dialectolalia to refer to the speech "pathology" suffered by many ghetto black children (Hurst, 1965, p. 2):

> ... dialectolalia involves such specific oral aberrations as phonemic and subphonemic replacements, segmental phonemes, phonetic distortions, defective syntax, misarticulations, mispronunciations, limited or poor vocabulary, and faulty phonology. These variables exist most commonly in unsystematic, multifarious combinations.

Recent investigation of ghetto speech by linguists has revealed a highly structured, regular, and systematic language system with none of the supposed aberrations noted by Hurst (see, for example, Wolfram, 1969).

Finally, linguists affirm that language is learned in the context of the community. To be sure, relatively little research will support exactly how the community affects this learning. We know that parents are influential and that if parents speak a particular social dialect, the child is apt to be influenced to a certain extent by it. We also know that once the child's peer group is established, it somehow takes precedence over the parents as an influence on his speech. Again, it is not clear exactly what the parameters of these influences are. It is small wonder, then, that linguists take a dim view of education programs which are built around the assumption that the parent is the effective speech model or, even less convincing, programs that assume that the surrogate parent or teacher is an active model or influence on child speech.

Thus the accesses to the study of language problems of disadvantaged children have been varied. As might be expected, different disciplines have approached the study when internal and external pressures seemed to require it, with surface eruptions preceding in the fields more immediate to the action. Educators and psychologists, who first felt the pressures, answered the call by applying the strategies and assumptions of their own disciplines. Once linguists, social scientists, and speech specialists entered the discussion they also tended to follow their own comfortable techniques. Even among linguists, however, access to the study of the speech of disadvantaged children was varied. Linguistic geographers, of course, have long been observing small group language dynamics based on geography and history. In addition, Hans Kurath (1939) introduced the dimension of the social group in the Handbook of the Linguistic Atlas of the United States and Canada, even though his criteria for social marking are hardly acceptable by current standards. Significant development in Atlas methodology and analysis was made by R. I. McDavid, who as early as 1948 observed that the data sometimes cannot be explained by geography or settlement history alone. His "Postvocalic -r in South Carolina: A Social Analysis" is an important contribution of linguistic geography to the study of social dialects. Whereas linguistic geographers rely heavily on the elicitation of citation forms of language, particularly lexicon and phonology, specialists in Caribbean languages (e.g., Stewart, 1967, 1968), have begun to see a relationship between Creole speech and the dialects of certain Negroes in the United States, particularly in matters of grammar. A third access has been from the field of linguistic theory, exemplified in the work of William Labov (1966, 1968), who approaches the study of language in society in order to solve linguistic problems such as the description of continuous variations, overlapping phonemic systems, and the mechanism of linguistic change. Some of Labov's work moves toward sociological phenomena per se, as, for example, the discreteness of socioeconomic stratification, the relation of normative values to social behavior, and the nature of social control.

THE PRESENT STATUS OF RESEARCH ON THE LANGUAGE PROBLEMS OF THE DISADVANTAGED

To this point we have observed briefly the emergence of concern for the language problems of the disadvantaged. It has been pointed out that the beginning research assumptions of the fields of psychology, education, speech, social science, and linguistics have more or less dictated the framework for research in these areas.

Harry Osser has recently observed that psychologists today are becoming less eager to interpret consistent discovery of differences in language performance between children of different backgrounds as deficiences in the lower-class group (Osser, 1971). This healthy tendency indicates that psychologists are beginning to be more concerned with the meaning of these differences. He points out a growing awareness that the comparatively poorer performance of lower-class children on experimental language tasks is frequently a reflection of procedural bias and that if, in speech samples obtained from both advantaged and disadvantaged children. only standard forms are noted, this is evidence of interpretive bias.

The type of contribution to our knowledge of the language of disadvantaged children which psychologists (or perhaps more accurately, psycholinguists) are currently providing has been labeled "studies of communicative competence." Williams and Naremore, for example, have shown that lower-class children tend to use the first person in discourse more than middle-class children, who tend to make greater use of the third person and employ a variety of perspectives (Williams and Naremore, 1969).

Hawkins, in his study of the speech of 5-year-old middle- and lower-class children observed that the middle-class subjects tended to use nouns more in discourse while the lower-class children rely more on pronouns (Hawkins, 1971). By using nouns, the middle-class child has greater flexibility in modification, opening up possibilities of linguistic expansion that lower-class children do not have. Hawkins also noted a greater use of anaphoric prounouns (i.e, pronouns that refer specifically to previously used nouns) by middle-class children. Lower-class children tend to use exaphoric pronouns (i.e., those which refer outward to a larger situational context). In other words, the speaker assumes that the listener knows what he means and, therefore, does not bother with the disambiguating specifics of anaphora.

One last example of the kind of information about the language problems of disadvantaged children which recent psycholinguistics has revealed relates to various types of hesitation phenomena. Osser (Osser, 1971) notes that middle-class children engage in a larger number of self-correcting hesitation markers (*He's wearing a hat/I mean a cap*) than lower-class children do.

The current research of educators concerning the language problems of the disadvantaged suffers greatly by being out of sequence. The educator's job is primarily to interpret for the classroom the analyses of some preceding descriptive studies. The problem is obvious. If the preceding description has not been made, analysis will not have been completed and sensitive interpretation will be impossible. It has been pointed out already that psychologists have faced the same kind of problem. An accurate ethnographic and linguistic description has to precede language analysis and prescription.

Despite this handicap, several programs for teaching Standard English to disadvantaged, especially black, children were developed during the 1960s. Such programs can be characterized as isolative, generally based on little or no descriptive data of the way their populations actually talk, and pedagogically generalized from foreign-language-teaching methodology.

In a recent study for the U. S. Office of Education, staff members at The Center for Applied Linguistics surveyed extant materials intended to teach oral Standard English to native speakers of English. An intensive survey over a period of a year's time turned up 31 full or partial sets of such materials (Shuy, 1970). The difficulties encountered in locating such programs and in extracting copies of the materials from the authors indicate the uncertainty of the field today. The fact that few materials developers could give accurate "leads" about competing programs supported the survey staff's informal evidence that material developers in this field have worked in almost total isolation from each other. These materials can be divided into three levels: primary (14 sets), secondary (10 sets), and adult (7 sets). Most were produced by special materials-development groups working in or closely with a school system. About half of them consist only of a teacher's manual, six programs include tapes, and four have student books as part of the instructional package. In almost every case, the materials lean heavily on foreign-language teaching techniques; student tests and general program evaluation were conspicuously weak throughout.

The general lack of input from linguistic research in most of these programs is evident in a number of ways. Over half of them fail to mention how the specific features dealt with were selected for inclusion. Those which deal primarily with pronunciation reveal that the authors are not familiar with the research, which demonstrates that grammatical features are more socially stigmatizing than various pronunciations.

Of the three commonly held approaches to teaching Standard English to speakers of various nonstandards—eradication, bidialectalism, and a difficult-to-label approach in which it is advocated that Standard English speakers be taught to know and/or appreciate nonstandard varieties of the language—most programs purport to be bidialectal. For a further discussion of these approaches see Shuy (1972). Still, one primary program refers to the dialect of a disadvantaged child as "an inadequate verbal system." Two of the adult programs call dialect *incorrect* and Standard English *correct*. Even among the supposedly bidialectal materials, however, one frequently gets the clear impression that the approach is really remedial.

In terms of pedagogical strategies, about half of the programs restrict their activities to audiolingual methodology; that is, pattern practice drills with repetition. This is particularly characteristic of secondary and adult programs but not so much on the elementary level, where this methodology is more apt to be combined with group games and other activities. Only five of the programs make any overt use of the student's dialect, despite the longheld educational principle of "starting with the child where he is." All five used nonstandard dialect to compare it with Standard English, opening the door to learning by contrast. Since these programs admit the possibility that nonstandard varieties are perfectly appropriate in certain language contexts (such as the football huddle), the emphasis in not on eradicating the nonstandard, but on teaching the student to recognize the appropriate contexts in which to switch from one system to another.

In addition to the teaching of Standard English to native English speakers, considerable discussion has taken place among educators concerning the role of nonstandard speech in the child's acquisition of reading skills. Concern for the possible interference of the speech of black working-class children on their learning to read was manifested in the Chicago Public Schools' Psycholinguistics Reading Program (Leaverton, Gladney, and Davis, 1968) in a collection of articles on the subject called Teaching Black Children to Read (Baratz and Shuy, 1969) and in the materials currently being developed by Joan Baratz and William A. Stewart.

There are currently at least four models of reading instruction which attempt to relate in some way to the child's nonstandard language (for further discussion of these models see Venezky, 1970; Shuy, in press):

1. First teach the child Standard English.

2. Accept the child's oral rendering in his own dialect of material written in Standard English.

3. Develop materials in Standard English which minimize dialect and cultural differences.

4. Develop materials which incorporate the grammar of disadvantaged black children.

At the moment, it is difficult to prove or disprove any of these models. Unlike the hard sciences, where a clear scientific base makes research more controllable, educational research suffers from galloping variables that make experimental control difficult, if not impossible. What we are left with is a series of hypotheses to be tested, then affirmed or rejected. Since we know relatively little about how humans acquire learning, how they process language input or control its output, and how their knowledge and use of language relates to all this, we are probably doing well to operate even at the level of hypotheses. What we are finally beginning to know something about, however, is the broad outline of the linguistic system of the target population. It would seem reasonable to try to utilize this small segment of what may be called a scientific base in connection with reasonable hypotheses about the acquisition of reading skills. All four models should be thoroughly tested.

The hypothesis of researchers who claim that speakers of Nonstandard English should be taught Standard English before they are taught reading should be thoroughly investigated with as much rigor as possible, despite the apparent contradictory positions of researchers concerning the ability of children to acquire such language skills at this age.

Those who advocate the development of beginning reading materials written in Standard English but which avoid the grammatical and cultural mismatch of Black English-speaking children with the printed page also work from a reasonable but unproved hypothesis but one which should certainly not be ignored.

The advocates of both the second and fourth models are already at work testing their hypotheses, and the early results appear to be positive in both cases.

A major reason for discouraging any of the hypotheses noted may come from the black community itself. In a time such as this, when it is commonplace to be suspicious of the motives of researchers, it is particularly difficult for them to address themselves to the problems of minority groups, whether in reading, welfare, or anything else. No matter what approach they take in examining these problems they run the risk of being called racists or empire builders. It is not likely that teaching strategies which grow out of any of these models will be any more harmful than the International Teaching Alphabet, the look-say method, or any number of current reading strategies, but the public-relations problem is intensified because a specific minority population is identified.

In general the current relationship of educators to the language problems of disadvantaged children was recently summed up by Courtney Cazden (1971), who observed that there is a vagueness about the locus of the children's problems in their use of language. This vagueness is so strong that knowledge of vocabulary is confused with knowledge of verb forms and a child's failure to produce Standard English is equated with his lack of intelligence. Educators, further, tend to err in equating performance on a test as evidence of ability, in urging conformity to school English regardless of whether or not communication is impaired, in assuming causation from correlation, and in arguing that because a program is good, the education process can be speeded up by offering it earlier.

Speech specialists have related somewhat to the language problems of the disadvantaged despite the fact that the major measurement instruments are biased to the grammar of Standard English and that there is a general confusion between socially induced language difference and genuine language pathology. Irwin's research on the relationship between social class differences and speech development in infant speech (Irwin, 1948) and the language development monographs by McCarthy (1930) and Templin (1957) all evidence some sensitivity to the existence of social difference in speech, albeit following the *deficit* rather than *difference* model. More recently Raph's study of the language problems of the disadvantaged child (Raph, 1967) was countered by Weber (1968) and Baratz (1968), who called attention to the lack of relativism in the long tradition of speech researchers. In addition to the disciplinary leavening brought to the field of speech of Baratz, the work of Williams seems most promising in terms of providing new insights to speech pathologists and researchers. Williams and Naremore, in a recent paper, make several cogent observations about the relationship between social class and ethnic differences in the functional use of speech by children (1969).

Linguists, sociolinguists in particular, have put forth a number of useful studies which, at least in part, deal with the language of disadvantaged people. The major thrusts of such studies have been on the systematic correlation of variations in dialect features, or stylistic consistency and shifting, and on subjective reactions to language variants.

In order to address themselves to these topics, sociolinguists have borrowed research techniques from other disciplines and have developed some new analytical styles of their own. It has been necessary, for example, to conceptualize speech as part of a continuum rather than as an isolated phenomenon. The occurrence of a grammatical feature, for example, can no longer be interpreted on a purely qualitative basis, as it once was. Realizing that speakers of a language, standard or nonstandard, exist on such a continuum, some sociolinguists find it useful to employ quantitative as well as qualitative analyses in order to determine the frequency with which any given form occurs in the speech of an individual. This concept of the linguistic continuum enables them to view groups of individuals with similar or identical continua as linguistically homogeneous.

The concept of the linguistic variable, first formulated by William Labov, enables sociolinguists to account for continuous, ordered variation within linguistic features (Labov, 1966). In the past it was commonplace to consider exceptions to the regular patterns as free variation, a term somewhat analogous to the remainder in a long-division problem. In formulating the linguistic variable, Labov sought to correlate matters formerly considered free variation with such social characteristics as social status, age, style, race, and sex. As long as language is viewed as code (as descriptive linguists generally treat it), free variation continues to be a valid analytical tool. But when language is seen as behavior (as sociolinguists view it), free variation can now be accounted for more adequately, thanks to the linguistic variable.

The linguistic situation is another of the concepts developed by sociolinguists. John Gumperz (1964), for example, utilized the concept of a communication network, particularly a friendship network, to investigate linguistic code switching between local and prestige dialects in India. Labov (1966) and Wolfram (1969) have made detailed analyses of the realization of certain grammatical and phonological features across speech contexts such as casual, formal, or oral reading.

From other disciplines, sociolinguists have been borrowing heavily, especially in matters of research design, cognition, statistical analyses, attitude measurement, and demography.

The sociolinguists who have been generally concerned with the social implications of the use of the language in urban areas have carried out basic research on language variation and acquisition among social groups (e.g., Wolfram, 1969), on standard language in relation to nonstandard varieties (Labov et al., 1968), and on attitudes toward the use of language by speakers of all social levels (Shuy, Baratz, and Wolfram, 1969). Some (e.g., Feigenbaum, 1969) are particularly interested in the Nonstandard English of the urban Negro and are preparing teaching materials for elementary and secondary schools, as well as participating in teacher training to provide the necessary skills for dealing with nonstandard speech.

Although it has not been common for linguists to correlate linguistic forms with social context, there is a rather strong current movement to expand the focus on linguistic form in isolation (idealized language) to linguistic form within a defined social context. An example of this sort of activity may be seen in the Detroit Dialect Study, in which the staff calculated a social status index for each informant (Shuy, Wolfram, and Riley, 1968). The distribution of assigned social status indexes was then quartiled. Having established a tentative social population, the next task was to extract relevant linguistic data from the interviews of randomly selected Detroit residents and to display these data along with the social classes in which they occurred. Figures noting such displays are found in Shuy, Wolfram, and Riley (1967) and in Wolfram (1969). Figure 1, modified from the former, is illustrative of these displays. For each informant, all instances of negatives co-occurring with indefinites were tabulated (e.g., *He didn't do nothing*). This procedure gave a total number of *potential* occurrences for *multiple negation.* From this total the number of actual occurrences of multiple negation was tabulated. The percentage of actual multiple negatives in relation to potential multiple negatives was then computed and displayed as in Fig. 1.

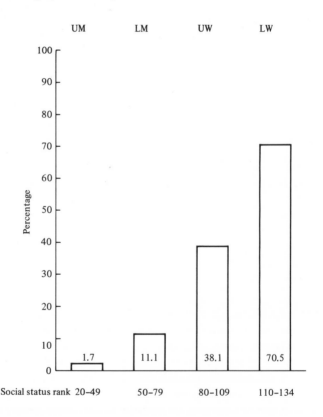

Figure 1. Multiple negation social stratification. UM, upper middle class; LM, lower middle class; UW, upper working class; LW, lower working class.

Many sociolinguists feel that most of the major linguistic differences across social class boundaries are more a case of relative usage than of some highly consistent presence or absence of a feature. Further research may reveal, however, some structural differences across dialects that would reflect such things as clear differences in rules, and the like, rather than simply relative frequencies.

The matrix of linguistic situation or style is tremendously important for any accurate assessment of the social stigmatization of a linguistic feature. Although very little more than exploratory and programmatic information exists in this area, it is obvious that people speak differently in different social contexts. Early research which attempts to obtain information of this sort has been done by Gumperz (1964) in India. There is considerable discussion on this subject by Hymes (1964) and Ervin-Tripp (1967).

With respect to this growing concern for stylistic matters in language analysis it has become clear that the major task of the English teacher is *not* just to teach his pupils their own language. It is, rather, to help students understand that a language has a number of different social dialects, each of which has acceptability within the sphere of its influence. In addition, students must be helped to use several different social dialects (or parts of these dialects) on different occasions, depending on such nonlinguistic phenomena as the speaker's emotional involvement, his real or conceptualized audience, his intention, his understanding of stylistic requirements, and other factors.

If the teacher is willing to accept the speaker's need to switch social dialects for different social involvements and stylistic requirements, he must discover not just the items which characterize social differences but also the processes by which this switching takes place. One of the important research questions in American urban sociolinguistics, then, is: How is language switching accomplished?

Extensive observation of style shifting and code shifting should yield a description of the process in relation to the social situations in which such switching takes place. We now know, for example, that people engage in style shifts within or crossing social dialects. A sudden shift in subject matter, for example, may bring about emotional overtones causing phonological or grammatical shifts. An example of this kind of research can be seen in Wolfram (1969), who computed the frequency distribution of various grammatical and phonological features across the styles of narrative and oral reading, observing, in each case, a greater tendency toward the mainstream norm in the reading style.

Although people make assumptions about other people on the basis of speech characteristics, there has been relatively little systematic research concerning the linguistic variables upon which the listener bases these assumptions. Language attitude studies have been done by Lambert and co-workers (1960-1968), Harms (1961), Labov (1966), Buck (1968), Williams (1969), and Shuy, Baratz, and Wolfram (1969). In these studies, listeners rate voices out of context along scales of intelligence, occupation group (with education level and income implied), race, ambition, honesty, and other factors. The methodologies of such tests tend to make use of questionnaires more than any other methods. The Shuy, Baratz, and Wolfram study may serve as an example. In this study the researchers were primarily concerned with the ability of Detroit residents to identify the race and socioeconomic status of adult males on the basis of a small sample of their speech. A part of the taped stimulus included 21 passages of discourse 20 to 30 seconds in length from three adult white males from the upper middle, lower middle, and upper working classes of Detroit.

Several research questions were asked in the study, but let us note only one or two examples. In response to the question, "Can individuals correctly identify the social class of a person from a sample of his spoken language?" the following results were obtained. The social class of the taped stimulus was correctly identified by all respondents as follows: upper middle classes 29.6 percent, lower middle classes 31.8 percent, the upper working classes 40.8 percent, and the lower working classes 60.8 percent. Thus it appears that overall ability to identify socioeconomic status from these speech samples appears to increase as socioeconomic status decreases.

Another research question asked in the preceding study was, "What is the effect of the socioeconomic status of the speaker?" Not surprisingly, lower-working-class speakers are most often correctly identified regardless of the socioeconomic status of the respondent and upper-middle-class respondents appear to perform significantly better than lower-working-class respondents on all identificiations.

Several other research questions were posed in this study, including the ability of individuals to identify ethnicity, the relationship of the sex of the respondent to his ability to make such identifications, the differences in the identification abilities of children and adults, the relative merits of the grammatical or phonological indices, and the utility of semantic differential testing in such studies.

One of the fundamental principles in sociolinguistics is that speech is context-sensitive, both in its realization and its norms. The ways in which people subjectively react to language can provide researchers with a number of clues about the relative appropriateness of language to situation and with a better understanding of how sensitive children are to these co-occurrence constraints.

If anything characterizes the present status of research on the language problems of disadvantaged children, it seems to be an increased awareness that future progress in the area requires the combined efforts of specialists from the several fields involved. Although the earliest, halting starts made by some psychologists and educators appeared to be headed in the wrong direction, more recent studies have made enough use of linguistic expertise to be more practical and, at least in some circles, there appears to be a long-awaited rapprochment between the various disciplines involved in the study.

THE LINGUISTIC PROBLEMS OF STUDENTS

Sociolinguists have assumed the primary responsibility for identifying and analyzing the linguistic features which set off one social group from another. Although there are currently available several "grocery lists" of features said to be characteristic of Nonstandard English, these lists generally tend to oversimplify and frequently they are downright misleading (Non-Standard Dialects, 1968, is a case in point).

An important question, of course, is: How much do teachers need to know about a linguistic feature in order to teach about it? In this respect, the "grocery lists" may be useful, for earlier research by Ann E. Hughes has clearly revealed the general inability of teachers even to identify the features which they consider problems in their students' speech (Hughes, 1967). Only 10 percent of the teachers in Hughes's study of Detroit Head Start teachers demonstrate any understanding that the so-called nonverbal child has a language which may be perfectly appropriate for certain, but not all, circumstances in life. From such data as these, it has become apparent that a simple listing of the features will not be enough. If materials developers had only the analysis found in Non-Standard Dialects, they would not know enough about the relationship between the environmental constraints and the social status of the speaker in order to focus and sequence the materials effectively. Much of sociolinguistic analysis is addressed specifically to these and other relationships.

Meanwhile, linguists have been slowly and painstakingly describing these linguistic features of the speech of disadvantaged people in detail. Labov's technical description of five phonological features in New York speech was published in 1966. Wolfram has recently completed an analysis of four phonological and four grammatical features of Detroit Negro speech (Wolfram, 1969). Shuy, Wolfram, and Riley dealt with two grammatical features and one phonological feature (in addition to some preliminary analyses of syntax) in the Detroit Dialect Study (Shuy, Wolfram, and Riley, 1967). Fasold had done preliminary research on the low vowel system of a cross section of Detroiters (Fasold, 1968) and is currently studying various features in Washington, D. C. Now Labov has extended his New York research to include several more features there (Labov et al., 1968), and Crockett and Levine have added to our knowledge of *r* in the Piedmont (Levine and Crockett, 1966).

Upon first reflection, it may seem that these features are really no different than those noted in the "grocery list" approach mentioned earlier. And, to a limited extent, this is true. One important type of difference, however, must be noted. In the New York City Board of Education's *Non-Standard Dialect* it is reported that for nonstandard speakers the *-st* cluster reduced to *-s* in words like *test, toast,* and *ghost* (p. 13). In fact, however, this reduction also characterizes Standard English speakers in the environment before consonants. Since speakers of Nonstandard English also reduce these clusters before vowels, the grocery list is partly right, but it does not tell the whole story.

In general, the grocery-list approach usually sacrifices adequacy in favor of simplicity while the technical description is frequently too complex and specific for the nonlinguist to understand. In an effort to counter the unfavorable aspects of both types of description, Fasold and Wolfram produced a description of some of the major features of Negro dialect "in non-technical language, but in sufficient detail to be useful, if not to teachers themselves, at least to those who would like to write teaching materials but do not feel secure in their knowledge of the features involved" (Fasold and Wolfram, 1970, p. 21). Since this description is readily accessible to the public, there will be no attempt made to repeat it here. Fasold and Wolfram address themselves to the following linguistic features:

A. Pronunciation
  1. Word-final consonant clusters (e.g., /st/ *test, missed;* and /nd/ *find, canned*)
  2. The *th* sounds (e.g., *think, nothing, tooth*)

3. *r* and *l* (e.g., *sister, nickel, help, four*)
4. Final *b, d,* and *g* (devoicing and deletion) (e.g., *pig, salad, good, mud*)
5. Nasalization (in the *-ing* suffix, nasalized vowels, and effect of nasal consonants on /I/ and /ɛ/) (e.g., *singin', run,* and *pen*)
6. Vowel glides (e.g., *time, boy, kite*)
7. Indefinite articles *a* and *an* (e.g., *an apple*)
8. Stress (e.g., *hótel, pólice*)
9. Other pronunciation features (e.g., *ask* ~ *axe, street* ~ *skreet*)

B. Grammar
1. The *-ed* suffix (e.g., *missed, started, said*)
2. Perfective constructions (e.g., *He gone home, He done it, I done forgot, I been had it*)
3. The third-person-singular present-tense marker (*He walk, He don't go, He have a car*)
4. Future (e.g., *He gonna go, I'ma go, He see you tomorrow*)
5. Invariant *be* (e.g., *Sometime he be busy*)
6. Absence of forms of *to be* (*He a man, You here*)
7. The use of *aint* (e.g., *He aint do that, He aint here*)
8. Multiple negative (e.g., *Nobody didn't know it didn't rain, Can't nobody do it*)
9. Possessive (e.g., *The boy hat, Jack's Johnson car, This he book, it mines*)
10. Plural (e.g., *five book, two deers, mens*)
11. Question formation (e.g., *I want to know did he go home*)
12. The absence of preposed auxiliaries (e.g., *He coming with us*)
13. Pronominal apposition (e.g., *My mother she came home early*)
14. Existential *it* (e.g., *It's a lot of people out there*)

The discussion accompanying each of the above topics reveals the most up-to-date research information on each feature. Fasold and Wolfram explain the feature in detail, indicating the effect of linguistic environment on the particular feature, the linguistic rules by which the speaker produces the particular pronunciation or grammatical form, and how such production contrasts with Standard English.

Much of the recent research of sociolinguists has pointed out, consistently, the importance of being able to determine the exact linguistic environments of the features which are said to contrast between Standard English and the variety used by disadvantaged people. This particular type of knowledge enables the teacher or materials developer to build lessons with desirable precision. For example, it is important to note that the frequently observed lack of the *-ed* past-tense marker in the speech of black children is not an indication that such children have no sensitivity to the past tense or are unable to conceptualize on a time dimension. Indeed, their use of irregular-verb past-tense forms is substantially similar to that of white people of similar socioeconomic status. What must be seen here is the working of the word-final consonant cluster. Since most regular past-tense formations are merely the addition of /t/ to verb bases ending in certain voiceless sounds (i.e., *jumped, picked*) and /d/ added to verb bases ending in voiced sounds (i.e., *pinned, hanged, zoomed, rubbed, begged*), and since these *t* and *d* sounds tend to be lost in certain kinds of word-final consonant clusters whether they are part of a past-tense formation or not, this past-tense reduction must be interpreted as directly related to phonological environment.

Fasold and Wolfram clearly point out how consonant cluster reduction operates both in Black English and in the colloquial speech of Standard English speakers. Both groups reduce the second member of the cluster when the following word or suffix begins with a consonant. Thus all normally say, *bes' kind* or *wes' side* in casual speech. The major difference between Black English and Standard English, however, occurs when the following sound is a vowel, as in *bes' one* and *wes' end*. Another aspect of consonant cluster reduction, noted earlier by Wolfram, is that it operates only when both members of the cluster are either voiced or voiceless. Where the consonants are of mixed voicing, as in *jump, colt,* or *belt,* this reduction does not take place. These two clarifications of the general nature of consonant cluster reduction in the speech of black children should prevent future material writers from producing lessons on the nonexistent problems involving clusters of mixed voicing (as in *jump, colt,* and *belt*) as well as wasting the time of black children by trying to get them to produce consonants in positions where even colloquial Standard English does not require them (as in *best* + *kind* and *west* + *side*).

It should be noted that most of the recent research cited herein relates to the disadvantaged black children of this country, particularly in the urban North. This is partly because the black child's problems have been considered greater than those of other groups and partly because of the development of black awareness and urban problems in the 1960s. The disadvantaged Caucasian child has probably suffered, as McDavid observes, because he is physically inconspicuous, just as the disadvantaged black child has suffered in the schools because he is conspicuous: ". . . his divergences from the teacher's dialect are likely to be ascribed to his innate ignorance, whereas the Negro's divergences are ascribed to his race" (McDavid, 1970, p. 136). The disadvantaged white child is often transplanted to the urban North from the South or South Midlands of America. McDavid points out that such speakers overgeneralize the tendency of American English toward word initial stress (as in *hótel, guítar*), strongly stress word-final morphemes such as *-ence, -ment,* and *-ent* (as in *settlemént, evidénce*), and shorten weak-stressed syllables (as in *borruh* for *borrow* and *Tuesdah* for *Tuesday*). The Southerner or South Midlander, as McDavid observes, has nearly all the significant pronunciation contrasts of the Northeasterner or Midwesterner plus a few more. He may distinguish among *dew, do,* and *due; marry, Mary,* and *merry; hoarse* and *horse;* and *wails* and *whales.* He is likely to simplify consonant clusters of the sort that make homonyms out of *six, sixth,* and *sixths,* especially where the base form of the noun ends in /-sp/, /-st/, or /-sk/ as in *pos* for *posts, cos* for *cost,* and *ris* for *risks.*

The field records of the Linguistic Atlas of the United States and Canada are a fruitful source of information about these and other aspects of the language of disadvantaged Caucasians, although considerable research remains to be done in many parts of the country, particularly concerning the assimilation and swamping of local norms by in-migration and the special characteristics of disadvantaged ethnic groups such as the lower income Polish residents in Detroit and Buffalo. Likewise, a major concern in this country is developing for the native English child of Spanish-speaking parents whose acquisition of Standard English is often inhibited by the local nonstandard variety. Thus, the Harlem Puerto Rican child is expected to learn Standard English even though the variety he hears most often is that spoken by the local black community.

THE LINGUISTIC PROBLEM OF TEACHERS

Just as the blame for a communication breakdown cannot be placed entirely on the listener (the sender might well be the source of the problem), so the language problems of the disadvantaged child cannot be viewed in isolation from the classroom. Little research has been done on the effect of teacher speech as a model for child speech or on how the teacher is capable of creating negative views toward language, standard or not, in his students. In fact, relatively little research has been done on what the teacher knows, feels, or thinks about the language of disadvantaged pupils. Considerable data have been gathered on how a teacher is trained, on whether or not he feels adequately trained, and on what he actually does in the process of teaching. But assessments of what teachers really know about the language used by children and how they feel about it are infrequent. We know from The National Interest and the Teaching of English (1961) that the linguistic preparation of prospective English teachers is woefully inadequate. It should not be surprising, then, that teachers find it difficult to describe accurately the language problems of their disadvantaged students. In the study by Anne Hughes, mentioned earlier, 30 Detroit teachers were randomly selected and asked to identify the language problems of their students who were designated, in one way or another, as disadvantaged.

About 80 percent of the teachers observed that their students have a limited vocabulary and many teachers offered reasons such as the following for this handicap (Hughes, pp. 78, 80):

> In the program, the children come with a very meager vocabulary. I think it's because of the background of the home and the lack of books at home, the lack of communication with the family, especially, if there are only one or two children in the family. Perhaps if there are more children in the family communication might be a bit better. They might have a few more words in their vocabulary.

> In the inner-city, the child's vocabulary is very limited. His experiences are very limited.

These comments are typical in that the atmosphere of the home is blamed for the child's limited vocabulary. None of the teachers gave any indication that the home environment might produce a *different* vocabulary. On the contrary, it was generally felt that lack of school vocabulary was equivalent to a lack of overall vocabulary.

The widely held but erroneous concept that disadvantaged children have limited vocabularies can be traced to earlier reports on the language of the disadvantaged child. Yet, nothing in the current research of sociolinguists supports this idea. Several different reasons can be given for the rise of the notion that children in disadvantaged homes have limited vocabularies. It may be that the investigators proved to be such a cultural barrier to the children that they were too frightened and awed to talk freely, that the investigators asked the wrong questions, or that the student's life style simply requires a different lexicon.

The interviewed teachers' misconceptions about the size of a disadvantaged child's vocabulary may be illustrated as follows (Hughes, p. 77):

> Some had a vocabulary of about a hundred and some words, I'd say; no more than that. They got along fine with what they knew. They didn't have any trouble expressing themselves. They knew the important words for them to get along okay. Some could talk your foot off. I mean, they just knew everything. The quieter ones were the ones who didn't have a large vocabulary.

The assumption that disadvantaged children use only a hundred words or so is one of the curious stereotypes of the teaching profession. What is more distressing than this exaggeration, however, is the assumption that quiet children are quiet because they have no vocabulary.

The responses of these teachers to the grammar problems of their disadvantaged students is equally naive. One third of the teachers characterized the child's greatest problem as his failure to communicate complete thoughts in complete sentences (Hughes, p. 81):

> I can't get them to make a sentence. Even if I have them repeat after me exactly, they don't do it. They repeat in sentences they are familiar with. They're not really sentences but fragments of sentences that are familiar to them, and they understand them. They don't realize that they aren't making a complete thought.

> Where we would use a sentence to convey a thought, they are in the habit of maybe using a phrase or just a few words to try to convey the same thought which I would presume would affect their communication to a great extent.

Of the grammar of their students, the teachers offered the following comments (Hughes, p. 83):

> The biggest problem that I've had so far is "I'm gonna."

> Because there is no real honest communication between parent and child, the child isn't taught to listen. He doesn't hear; he doesn't enunciate, you see.

> These children cut words off: *could* would be *ould*, such as in "Ould you like to do this?" Too, their "l's" were often missing.

Even when the teachers' responses reflected a clear distinction between phonology and grammar, the description was often not accurate enough to be diagnostically useful.

> Their grammar problems are many because they use substitutions, this for that.

> They use too many personal pronouns.

Although the teachers generally had more to say about pronunciation than vocabulary or grammar, there were many overgeneralizations, such as (Hughes, p. 87):

> They do have trouble with pronunciation for they fail to use their teeth and tongue and their lips. This is necessary for getting the correct sound.

> I have one child who mispronounces almost every word, but they say he does not have a speech problem.

> Many times they mispronounce because they do not know the sounds.

> Their trouble was the use of dialect for they said *hal* for *how*. It was southern dialect among some of the children which caused them to use the wrong words.

> Pronunciation is poor. Things like, "I wanna go," or *punkin* for *pumpkin* and things like that. Their dialect is just hard to understand for most teachers. We were born and raised in the Midwest, for the most part.

It is indeed difficult to imagine anyone using language who fails to use his teeth and tongue and lips. The supposed substitution of *hal* for *how* indicates an awareness of the *l* problem in Nonstandard English but a confusion about the nature of the problem (the *l* is not inserted, it is deleted). The parochialism of the last quotation is unsound, because it is an easy matter to cite pronunciations of *wanna* for *want to* in the speech of almost any speaker of Standard English.

As for specific kinds of pronunciation problems, the teachers agreed rather clearly that disadvantaged children delete word-final consonant sounds (Hughes, p. 89):

> They leave off last sounds, leave off beginning sounds some times. But then I have that trouble now even with the other children. I keep saying to them to put in all the letters for that's why they're there.

> Some of the children had problems with their consonants, particularly at the ends of words.

> They leave off the endings of words; instead of *going* it's *goin*. (Also the *d*'s and *t*'s give them trouble.) Even at the beginning of words you often cannot hear the beginning letter.

> I think that they're in the habit of not saying the things as clearly as we do and they say a word as *looking* by leaving the *g* off.

The teachers' confusion of sounds and orthography is perhaps to be expected (for it seems widespread in this country), but it may be confusing to a first-grade child to be told to add a *g* when the *ng* combination stands for the single sound, /ɔ/.

On the other hand, these came a bit closer to some of the significant problems of disadvantaged pronunciation than they did for vocabulary or grammar. In general, however, the analyses were too vague to be diagnostically useful. The major point that the teachers did not perceive is that there is a pattern in inner-city speech—just as there is pattern in every kind of speech. These teachers neither described the problem accurately nor understood its pattern.

One of the most important aspects involved in the language problems of disadvantaged children, therefore, focuses on the teachers' imprecise descriptions of the problem, their ignorance of how to make such descriptions, and on their imperfect knowledge about a vastly neglected and underprivileged group of human beings. It is not inappropriate to observe that the linguistic sophistication of teachers is currently quite limited.

It seems very clear, then, that teachers need to learn about the current research in urban language problems, why the research is being done, how it is carried out, what is known at the moment and, every bit as important, what is not known. Further, teachers need to take cognizance of their own language in relation to that of their pupils. They need to understand language variation—the reasons underlying it and the attitudes of various subcultures toward it. Teachers should learn to listen to the language of their students. They should find out how systematic the language of disadvantaged children can be and they should develop a sensitivity to the editing processes that take place as one person listens to another.

In short, the preparation of language arts teachers must be overhauled to put language at the center of the program, accompanied wherever possible by courses in administration, techniques, and evaluation. It is an indisputable fact that the most important tool for survival, for communicating, and for obtaining knowledge and skills is language. This is as true for middle-class children as for disadvantaged socioeconomic groups. But if the circumstances under which disadvantaged children acquire this tool militate in some way against their acquiring middle-class language patterns, some kind of special attention must be given them. This special attention requires the teacher to develop an ability to learn how to deal with the child's language, how to listen and respond to it, how to diagnose what is needed, how to best teach alternative linguistic systems, and how to treat it as a positive and healthy entity.

THE FUTURE OF LANGUAGE PROBLEMS OF THE DISADVANTAGED CHILD

The most important focus in the child's early education centers around language. It is his only tool for communicating with the adult world, thereby enabling teachers to evaluate him and teach him. One of the most logical subjects for teachers to study, therefore, is the language of children. In order to study the language of children, it is important for teachers to study language in a broad sense, especially as linguists see it. The following areas of preparation should form the core of a revised training curriculum for teachers of disadvantaged children.

1. *The nature of language.* Teachers need to know about the systematic nature of language, how languages differ from each other, how they change, the difference between oral and written symbolization, and the structure of communication. They should be made at least minimally aware of current theoretical views of linguistics. No extant college linguistics courses meet this need exactly. Courses called "Introduction to Linguistics," as they are now conceived by linguistics departments, are not what future teachers need. Nor are the college courses in the structure and history of the English language immediately applicable. If linguists have not developed a course which suits the need of future elementary teachers, it is high time they were made to develop such a course *along with knowledgeable specialists in education.* Students with special abilities in this course should, upon completion, be encouraged to take further work in general linguistics courses.

2. *The nature of Nonstandard English.* This course should include a contrastive grammar and phonology. It should reflect the recent research of Labov, Wolfram, Fasold, Stewart, McDavid, and Shuy on nonstandard varieties of English. It should contain a unit on the historical origins of current nonstandards, a unit on grammatical features including the correlations with social stratification, frequency of occurrence, and social diagnosticity of the feature. The concepts of the linguistic variable, the linguistic continuum, and the linguistic situation must be seen in relation to language data.

3. *Field work in child language.* After studying current approaches to the study of oral language (Slobin, 1967; Shuy, Wolfram, and Riley, 1968), teachers should be guided in gathering language data within a disadvantaged group.

Then the teachers should be asked to focus on several major phonological features which seem nonstandard, describe them thoroughly, and search the literature for their use elsewhere. They should do the same for several grammatical features.

4. *Teaching oral language to the disadvantaged child.* Focus should begin with a question of the relevance of foreign-language-teaching techniques to second dialect learning (Feigenbaum, 1969). It should review foreign-language techniques (see Lado, 1964; Rivers, 1969) and discuss problems of defining Standard English, social dialect, and so forth. Teachers should then be guided in an examination of extant oral language materials for nonstandard speakers (Golden, 1965; Lin, 1965; Hurst, 1965; Leaverton et al., 1968; Feigenbaum, 1969). They should be helped to set up criteria for evaluating such materials.

5. *Oral language and reading.* As they examine the relationship of a child's oral language to his acquisition of reading skills, teachers should examine problems of dialect interference through phonology, grammar, and orthography (see Baratz and Shuy, 1969). They should examine current reading materials to determine how well they adjust to the linguistic features observed in areas 2 and 3.

However, these units are presented (as areas, fields, courses, or workshops), teachers of the disadvantaged should have primary training in the nature of language, in the characteristics of Nonstandard English, in foreign-language-teaching techniques, and in the potential interference of one dialect on another in the reading process. In addition, they should have a significant exposure to child language brought about by actual contact with such children. The core should be seen first, and all other things revolve around it.

In addition to a revised program for training teachers of the disadvantaged, the future requires continued research in language attitudes, on linguistic descriptions of the speech of various subcultures, and in the development of pedagogical materials. Perhaps most important of all, however, is the need to develop means of assessing the usefulness of programs and materials developed with the language problems of disadvantaged children in mind.

As research into these problems is continued, however, several important questions must be asked. How generalizable are any of these linguistic descriptions from one area to another? Although most of the aforementioned sociolinguistic research deals with a broad section of the population, the clear focus has been on the speech of minority groups, and further research must be done on the speech of the middle classes, Southern whites, and rural Negroes, to mention only a few groups, in order to get a clearer focus of the target group in a realistic linguistic context.

Despite the recent research by linguists and psychologists concerning language acquisition of children, practically nothing is yet known about contrastive rates of acquisition caused by dialect or language interference. What effect does a Nonstandard English home environment have on this acquisition? Can this effect be quantified? What effect does the sex of the child have on his rate of acquiring Standard English? Who are the language models of children of different ages, race, sex, and socioeconomic status? What is the role of the teacher as a language model? What is the role of Nonstandard English as a tool of instruction? At what age can adult norms of Standard English be best learned? If a certain feature is more efficiently learned at one age than another can the school tolerate the nonstandard form until the standard feature is more efficiently learned?

These and many other such questions should be answered in the near future if we are serious about research in the relationship between the child's oral language and the classroom.

REFERENCES

Baratz, J. C. 1968. Reply to Dr. Raph's article on speech and language deficits in culturally disadvantaged children. J. Speech Hearing Dis., 33:299-300.
—— and R. W. Shuy, eds. 1969. Teaching Black Children to Read. Washington, D. C., Center for Applied Linguistics.
Bereiter, Carl, et al. 1966. An academically oriented pre-school for culturally deprived children. In Hechinger, F. M. ed., Pre-School Education Today. Garden City, N. Y., Doubleday.
Buck, J. F. 1968. The effects of Negro and white dialectal variations upon attitudes of college students. Speech Monogr., 35:181-186.
Cazden, Courtney. 1971. Approaches to social dialects in early childhood education, In Shuy, R., compiler. Social Dialects and Interdisciplinary Perspectives (in preparation). Washington, D. C., Center for Applied Linguistics.

Ervin-Tripp, S. 1967. Sociolinguistics. Working paper No. 3, Language Behavior Research Laboratory, University of California at Berkeley.

Fasold, R. W. 1968. A Sociolinguistic Study of the Pronunciation of Three Vowels in Detroit Speech. Washington, D. C., Center for Applied Linguistics. (mimeographed)

—— and Walt Wolfram. 1970. Some linguistic features of Negro dialect. *In* Fasold, R. W., and R. W. Shuy, eds., Teaching Standard English in the Inner City, pp. 41-86. Washington, D. C., Center for Applied Linguistics.

Feigenbaum, Irwin. 1969. Using foreign language methodology to teach standard English: evaluation and adaptation. Florida FL Reporter, 7(1):116-122, 156-157.

——1970. Using nonstandard to teach standard: contrast and comparison. *In* Fasold, R. W., and R. W. Shuy, eds., Teaching Standard English in the Inner City. Washington, D. C., Center for Applied Linguistics.

Fishman, Joshua. 1968. The sociology of language. *In* Fishman, Joshua, ed., Readings in the Sociology of Language. The Hague, Mouton and Co.

Golden, Ruth. 1965. Instructional Record for Changing Regional Speech Patterns. Folkway/Scholastic, No. 9323.

Gumperz, John. 1964. Linguistic and social interaction in two communities. *In* Hymes, D., ed., The Ethnography of Communication. Amer. Anthropol., 66(no. 6, pt. 2):137-153.

Harms, L. S. 1961. Listener judgments of status cues in speech. Quart. J. Speech, 47:164-168.

Hawkins, P. R. 1971. Social-class, the nominal group and reference. Lang. Speech. (in press)

Hughes, A. E. 1967. An Investigation of Some Sociolinguistic Phenomena in the Vocabulary, Pronunciation and Grammar of Detroit Pre-School Children, Their Parents and Teachers. Ed. D. dissertation, East Lansing, Mich., Michigan State University.

Hurst, Charles. 1965. Psychological Correlates in Dialectolalia. Washington, D. C., Howard University.

Hymes, D., ed. 1964. The Ethnography of Communication. American Anthropol., 66(no. 6, pt. 2).

Irwin, O. C. 1948. Infant speech: The effect of family occupational status and of age on use of sound types. J. Speech Hearing Dis., 13:224, 226.

Kurath, H. 1939. Handbook of the Linguistic Atlas of the United States and Canada. Providence, R. I., Brown University Press.

Labov, William. 1966. The Social Stratification of English in New York City. Washington, D. C., Center for Applied Linguistics.

—— et al. 1968. A Study of the Non-Standard English of Negro and Puerto Rican Speakers in New York City. Cooperative Research Project No. 3288, Columbia University.

Lado, Robert. 1964. Language Teaching: A Scientific Approach. New York, McGraw-Hill.

Lambert, W. E., R. C. Hodgson, R. C. Gardner, and A. Fillenbaum. 1960. Evaluational reactions to spoken language. J. Abnorm. Social Psychol., 60:44-51.

Leaverton, Lloyd, Mildred Gladney, Melvin Hoffman, Zorenda Patterson, and O. J. Davis. 1968. Psycholinguistic Oral Language Program. Chicago, Chicago Public Schools.

——Mildred Gladney, and Olga Davis. 1968. Psycholinguistics Reading Program. Chicago, Chicago Public Schools.

Levine, Lewis, and Harry Crockett. 1966. Speech variation in a Piedmont community postvocalic r. Sociol. Inquiry, 36:204-226.

Lin, San-su. 1965. Pattern Practice in the Teaching of Standard English to Students with a Non-Standard Dialect. New York, Teachers College, Columbia University.

McCarthy, Dorothea. 1930. The language development of the pre-school child. Institute of Child Welfare Monograph Series, No. 4. Minneapolis, University of Minnesota Press.

McDavid, R. I., Jr. 1948. Post-vocalic r in South Carolina: A social analysis. American Speech, 23 (Oct.-Dec. 1948):194-203.

———1970. Language Characteristics of Native Whites. In Horn, Thomas, ed., Reading for the Disadvantaged, pp. 135-139. New York, Harcourt Brace Jovanovich.

Non-Standard Dialects. 1966. Champaign, Ill., National Council of Teachers of English,

Osser, Harry. 1971. Developmental studies of communicative competence. In Shuy, R., compiler, Social Dialects and Interdisciplinary Perspective. Washington, D. C., Center for Applied Linguistics.

Raph, J. B. 1967. Language and speech deficits in culturally disadvantaged children and their implications for the speech of children. J. Speech Hearing Dis., 32:203-214.

Rivers, W. M. 1969. Teaching Foreign Language Skills. Chicago, University of Chicago Press.

Shuy, R. W. 1969. Bonnie and Clyde tactics in English teaching. Florida FL Reporter, 7(1):81-83, 160-161.

———1970. Sociolinguistic Theory, Materials and Training Programs. Final report OEC-3-9-180357-0400 (010) (September 1970), Part II, pp. 155-175.

———1972. Speech differences and teaching strategies: how different is enough? In Hodges, R. E., and H. Rudorf, Language and Reading. Boston, Houghton Mifflin.

———J. C. Baratz, and W. A. Wolfram. 1969. Sociolinguistic factors in speech identification. Bethesda, Md., National Institutes of Mental Health Research Project No. MH-15048-01.

——— W. A. Wolfram, and W. K. Riley. 1967. Linguistic correlates of social stratification in Detroit speech. Washington, D. C., U. S. Office of Education Cooperative Research Project No. 6-1347.

——— W. A. Wolfram, and W. K. Riley. 1968. Field Techniques in an Urban Language Study. Washington, D. C., Center for Applied Linguistics.

Slobin, Dan, ed., 1967. A Field Manual for Gross Cultural Study of the Acquisition of Communicative Competence. Berkeley, University of California.

Stewart, W. A. 1967. Sociolinguistic factors in the history of American Negro dialects. Florida FL Reporter, Spring, 1967.

———1968. Continuity and change in American Negro dialects. Florida FL Reporter, Spring, 1968.

Templin, Mildred. 1957. Certain Language Skills in Children: Their Development and Interrelationships. Institute of Child Welfare Monograph Series, No. 26. Minneapolis, University of Minnesota Press.

The National Interest and the Teaching of English. 1961. National Council of Teachers of English, Champaign, Ill.

Venezky, Richard. 1970. Nonstandard language and reading. Elem. English, March, 1970:334-345.

Weber, J. L. 1968. Conspicuous Deficits. J. Speech Hearing Dis., 33:96.

Williams, Frederick. 1969. Psychological correlates of speech characteristics: sounding "disadvantaged." Unpublished report, Institute for Research on Poverty. Madison, Wis., University of Wisconsin.

―――― and Rita Naremore. 1969. On the functional analysis of social class differences in modes of speech. Speech Monogr., 36:77-102.

Wolfram, W. A. 1969. A Sociolinguistic Description of Detroit Negro Speech. Washington, D. C., Center for Applied Linguistics.

――――1971. Social Dialects from a Linguistic Perspective: Assumptions, Current Research and Future Directions. *In* Shuy, R., compiler. Social Dialects and Interdisciplinary Perspectives. Washington, D. C., Center for Applied Linguistics.

8: Language disabilities of cognitively involved children

Richard Schiefelbusch

The past ten years has seen a surge of interest in the language of cognitively involved (retarded) children. This increasing productivity is reflected in comprehensive reviews by Spradlin (1967), Spreen (1965a, b), Jordan (1967), Schiefelbusch (1969), and McCarthy (1964). In addition, Fulton and Lloyd (1969) have provided a special compilation of hearing research, and Peins (1970) has published a compilation of bibliographic references.

An apparent characteristic of recent studies has been increasing care in delineating the issues treated. In so doing, the authors have specified the frames of reference they have used; and they have also referred to the applied and basic literatures from which the methods described have been drawn, the relative nature of the subject groups described, the parameters of the language content that they index, and the definitional nature of their areas of discussion.

Recent developments in the fields of cognition, psycholinguistics, and behavioral assessment and management have been of special importance. These areas provide an important conceptual base for much of the recent work in language of the retarded. Consequently, these areas have received a prominent place in this chapter. From these new conceptual frames of reference, we are able to evolve valid, realistic approaches to the study of language of the cognitively involved child.

COGNITION AND LANGUAGE

To an increasing number of professional workers, the term cognition suggests a structure of behavior and lends itself to considerations of hierarchies of functioning (cognitive stages). Further, for many workers it avoids the issue of fixed capabilities and anticipates additional stages of cognitive development. In this sense a cognitive deficit may be regarded as a failure on the part of the child to learn some antecedent, cognitive feature that is essential for the learning task or program which the professional worker and the child are now undertaking. The assumption is that, if necessary to avoid failure, the teacher and the child can move back to an antecedent point, learn the requisite features, and again resume the learning activities leading to the higher cognitive level. The stages delineated by Piaget and colleagues provide a set of guidelines for planning or evaluating such a program of training.

However, children diagnosed as having low intelligence or as mentally retarded may or may not be placed in a learning environment designed to teach antecedent cognitive behaviors. Consequently, it may be said that a cognitively involved child is often placed in a wrong (for him) program of learning. The corrective procedure may simply be to move him to a lower level. For instance, children at the lower end of the cognitive range who show marked impairment in task performance should first be placed in a learning environment designed to teach preparatory, sensory-motor skills. Also, since instructional programs are heavily dependent upon language functions, cognitively involved children often are judged as having learning deficiencies, at least according to the demands of the school environment. Thus language training may provide a means for improving the cognitive deficiencies.

In seeking a realistic orientation we should emphasize also the relative nature of the performances implied by the term *language disorders of cognitively involved children*. This emphasis is in contrast to dependence upon absolutes in definition or measurement that can do little more than label the child. (The designation "retarded" has little descriptive value for an educator or a speech and language clinician.) It should be equally apparent that one cannot examine the basic issues of *language disorders* and *cognitive involvement* in terms of *levels of functioning* without careful consideration of the relationship of cognition and language. In other words, before describing the speech and language of cognitively involved children, perhaps we should consider the nature of cognition and the nature of language.

Cognitive development is assumed to progress through stages from early perceptual motor functioning (infancy) to formal operations beginning at about 12 years and extending into the period of adolescence. Between the sensory-motor level and the abstract-thinking level is a period of concrete operations during which time the child develops the concepts of classes, relations, and numbers. This period is assumed to extend from about 18 months to adolescence. Consequently, it spans the periods of preschool and elementary education for normal children and the special class placement years for the retarded. It also includes the period during which the child develops a language code structure, communication and social functions, and the language performance skills used in formal learning.

Piaget, whose work forms the basis for the cognitive-developmental view, subdivides the concrete operations stage into two substages. The period II_A from about 18 months to about 7 years is a preoperational stage. It is again subdivided into two stages: the first, the preconceptional stage, extends to about 4 years; the second is the intuitive stage. Period II_B, which extends roughly from 7 years to adolescence, is the period of concrete operations. Several excellent descriptions of cognitive stages of development are now available; see Beard (1969), Bruner et al. (1967), and Flavell (1963).

The period we are most concerned with here extends roughly from about 2 to 9 years or normal children. Most children designated as retarded may not progress beyond this level. It is bounded at the lower end by the period of sensory-motor intelligence and the development of a simple syntactical structure. Probably it is the onset and development of speech which sets the stage for the structural changes to follow in the formation of concrete operations, as Piaget conceives them. At the upper end of this period the child will have learned the concepts of classes and relationships and will also have attained the number concept. These concepts are considered by Piaget to be the foundations for more abstract intelligence that follows for normal children at a later period.

Piaget's position is somewhat as follows (Flavell, 1963). During the prelanguage phase the infant utilizes primarily a form of sensory-motor imagery, which is evoked by imitative experiences. As these images evolve in number and complexity, he acquires words or *signifiers*. These signifiers are tied to concrete events or objects—*his* events, *his* objects. The ability to associate a word and an object Piaget designates as a *symbolic function*. However, the infant cannot evoke a signifier which symbolizes a perceptually present event (the significate) from which the signifier is clearly differentiated. Nevertheless, he considers these reference giving cues to be the functional predecessors of the "true" signifiers which come later. What happens, Piaget reasons, is that with the growth and refinement of the ability to imitate, the child is eventually able to make "internal" imitations as well as externally visible ones. At first, these internal imitations are the child's private symbols. Consequently, the child is egocentric with respect to presentations.

At about this time the child repeatedly demonstrates a relative inability to take the role of the other person—at least, he seems to make little real effort to adapt his speech to the listener. After about seven years of age, Piaget contends that the child begins a phase involving more socialized operations. Through repeated and often frustrating interchanges with his peers, the child has come to grips with other viewpoints and perspectives which differ from his own. From such repeated encounters he also gradually moves from "a static and centrated egocentrism . . . " Flavell (1963, p. 201). This social or interpersonal language skill apparently derives from social experiences. In turn it provides the means for increasingly effective social uses of language.

Whereas Piaget continues the study of egocentric language by shifting to social language, Vygotsky (1962), whose work was contemporary to this phase of Piaget's work (1930's), chose to regard egocentric speech as the precursor of "inner speech." He believed that egocentric speech is social in character and that it is gradually transformed into a private language (as the child gains sufficient practice and experience). He further believed that, when egocentric speech becomes inner speech, significant changes occur. Most importantly, speech no longer is tied to a concrete situation or to a social context. Perception changes from wordless perception of objects to the perception of objects aided by and expressed in words, and finally to the ideation of objects represented by word symbols which do not require the object to be present. Thus the word which was originally a property of the object now becomes a symbol of it.

Vygotsky also assumed that the ability to think, reason, remember, plan, and organize has its basis in meaningful language. If children are inadequately trained in word

meanings, they will likely be retarded. Logically, the reverse is also true, and the Russi
view offers promise by demonstrating that these disorders can be corrected i
appropriate re-education of word meanings. Some examples are reported by Luria (196
and by Luria and Yudovich (1959).

Although the most common approach to cognition is developmental in nature, t
sequences in the development are not fully outlined. The same statement may be ma
for language development. Also, the two systems have not been carefully related. At be
the literature on these subjects permits us to present two developmental pictures in
somewhat parallel fashion. Hence the description of cognitive involvement and langua
disabilities must be presented against an incomplete background of general developmer

Even this general acknowledgment, however, does not entirely explain the difficulti
of the comparison. As Wohlwill (1964) has pointed out, Piaget presents essentially
structural analysis of children's performance in cognitive tasks at different levels of the
development. His treatment of the *functional* side of the problem (i.e., the nature of tl
processes by which these changes take place) is much less complete.

The evaluations of language development are apparently following the san
emphasis. The linguists are attempting to write linguistic codes for children at various a
levels. The functional side of the problem is left largely to the psycholinguists and tl
sociolinguists who are interested in how language is acquired and to the clinicians and tl
educators who are interested in how it can be taught.

Kessen (1962) suggests that what is needed is a concern for the rules of transitic
that specify the conditions governing a child's change from one stage to the next.]
Kessen's view it is the psychology of learning which has most actively concerned itse
with the study of such rules. He points out, however, that the real question is whether tl
conceptual apparatus of the learning theorist is compatible with the structural analysis
developmental stages such as Piaget's so as to make possible a complete model
development.

PSYCHOLINGUISTICS AND CHANGING BEHAVIOR

Recently a large body of literature has emerged which bears directly upon the functio
of change, especially the factors which presumably control change (Schiefelbusch, 196
Bricker and Bricker, 1969; Girardeau and Spradlin, 1970; Staats, 1968; Schiefelbusch
al., 1967; Sloane and Macaulay, 1968). Language change may well be guided b
contingent events which shape the social behavior of the child. The general assumption
that language acquisition is strongly influenced by a system of discriminated, differer
tiated operants that may be grouped into functional classes and studied for their effec
upon the rates and topographies of behavior that represent the performance of languag
The performance features, both the levels of performance and the changes i
performance, can be described as syntactic, phonological, and semantic data.

However, these views about the shaping influence of contingent events, and abou
environmental influences in general, are challenged by many linguists, especially by thos
who adhere to the generative grammar concepts of Noam Chomsky. By generativ
grammar Chomsky (Aspects of a Theory of Syntax, 1965, p. 8) means:

... simply a system of rules that in some explicit and well defined way assigns structural descriptions to sentences. Obviously, every speaker of a language has mastered and internalized a generative grammar that expresses his knowledge of his language. This is not to say that he is aware of the rules of the grammar or even that he can become aware of them, or that his statements about his intuitive knowledge of the language are necessarily accurate. Any interesting generative grammar will be dealing, for the most part, with mental processes that are far beyond the level of actual or even potential consciousness; furthermore, it is quite apparent that a speaker's reports and viewpoints about his behavior and his competence may be in error. Thus, a generative grammar attempts to specify what the speaker actually knows, not what he may report about his knowledge.

Chomsky further explains that a generative grammar is not a model for a speaker or a listener, but an attempt to characterize in the most neutral possible terms the knowledge of the language that provides the basis for actual use of language by a speaker-hearer. A particular generative grammar says nothing about how the speaker-hearer might proceed in some practical or efficient way to construct such a derivation. These questions belong to the theory of language use—the theory of performance.

Cazden (1967) and McNeill (1967) have drawn further linguistic distinctions between language competence and language performance. Perhaps the distinction may provide a useful way to approach this difficult area (linguistic description). In McNeill's view competence is the knowledge of syntax, meaning, and sound that makes performance possible. Linguistic research on the development of competence explains the progressively more complex system of rules with which children comprehend and produce speech. However, as McNeill explains, a grammar is concerned with knowledge, not behavior; consequently, factors which affect speaking and listening can be disregarded when thinking about competence.

Cazden discusses current research on individual differences in competence as undertaken by transformational linguists. According to their views, performance varies to much greater degree among speakers than does competence. She describes two types of performance. Performance A is defined as verbal ability performed by a person in a prescribed setting where behavior is affected primarily by such interpersonal factors as attention and memory. The emphasis is upon what the speaker *can do* presumably under eliciting or carefully arranged conducive situations.

In contrast, performance B refers to what a person *does do*. The emphasis here is upon natural speech situations and pertains to behavior affected by such interpersonal factors as the setting, the topic, the participants, and the language function. One may question the functional delineation between the *can do* and the *does do* aspects of performance. However, insofar as the distinctions are practical, there may be value in assigning the first of these to psycholinguists and the second to language clinicians. In any event, the empirical value of the distinction must rest with the clinician who must manipulate the functions which influence performance.

Cazden (1967, 1971), E. Carrow (1970), and Berry (1969) present ways to assess language performance. They document and analyze most of the tests and other information now available. Their treatment of the material is especially valuable for teachers and clinicians who seek to evaluate language as a means for planning training programs. In the following pages an attempt will be made to relate meaningfully to these areas in considering the speech and hearing, the language, and the communication disorders of cognitively involved children.

DEFINITIONS OF SPEECH, LANGUAGE, AND COMMUNICATION

In a previous publication (Schiefelbusch, 1969) the author divided the general language problems of the retarded into three delineations: *speech and hearing*—the speaking and/or listening behavior of a single speaking individual; *language*—the system or code that speakers have learned to use including sounds, words, and grammatical patterns; and *communication*—the language event including verbal and gestural behavior that is interpersonal.

Speech behavior was further delineated into four broad categories: (1) articulation—the way sounds are formed, (2) rhythm—the time relationship between sounds in a word and between words in a sentence, (3) voice—the sounds produced by the vibration of vocal folds and modified by resonators, and (4) speech usage—comprehension of the speech of others and/or the projection of ideas through the medium of speech. The last category might also be called *speech performance* since it refers to the child's probable behavior in speech situations.

Hearing refers to the auditory performance in regard to loudness features and in relation to comprehension, to the ability to detect the signal in both simple and complex forms, and to the ability to understand and/or respond appropriately. The auditory function has a decisive effect upon the speech behavior of the speaker and, indeed, cannot be separated from speaking. The speaker monitors himself while speaking and is dependent upon auditory feedback in performing a variety of expressive speech functions.

Language has been defined by Carroll (1967) as a code or system which speakers have learned. The code includes four distinct aspects: (1) phonology—the specification of units of sound (phonemes) which go to compose words and other forms in language; (2) morphology—the listing of words and other basic meaningful forms (morphemes) of the language and the specification of the ways in which these forms may be modified and placed in varying contexts; (3) syntax—the specification of the patterns in which linguistic forms may be arranged and the ways in which patterns may be modified or transformed in varying contexts; and (4) semantics—the specification of the meanings of linguistic forms and syntactical patterns in relation to objects, events, processes, attributes, and relationships in human experience.

The model of communication behavior used is taken from Glucksberg et al. (1966). They describe a communication unit that is divided into four parts: (1) the initial verbal instruction of the speaker (message), (2) the discrimination of the listener, (3) the response (feedback) provided by the listener to the speaker, and (4) the modified response of the speaker. This four-part communication system is assumed to be a natural stimulus-response relationship between two or more people in which the listener and the peaker are recurrently contingent stimuli for each other. In this sense the two are assumed to be under each other's stimulus control and are affected by the responses provided by each recurrently. Perhaps this orientation may be useful for clinicians who relate to the communication disorders of the cognitively involved child.

SPEECH AND HEARING IMPAIRMENTS

Spreen (1965a) points out that the higher incidence figures for *speech impairment*, in general, are found for children with quite low intelligence scores and that incidence figures drop as the intelligence level increases. The highest incidence figures are found among institutionalized retardates: Gens (1951) reported 70 to 75 percent; Bibey (1951), 56 percent; and Schlanger and Gottsleben (1957), 79 percent. In contrast, Donovan (1957) found only 8 percent of 2,000 educable mentally retarded public school children to have severe speech defects.

These figures in this form, of course, are not definitive. They neither tell the nature of the problem as to category—for example, articulation, voice, or rhythm—nor the criteria used to judge incidence. Bangs (1942) found that institutional children made more articulation errors than do normal children, but that in general they make about the same type of errors as do normal children. There were two possible exceptions in that the retardates seemed to have a higher incidence of omissions of final sounds and sometimes seemed to show errors that were bizarre and not of the sort ever found among normal children. Karlin and Strazzula (1952) found the order of difficulty of consonant sounds for retardates to agree closely to the order found for normal children. Matthews (1957) concludes his review of studies pertaining to the mentally retarded with this statement: "There is no evidence to suggest that the speech defects of the mentally retarded differ in kind from those of non-retarded speech defective populations."

A different interpretation is suggested in a recent review by Dever (1966). He concludes that the phonological deficits among the mentally retarded are a prominent feature of a possible structural deficit. He suggests further that structural linguistics provides the tools for a definitive study. The work he urges should not be to list or catalog mistakes, but to describe the "dialect" of retarded subjects living in certain environments. These descriptions then can be used to evaluate the dialect in terms of similarities or differences from the standard dialect. [This suggestion has since been carried out by Lachner (1968) who wrote grammars for five mentally retarded children. The study is described briefly in the language section.]

Another approach that might be useful in evaluating the speech of retarded children would be to determine the intelligibility of the child's pronunciation. This can be done in both formal and informal situations. The formal situation would involve the administering of a formal articulation test such as the Templin-Darley Screening and Diagnostic Tests of Articulation, the Goldman-Fristoe Articulation Test, the Deep Test of Articulation (McDonald), or the Developmental Articulation Test (Hejna). Of course there are some practical limitations of such tests. There may be children whose articulation of individual sounds is acceptable, but whose speech disintegrates when they have to formulate complex ideas, and the organizational load becomes too heavy—as in telling a story or describing an experience in front of a group. This issue is treated by de Hirsch et al. (1964).

In real life intelligibility must meet a shifting criterion. At any one time an utterance is either understood by the listener or not. But identical pronunciations might be intelligible to one listener and not to another, depending upon the listener's familiarity with the child and the degree of shared information. The Sapon Intelligibility Function Test (SIFT) has been designed to take these issues into account. The test can yield several scores of intelligibility with or without a shared environment and for either a familiar adult or a stranger. Intelligibility assumes importance in light of the difficulty of the cognitively impaired child in establishing effective communicative relationships with adults—especially adult strangers.

This leads into a complex and practical issue of the speech of the cognitively impaired child which may be listed as "speech usage." Usage can be sampled (recorded) by having the child describe what he sees in a picture, tell what he remembers from a recent experience, or describe his favorite game. The speech sample can then be analyzed by a systematized procedure which contains the usage functions deemed to be important.

Loban (1963) classifies usage according to fundamental units—that is, phonological units, communication units, and mazes. Other evaluators use such measures as rate of speaking, loudness, amount of speaking, pitch, and length of response (Johnson et al. 1952). The relevant aspects of speech usage are suggested by criteria pertaining to the effect on listener behavior. If so, the functions are similar in nature and could be classified also under the headings of language usage or communication behavior. In this sense, it is important to note that speech impairments are not usually detected by instrumentation, but by listener evaluations. That is, speech is considered to be impaired when its variants call attention, distract, or confuse. Again this is the central speech problem of the cognitively impaired child because he has difficulty in establishing and holding the attention of adults. Cazden (1967) suggests several practical arrangements for sampling the speech usage of children. Resourceful clinicians and teachers can easily design other arrangements for sampling the base-line speech behaviors of children that are included in their clinic load or in their classroom.

Incidence figures for hearing loss among retardates suffer from criteria difficulties, which similarly make evaluation and comparisons tenuous. Webb et al. (1964) report that a 15 decibel loss level in two or more frequencies produces an incidence figure of 40.5 percent, whereas a 20-decibel loss level in two or more frequencies produces an incidence of 24 percent. Other studies suggest that loss figures apparently vary according to the level of retardation of the subjects and the testing techniques employed.

Again, as with aspects of speech production, the incidence figures of hearing loss may give us little useful information. Webb et al. (1964, p. 117) conclude:

> The major point here is that many test procedures as evaluated . . . do not appear to result in valid estimates of hearing ability when applied to this population. The procedure recommended [Electroencephalic Response Audiometry—EER], although statistically useful in this study, appeared capable of similar error unless the discrimination ability and extent of judge error is previously determined on a known population.

Schlanger (1961, pp. 82-83) also offers a note of caution, but relates to somewhat different issues:

> Not understanding what is required of him in terms of stimulus-response patterns leaves the subject no choice but to respond to sound stimuli of high intensity, not respond at all, react when urged, or respond when he feels like it. To overcome this attitude and negate some of the behavioral and physiological factors which inhibit responses to auditory stimuli, it is recommended that a training program especially geared to condition a child to hearing testing (may result in) improved stimulus-response patterns.

Fulton and Lloyd (1969, pp. xii-xiii) state that audiology with the mentally retarded has progressed through three phases. The first phase focused upon incidence of hearing loss among retarded populations.

> ...unfortunately most of these findings were based upon incomplete or inappropriate assessment techniques. Subsequently, however, investigators realizing that standard pure-tone techniques were not wholly adequate, devised new techniques. Several looked to classical conditioning principles which emphasized electrodermal or galvanic skin response techniques. These classical conditioning procedures usually resulted in limited or questionable results . . . However, this experimental period, with its attention to variation in reinforcers, permitted more sophistication in selecting and utilizing reinforcers in later instrumental conditioning programs which controlled the stimulus, the response, and the reinforcer.

Fulton and Lloyd further indicate that subsequent reliability and validity studies have resulted in more stringent control over the critical variables with consequent improvements in the assessment data. This represents the beginning of a systematic approach to clinical audiology with the retarded. They feel that a fourth period is now emerging in which an increasing number of audiologists are fully aware of the diagnostic, treatment, and rehabilitation needs of the mentally retarded and the assessment problems they pose. "The development of improved methods for applying advanced electronic instrumentation and human engineering principles to audiological procedures [for the retarded] is the foremost concern in this contemporary phase" (1969, p. xiii).

In subsequent publication Lloyd and Fulton (1970) describe a procedure for speech audiometry for the severely retarded. Their work also outlines procedures for a full-blown program of audiologic differential diagnosis with the retarded. (See Fig. 1.)

LANGUAGE IMPAIRMENTS

Factual information about the language of the retarded before 1960 was traditionally general in nature. That is, the data pertained to naming and labeling, comprehension of words, speech sounds, and "grammar." Items usually were taken from verbal subtests of standardized tests of intelligence (Lyle, 1959, 1960a, b, c, 1961a, b; Goda and Griffith, 1962; O'Conner and Hermelin, 1963; Mein, 1961). This practice, in part at least, tends to

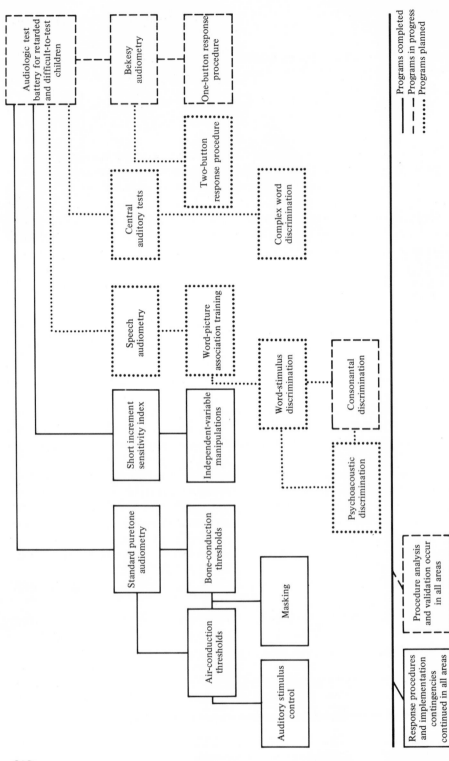

Figure 1. Program of audiologic differential diagnosis.

218

explain the high correlation between intelligence and language of the retarded. Several, but not all, of the studies found a small lag in the language of retardates as compared to normal children with matching mental ages. Other studies have a strong inverse relationship between language handicap and intelligence. Frequencies reported are usually around 100 percent in groups with IQs below 20, around 90 percent in the 21 to 50 IQ groups, and around 45 percent in the mildly retarded groups. These observations are based upon a number of studies including those of Karlin and Strazzula (1952), Schlanger and Gottsleben (1957), and Sloan and Cutts (1947). Unfortunately, the aptness of these observations is somewhat confused by the difficulties in interpreting the results of standardized tests. In many instances it seems apparent that a high correlation between language and intelligence could be assured by the inclusion of similar items on the tests employed. Thus, the relationships are obscured by the selection of tests and test items.

Perhaps a better indication of the intelligence-language issue may be derived from studies of abstraction. These studies seem to indicate that a close relationship exists between language and thought processes and that some kind of inner language or verbal mediation may be essential to intelligent behavior. If this assumption is correct, retarded language development alone would be a severe handicap to adequate intellectual functioning. Luria, a Russian psychologist (1961), has been concerned primarily with the highly intricate role of speech and language in regulating the child's behavior. Higher mental functions are developed in the course of social interaction of a verbal nature. To provide empirical support for his position, he has examined the role of both the adult and the child's speech in regulating—that is, initiating and/or inhibiting—certain motor reactions of the child. Luria has conceptualized a number of stages of regulatory development. During the initial stage, the child's own speech is insufficient to control his motor reaction, although adult verbal instructions can serve to initiate or to impel such behavior and later to inhibit it. In the second stage, the child's own speech begins to play a regulatory role in that he can initiate, although not inhibit, an action in response to his own verbal command. In the third stage, the impellent action of speech recedes into the background and a regulatory function which now includes a system of meanings becomes predominant. The final stage is characterized by reduction in the role of the externally developed forms of speech, and the regulatory influence is exerted by a higher form of internal speech which constitutes an essential component of thought and volitional action.

In a study of retarded children, Luria has demonstrated that the behavior of retardates resembles that of chronologically younger normal children in that the verbal instructions do not result in the smooth regulation of motor behavior. These findings clearly indicate that retarded subjects have considerable difficulty in all tasks requiring verbal mediation. In light of these behavioral data, Luria has inferred the major defect in the retarded child involves both an underdevelopment of the verbal system and a disassociation of this system from motor action. A thorough discussion of this issue may be found in publications by Zigler (1964) and Spreen (1965a). These discussions may be considered a subpart to the general concept of abstraction and abstract behavior.

The assumption is that the mentally retarded do not handle abstract language effectively and are thus not able to complete tasks calling for abstract concepts. The abstract—concrete dimension has been shown to be of some value in differentiating retardates and normals of matched mental age. Although the controversy is still not settled, it is generally believed that the retarded are not able to perform certain language tasks as well as their matched mental-age equivalents.

Milgram (1966) states emphatically that mentally retarded children are especially deficient in learning by verbal channels to a degree above and beyond that which they are retarded in other spheres. His opinion is based in part on a study he conducted using classification tasks with groups of normal and retarded children. These tasks included both verbal and nonverbal stimulus presentation and response conditions. He found that under nonverbal conditions the performance of normal and retarded subjects of equal mental age showed no significant difference, whereas the retarded performed significantly poorer than their normal controls as verbal elements were added to the task.

Considerable support for Milgram's position seems to emerge from recent studies of retarded children involving the Illinois Test of Psycholinguistic Abilities (ITPA) (Mueller and Weaver, 1964; Bilovsky and Share, 1965; Ensminger and Smith, 1965). The severely retarded subject is found to be impaired in his ability to use auditory and vocal mechanisms in a sequencing manner. The problem of coordinating these two systems seems to contribute the largest part to the relative deficiency found for these subjects on language tasks. Ensminger and Smith note that approximately 80 percent of all retardates have similar stable ITPA profiles. They recommend that auditory vocal sequencing receive the major attention in planning group language programs.

Carroll (1967) has suggested that the linguistic model should be given increased attention in studying the language development of retarded children. More specifically he is advocating studies of the phonology, morphology, syntax, and semantics of retarded children at various age levels. Both Carroll (1967) and Lenneberg (1964) have speculated that mentally retarded children undergo a "slow-motion" language development. Thus the speculation is that the mentally retarded (MR) will have linguistic codes that correspond generally to younger normal children.

Lachner (1968) used this assumption in studying language development of the retarded. He wrote grammars for five MR children ranging in MA (mental age) from 2 years 3 months to 9 years 10 months and five normal children with CAs (chronological ages) from 2 years 8 months to 5 years 9 months. From his study he concluded that language behaviors of normal and retarded children are not qualitatively different. He found that both groups follow similar developmental trends.

A strikingly different research strategy was used by Semmel in studying the grammatical skills of retarded and normal children. He used the earlier work of Brown and Berko (1960b) and Ervin (1961), which suggested that as children grow older there is a shift from primary sequential responses (syntagmatic responses) to responses from the same grammatical form class (paradigmatic responses). This progression from syntagmatic to paradigmatic word associations was suggested as evidence for an increasing grammatical competence in language functioning (Jenkins and Palermo, 1964). Semmel conducted a series of studies to investigate this general hypothesis (Semmel, Lefson, and Sitko, 1967;

Semmel and Herzog, 1966; Semmel, 1967; Semmel, Barritt, Bennett, and Perfetti, 1968).
He found that educable mentally retardates (EMRs) did indeed produce significantly
fewer paradigmatic responses than did their normal peers; however, they did not differ
from younger normal children of comparable mental ages.

McNeill (1965) has suggested that the paradigmatic shift described by previous
researchers in fact may not constitute a change in grammatical form-class usage. Semmel,
Barritt, et al. (1968, p. 575) summarize McNeill's position.

> Paradigmatic responses consist of minimal contrasts between 'dictionary
> entries', i.e., possibly because a child hears words used in many different
> contexts, he learns more and more of these words. The more semantic
> "markers" applied to words by the child, the more likely that word
> associations will be of the same form-class as the stimulus words.

McNeill also points out that the rules required for the paradigmatic association probably
occur by MA of 3½ or 4. Thus, the implicit grammatical rules which we suppose to form
the basic "motor" for paradigmatic association are mastered by children at least 3 years
before they show the paradigmatic shift. Perhaps the implication to be drawn from
Semmel's research and McNeill's observations is that a high percentage of the mentally
retarded who make infrequent use of paradigmatic associations are simply less familiar
with noun and other semantic features of the language and, in this regard, may have had
less experience with interpersonal language.

Beier et al. (1969, p. 933) summarize their work on vocabulary usage of the low
mentally retarded by stating that they had

> ... a poor sentence structure and used their time to enumerate many simple,
> uncorrelated words rather than to speak in sentences ... there is no particular
> deficit in the type of memory function needed to retain a vocabulary, but the
> mentally retarded deficit is likely to be found in conceptualization,
> organization, language structure, grammar and syntax. It is believed that this
> finding ... [should] emphasize training in conceptualization in addition to
> word training ....

Bloom (1970) points out that every study of emerging grammars confirms the
conclusion that children learn the syntax of language—the arrangements of words in
sentences—before they learn the morphological inflections of noun, verb, and adjective
forms. This observation suggests in a predictive way that mentally retarded children
would perform poorly on tests of morphology. This has indeed been the case in studies
by Newfield and Schlanger (1968), Spradlin and McLean (1967), and Lovell and
Bradbury (1967). In each case the authors found that the mentally retarded children did
not perform as well as Berko's first-grade children; in one study, Spradlin and McLean,
who tested mildly retarded institutionalized subjects, found they did not score as well as
her preschool children.

Using the Berko test, Lovell and Bradbury (1967) tested 160 EMR equivalent
children between 8 and 15 years of age and found that even those children who were

approaching "school leaving age" do less well than Berko's (1958) first graders. Furthermore, they found that these children make little progress in inflecting either lexical or nonsense words as they progress through school. Lovell and Bradbury found a limited increase in the ability to inflect at the chronological age of 8 to 15 years. They did not assume from their work that language teaching in the schools is of no avail; rather they feel that their findings suggest that special school children need a wide range of language experience embracing all aspects of morphology. They feel that lexical words will continue to be inflected as much by usage and memory as by generation. The implication from their work is similar to findings by Newfield and Schlanger (1968), but it is apparent that children learn specific morphological usages derived from memory and from direct experience and are slower than normal children in developing generative uses for less familiar words and forms. Lovell and Bradbury assume that the special-class children experience some difficulties because of their less favorable social class background, where they experience less often the complex usages displayed in middle-class homes. They also postulate, however, that special-class children at the preoperational stage of thought do not possess schemata as complex or as flexible as those of normal children. They also speculate that when the special-class child reaches a state of concrete operational thought, his schemata once again do not increase in range and flexibility as in the case of normal 8- to 12-year-old children.

Newfield and Schlanger studied 30 retarded and 30 normal elementary school children in Columbus, Ohio. Although of different chronological ages, the children were of approximately the same mental age, with the retarded subjects having a mean chronological age of 10 years 4 months and a mean mental age of 6 years 2 months, and the normal subjects having a mean chronological age of 6 years 10 months with approximately matching mental ages. They concluded that retarded children appear to learn morphology in a manner comparable to normal children but at a much slower pace. The differences were quantitative rather than qualitative. Normal children were ahead of the selected retarded children with equivalent MAs on all counts, both with nonsense and lexical forms. As an introduction to their work, they point out that errors of omission in every area of language are in line with the principle that the child learns the coarse pattern first and later refines it by development of subcontrasts and formal distinctions. The child's hazy outline becomes sharper as he matures. However, in contrast to the normal child, the retarded child seems to retain an unrefined pattern of language development as he matures. Perhaps this observation explains in part the slower and less precise development of morphological forms among special class, public school, and institutionally based mentally retarded children.

Since these studies are based upon the 1958 Berko test, it might be well to bring in a note of caution expressed by Dever (1968), who has shown that the test instrument (Berko test) does not predict morphological errors in the free speech of mentally retarded children. The test does not appear to possess predictive validity. Other tests of morphology or syntax that can be used effectively to determine linguistic development of the mentally retarded are an Exploratory Test of Grammar (Berry and Talbot), an Auditory Test of Language Comprehension (Carrow), the Northwestern Syntax Screening Test (Lee), and a Grammatical Comprehension Test (Bellugi-Klima). In addition, for measurements of comprehension or vocabulary there are other tests: for example, the Basic Concept Inventory (Engelmann), the Peabody Picture Vocabulary Test (Dunn), the Full-Range Picture Vocabulary Test (Ammons), and the Illinois Test of Psycholinguistic Abilities (McCarthy and Kirk).

COMMUNICATION DISORDERS

There is some evidence that the linguistic and nonlinguistic behavior of an individual is affected systematically when he interacts with some one who displays a communication disorder. It has been shown, for example, that normal adults restrict the diversity of language they use when talking with retarded children (Siegel, 1963; Spradlin and Rosenberg, 1964). Also the more retarded the child, the less likely are other persons to interact with him (Rosenberg et al., 1961). Chronic social isolation or restriction in the diversity of language to which he is exposed can, of course, deprive the retarded of the kinds of stimulation he might require for more nearly normal development. The dynamic properties of social interaction make it difficult to analyze in detail the communication skill in which the retardate is deficient. However, his communication pathology may be studied in terms of defects of one or more of the skills involved in the total communication process.

In reference to the model of communication presented earlier, we can analyze each of the four parts of the process[1] in terms of behavioral disorders which might interfere with communication between a child and an adult. The initial message presented by the adult might be too complex or difficult for the retarded child to understand. In such cases there is of course an incomplete or nonfunctional communication. In many instances of this kind the child simply will present the appearance of a nonspeaker. That is, he shows a kind of incomprehensible behavior which is associated with "being retarded." We might infer from this that a common problem in the communication experiences of the retarded child is in receiving messages that are not appropriate for his level of comprehension. This is, of course, not to say that he has no functional level of comprehension or that he is not an effective listener under other circumstances. We may say also that the discrimination of the listener (the retarded child) is dependent upon an effective message presented by the speaker. We might infer from this that, if the message is appropriate, the discrimination of the listener is likely to be effective and he is thus more likely to respond appropriately. If so, we might then assume that he is likely to provide a response to the speaker which will have communication value. That is to say, he will provide cues to guide the speaker in presenting a modified message. In such instances the behavior of the retarded child will be functional to the speaker and therefore more likely to provide for a continuation of the communication exchange. If we analyze this arrangement carefully, we can assume that the speech of the adults who function with retarded children—whether these adults be parent, teachers, aides, or clinicians—is important to the outcome of the communication experiences of retarded children.

[1](1)The initial verbal instruction or message, (2) the discriminative response, (3) the verbal feedback, and (4) the modified response of the speaker.

The importance of their behavior may be indicated by means of a three-term contingency, which can be described symbolically as follows:

$$S^D\text{-}R\text{-}S^R$$

As applied to the speaker, S^D represents a stimulus (probably the listener), R is the response (the speaker's message), and S^R is the reinforcing stimulus (the feedback which the speaker gets from the listener). As applied to the listener, the S^D is the message he receives from the speaker. The R is the response he provides (feedback). The S^R is an altered message. If the contingency system is viewed in this manner, it appears to be a reciprocal contingency arrangement which either positively reinforces and increases the rate of functional communication or negatively reinforces it and thus decelerates the functional communication. Rosenberg and Cohen (1967) provide a more elaborate delineation of speaker and listener variables involved in a similar communication segment.

It should be apparent in light of this discussion that a speaker and listener in a communication arrangement exchange contingent stimuli in a rapid sequence of message exchanges. Either or both participants in the experience can fail in some manner and thus will render the exchange nonfunctional. It should also be apparent that certain probabilities exist for failure in the exchange. We have already suggested one probability—that the adult message (request, explanation, command, or instruction) will not be appropriate to the comprehension level of the retarded child. One way to correct this problem, of course, would be to preinstruct the adult. Another way would be to improve the comprehension level of the child through language training.

A second probable kind of failure is through inappropriate expressive behavior of the child. Perhaps he does not provide comprehensible messages to which the adult may respond effectively. Again we have two choices: we may train the adult to be more effective in comprehending inappropriate messages, or we can teach the child to speak more effectively.

The assumptions that guide the planning of training programs of the retarded, of course, are that the child must become more effective. This means that he must listen, comprehend, and speak more like the adults in his community. His success in community living, except in the most sheltered of environments, depends upon his achieving skills that more nearly match those to whom he will be communicating.

APPROACHES TO TRAINING

Spradlin and co-workers (1970) are currently endeavoring to develop a composite program for studying and for modifying the language of retarded children. Their approaches are based directly upon several years of work at Parsons State Hospital and Training Center and other settings under the auspices of the Bureau of Child Research, University of Kansas. In a more general sense, however, the work is based upon the advances in research that have evolved in the areas of systems analysis and programming, functional analysis of behavior, and psycholinguistics. The work is designed to unify the structural and functional aspects of linguistic performance with principles of behavior modification. They seek to show that a functional program can be devised for teaching increasingly complex language. The recognition of the increasing developmental complexity requires the construction of a program of sequential steps in which later behavioral (linguistic) forms are dependent upon previously established repertoires.

With the aid of a systems analyst, the researchers have planned a training lattice (see Fig. 2) which represents a first attempt to fix the extremely complex processes of language training into an organized framework. Although the diagram is considered to be tentative in nature and will be changed as a function of further planning and research, it nevertheless serves as an overall scheme for organizing language processes in an attempt to develop a language training program. The diagram also can be used to locate gaps in our current knowledge of language acquisition as the program proceeds. The staff anticipates that a number of functional improvements will be made in the system represented by the diagram and that changes in the diagram per se will be made throughout the several years of anticipated research.

Longitudinal empirically derived language programs for low-functioning children are virtually nonexistent. Only three programs for severely and profoundly retarded children (Kirk, 1958; Lyle, 1960a,b; Bricker and Bricker, 1969) which have an emphasis on language and which have continued for a period of 15 months or longer are known to the author.

Both Kirk and Lyle were interested primarily in the general effects of an improved and stimulating environment. They used several language measures in an attempt to index the success of the program. The Bricker and Bricker project, which extended over a period of 2½ years, focused on a group of 50 severely and profoundly retarded children. Investigations were made on auditory control, motor and verbal imitation, receptive vocabularies, and various aspects of sensory-motor development. Other short-term investigations of language training with low-functioning children have been reviewed by Kirk (1964) and Spradlin (1963). As indicated by these reviews, generalizations about training procedures, training sequences, or the content of instruction are impossible to derive from these investigations because of the lack of sufficiently specific descriptions of the intervention procedures.

Language programs for moderately retarded children are more numerous, but again few have been of a long-term nature. One such long-term program has been undertaken in the Mimosa Cottage project at Parsons State Hospital. Residents of this cottage receive systematic intensive training in a variety of skill areas aimed at preparing them for life in the community (Lent, 1968). Demonstration, role playing, and practice have been the primary modes of presentation and acquisition. The purpose of the project is to develop language in children which is functional, flexible, relatively durable, and contributive to community adjustments.

Kent and co-workers (1970) have developed a language-acquisition program for severely retarded children at Fort Custer State Home in Michigan. Working under the auspices of Michigan State Department of Health and Western Michigan University, the team has attempted to synthesize the contributions of many research efforts in developmental psycholinguistics with the principles of reinforcement theory and programmed instruction. The content of their program consists of a variety of preverbal

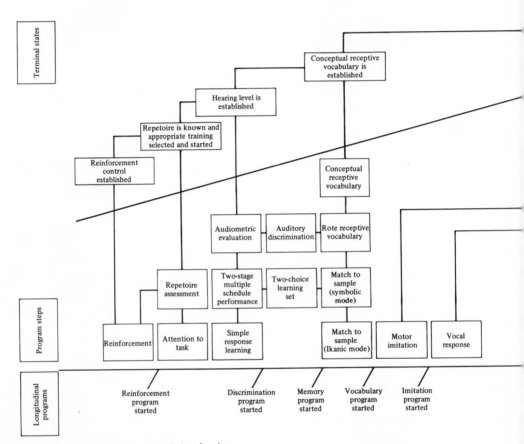

Figure 2. Language training lattice.

and beginning verbal tasks, some to be taught sequentially and some to be taught concurrently with respect to others. The program is divided into two major sections, preverbal and verbal. The preverbal section stresses the acquisition of appropriate attending behavior, motor imitation, and vocal imitation. In addition, it introduces a structured-group-play phase. The verbal section stresses the acquisition of receptive linguistic repertoire and a prelinguistic expressive repertoire. Each section (preverbal and

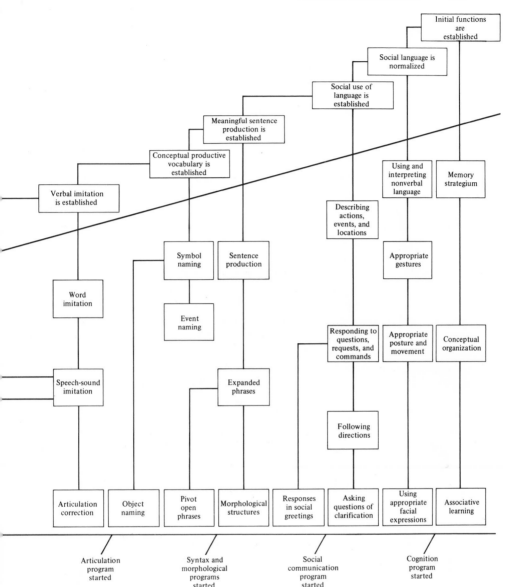

verbal) of the program is divided into phases; each phase is divided into parts; and some parts contain subparts. Each part has an initial inventory which allows the trainer to assess the child's performance of tasks he learned in that part and to discover which, if any, of the tasks to be learned in that part are already in the child's repertoire. The trainer then proceeds to attempt to teach the child those tasks on which he performed inadequately in the initial inventory. When the child appears to have mastered a particular part of a phase, the trainer administers a final inventory or test. Depending upon the child's performance, the trainer resumes or concludes training on that particular part. The child must meet criterion on the final inventory on each part before proceeding to the next.

Marshall and Hegrenes (1970) have developed a communication therapy model for "cognitively disorganized children." Their system can be applied to a variety of communication disorders seen in "cognitively disorganized children." They utilize a plan that includes four organizational areas: spatial, proprioceptive, transmission, and identity. Other authors—for instance Sommers (1969), Raymore and McLean (1970), and Miller and Yoder (1970)—have undertaken to develop training programs of a more specialized nature for retarded children. Although Sommers reported definite improvements in articulation therapy for retarded children should attempt to utilize a series of different basis of his findings, he suggested that future research concerning the efficacy of articulation therapy for retarded children should attempt to utilize a series of differnt types of carryover activities at important junctures of the therapy process. The program described in the articulation training by Raymore and McLean is in effect an effort to provide a stimulus shift program to achieve this recommended carryover. McLean (1970) points out that generalization across various stimulus types may be a major factor in the "carryover" of new responses from training situations into spontaneous speech situations. Raymore and McLean point out four dimensions of carryover with which the clinician must be concerned: (1) carryover from one stimulus condition to another stimulus condition which has less information regarding the topography of the trained response, (2) carryover of correct phoneme responses into all word positions, (3) continuation of inappropriate carryover to phonemes which are highly similar to the trained phoneme, and (4) carryover to novel situations. Their program extends stimulus control of new phoneme responses and trains the child in the initial, final, and medial word position. Their procedures are now available on film entitled *Shift of Stimulus Control*. It is available from the University of Kansas Bureau of Visual Instruction, Lawrence, Kansas.

Miller and Yoder (1970) have developed a syntax teaching program in which they make use of developmental stages which have been found operative in the acquisition of language in the normal child (Bloom, 1968). They attempt to present a developmental strategy to the child in an organized and sequential manner for constructing syntax. They employ the use of imitation, expansion of responses, and modeling of responses. In this manner they attempt to teach single words, word strings, syntactic constructions, and three-word utterances in that order. Their single-word program includes relational term substantives (referent terms). Word strings are related to topic and comment. Syntactic constructions include verb-object, subject-object, and subject-verb; and the three-word utterances include subject-verb-object and development of noun-phase instructions. The children undertaken for training in their program are those for whom there is a marked delay in the development of normal syntax functions. The teaching environment is structured to deal with those experiences which aid the child to learn and to talk about his most relevant needs and interests. The materials within the teaching environment are those which the child can handle and manipulate personally. They select words for use in the program that are taken directly from the child's comprehension repertoire. The training programs referred to briefly in this section are simply samples or examples of programs now being developed in realistic and comprehensive ways to provide stimulation, structured experiences, and long-term developmental opportunities for children with limited or severely deficient language. The general purposes of the programs obviously are to facilitate and to stimulate the acquisition of specific categories of responses or specific features or functions of language. The assumptions are that these will facilitate the acquisition of other more complex responses in subsequent periods of acquisition.

SUMMARY

The content of this chapter suggests that cognitively involved children have predictable language deficits and that these deficits are positively correlated with the involvement. The literatures on cognition and psycholinguistics are mutually relevant. Also the stages or levels can be compared and the results used to plan for language training. However, neither literature yields more than a gross picture of the structure of development. The functions for generative change from deficient levels can be sought in the fields of interpersonal learning theory and functional analysis of behavior. These areas provide the basis for behavioral assessments and management which are requisite to effective programs of training. Controversies regarding the extent of cognitive and linguistic changes that ideally can be effected have not been resolved. Programs of training now underway may possibly contribute valuable information both to the theories of cognitive and linguistic process and to the further planning of intervention strategies.

REFERENCES

Bangs, J. L. 1942. A clinical analysis of the articulatory defects of the feeble minded. J. Speech Hearing Dis., 7:343-356.

Beard, R. M. 1969. An Outline of Piaget's Developmental Psychology for Students and Teachers. New York, Basic Books.

Beier, E. B., J. A. Starkweather, and M. J. Lambert. 1969. Vocabulary usage of mentally retarded children. Amer. J. Ment. Defic., 73:927-934.

Bellugi, Ursula, and Edward Klima. 1970. Grammatical comprehension tests. In Development of Language in the Normal Child, paper presented at the Conference on Clinical Service in Speech, Language and Hearing for the Mentally Retarded held at Birmingham, Ala. March 1970.

———1958. The child's learning of English morphology. Word, 14:150-177.

———1961. The child's learning of English Morphology. In Soporta, S., ed., Psycholinguistics, p. 359-376. New York, Holt, Rinehart and Winston.

Berry, M. F. 1969. Language Disorders of Children. New York, Appleton-Century-Crofts.

———and R. Talbott. 1966. Exploratory Test of Grammar. 4332 Pine Crest Road, Rockford, Ill. 61107.

Bibey, M. 1951. A rationale of speech therapy for mentally deficient children. Training School Bull., 48:236-239.

Bilovsky, D., and J. Share. 1965. The ITPA and the Down's syndrome: An exploratory study. Amer. J. Ment. Defic., 70:78-82.

Bloom, Lois. 1968. Language development: form and function in emerging grammars. Doctoral Dissertation, Columbia University.

———1970. Semantic features in language development. Presented at the Conference on Language of the Mentally Retarded, University of Kansas, Lawrence, Kansas, January 1970.

Bricker, W. A., and D. D. Bricker. 1969. Four operant procedures for establishing auditory stimulus control with low functioning children. Amer. J. Ment. Defic., 73:(6):981-987.

Brown, R., and J. Berko. 1960a. Psycholinguistic research methods. In Mussen, P. H., ed., Handbook of Research Methods in Child Development, pp. 517-560. New York, John Wiley & Sons.

——— and J. Berko. 1960b. Word association and the acquisition of grammar. Child Develop. 31:1-14.

Bruner, J. S., R. R. Oliver, and P. M. Greenfield, 1967. Studies in Cognitive Growth. New York, John Wiley & Sons.

Carroll, J. B. 1967. Psycholinguistics in the study of mental retardation. In Schiefelbusch, R. L., R. H. Copeland, and J. O. Smith, eds., Language and Mental Retardation. New York, Holt, Rinehart and Winston.

Carrow, Elizabeth. 1970. Assessment of speech and language in children. Paper presented at the Conference on Clinical Service in Speech, Language and Hearing for the Mentally Retarded held at Birmingham, Ala. March 1970.

Carrow, Elizabeth, and Southwest Educational Development Laboratory. 1969. Auditory Test for Language Comprehension. Austin, Texas, Southwest Educational Development Corporation.

Carrow, M. A. 1968. The development of auditory comprehension of language structure in children. J. Speech Hearing Dis., 33:99-111.

Cazden, C. B. 1967. On individual differences in language competence and performance. J. Special Educ., 1:135-150.

——— 1971. Evaluation of learning in early language development. In Bloom, B. S., J. T. Hastings, and G. Madaus, eds., Formative and Summative Evaluation of Student Learning, New York, McGraw-Hill.

Chomsky, N. 1965. Aspects of a Theory of Syntax. Cambridge, Mass., The MIT Press.

de Hirsch, K., J. Jansky, and W. Longford. 1964. Oral language performance of two groups of immature children. Folia Phoniat. (Basel), 16:109-122.

Dever, R. B. 1966. A new perspective for language research. Ment. Retard., 4:20-23.

———1968. A comparison of the results of a revised version of Berko's test of morphology with the free speech of mentally retarded children. Doctoral dissertation, Madison, University of Wisconsin.

Donovan, H. 1957. Organization and development of a speech program for the mentally retarded children in the New York City Public Schools. Amer. J. Ment. Defic., 62:455-459.

Engelman, S. 1967. The Basic Concept Inventory. Chicago, Follett Publishing Co.

Ensminger, E. E., and J. O. Smith. 1965. Language development and the ITPA. Training School Bull., 62:97-107.

Ervin, S. 1961. Changes with age in the verbal determinants of word association. Amer. J. Psychol., 74:361-373.

Flavell, J. H. 1963. The Developmental Psychology of Jean Piaget. (The University Series in Psychology) New York, Van Nostrand Reinhold.

Fulton, R., and L. L. Lloyd. 1969. Audiometry for the Retarded. Baltimore, Williams & Wilkins.

Gens, G. W. 1951. The speech pathologist looks at the mentally retarded child. Training School Bull., 48:19-27.

Girardeau, F. L., and J. E. Spradlin. 1970. A functional analysis approach to speech and language behavior. Mongr. Amer. Speech Hearing Assoc.

Goda, S., and B. C. Griffith. 1962. Spoken language of adolescent retardates and its relation to intelligence, age and anxiety. Child Develop., 33:489-498.

Goldman, R., and M. Fristoe. 1969. The Goldman-Fristoe Test of Articulation. Circle Pines, Minn., American Guidance Service.

Hejna, R. 1955. Developmental Articulation Test. Storrs, Conn., R. Hejna.

Jenkins, J. J., and D. S. Palermo. 1964. Mediation processes and the acquisition of linguistic structure. Mongr. Soc. Res. Child Develop., 29:141-168.

Johnson, W., F. Darley, and D. Spriestersbach. 1952. Diagnostic Methods in Speech Pathology. New York, Harper & Row.

Jordan, T. E. 1967. Language and mental retardation: a review of the literature. *In* Schiefelbusch, R. L., R. H. Copeland, and J. O. Smith, eds., Language and Mental Retardation, Empirical and Conceptual Considerations. New York, Holt, Rinehart and Winston.

Karlin, I. W., and M. Strazzula. 1952. Speech and language problems of mentally deficient children. J. Speech Dis., 17:286-294.

Kent, L. R., and C. Kuhlmann, eds. 1962. Thought in the Young Child. Monogr. Soc. Res. Child Develop., 27:65-82.

———D. Klein, A. Falk, and H. Guenther. 1970. Fort Custer State Home, Language Acquisition Program, 1970 revision, presented at the Conference on Innovative Treatment Programs at the University of Oregon Medical School, Portland, Ore., April 1970.

Kessen, W., 1962. Stage and structure in the study of children. *In* W. Kessen and C. Kuhlman, eds. Thought in the Young Child. Monogr. Soc. Res. Child Develop., 27(2):Serial Nov. 83.

Kirk, S. A. 1958. Early education of the mentally retarded: an experimental study. Urbana, Ill., University of Illinois Press.

———1964. Research in education. *In* Stephens, H. A., and R. Heber, eds., Mental Retardation: A Review of Research. Chicago, University of Chicago Press.

Lachner, J. R. 1968. A developmental study of language behavior in retarded children. Neuropsychologia, 6:301-320.

Lee, L. L. 1969. Northwestern Syntax Screening Test. Evanston, Ill., Northwestern University Press.

Lenneberg, E. H. 1964. A biological perspective of language. *In* Lenneberg, E. H., ed., New Directions in the Study of Language, p. 65-88. Cambridge, Mass., the MIT Press.

Lent, J. R. 1968. Mimosa Cottage: experiment in hope. Psychol. Today, June 1968:51-58.

Lloyd, L. L., and R. Fulton. 1970. Assessing the hearing of the retarded and other difficult to test children. Paper presented at the Conference on Clinical Services in Speech, Language and Hearing for the Mentally Retarded, p. 23-24. Birmingham, Ala., March 1970.

Loban, W. D. 1963. The language of elementary school children. NCTE Research Report No. 1. Champaign, Ill., National Council of Teachers of English.

Lovell, K., and B. Bradbury. 1967. The learning of English morphology in educationally subnormal special school children. Amer. J. Ment. Defic., 71:609-615.

Luria, A. R. 1961. The Role of Speech in the Regulation of Normal and Abnormal Behavior. New York, Liveright Publishing Corporation.

—— and F. I. Yudovich. 1959. Speech and the Development of Mental Processes in the Child. London, Staples Press.

Lyle, J. G. 1959. The effect of an institution environment upon the verbal development of imbecile children: 1. Verbal intelligence. J. Ment. Defic. Res., 3:122-128.

—— 1960a. The effect of an institution environment upon the verbal development of imbecile children: 2. Speech and language. J. Ment. Defic. Res., 4:1-13.

—— 1960b. The effect of an institution environment upon the verbal development of imbecile children: 3. The Brooklands residential family unit. J. Ment. Defic. Res., 4:14-23.

—— 1960c. Some factors affecting the speech development of imbecile children in an institution. J. Child Psychol. Psychiat., 1:121-129.

—— 1961a. Comparison of the language of normal and imbecile children. J. Ment. Defic. Res., 5:40-51.

—— 1961b. A comparison of the verbal intelligence of normal and imbecile children. J. Genet. Psychol., 99:277-334.

Marshall, N. R., and J. R. Hegrenes. 1970. A communication therapy model for cognitively disorganized children. Presented at the Conference on Innovative Treatment Programs at the University of Oregon Medical School, Portland, Ore., April 1970.

Matthews, J. 1957. Speech problems of the mentally retarded. In Travis, L. E., ed., Handbook of Speech Pathology, pp. 531-551. New York, Appleton-Century-Crofts.

McCarthy, J. J. 1964. Research on the linguistic problems of the mentally retarded. Ment. Retard. Abstr., 2:90-96.

—— and S. Kirk. 1968. Examiners Manual, Illinois Test of Psycholinguistic Abilities (revised). Urbana, Ill., University of Illinois Press.

McDonald, E., 1964. A Deep Test of Articulation (Picture and Sentence Forms). Pittsburgh, Stanwix House.

McLean, J. E. 1970. Extending stimulus control of phoneme articulation by operant techniques. In Girardeau, F. L., and J. E. Spradlin, eds., A Functional Approach to Speech and Language. ASHA Monogr. 14:61-74.

McNeill, D. 1965. A study of word association. Unpublished paper. Cambridge, Mass., Center for Cognitive Studies, Harvard University.

—— 1967. The development of language. In Lane, H. L., and E. M. Zale, Studies in Language and Language Behavior. IV. Ann Arbor, Mich., Center for Research on Language and Language Behavior, University of Michigan.

Mein, R. 1961. A study of the oral vocabularies of severely subnormal patients. J. Ment. Defic. Res., 5:52-59.

Menyuk, Paula. 1964. Comparison of grammar of children with functionally deviant and normal speech. J. Speech Hearing Res., 7:109-121.

Milgram, N. A. 1966. Verbalization and conceptual classification of trainable mentally retarded children. Amer. J. Ment. Defic., 70:763-765.

Miller, J. F., and D. E. Yoder. 1970. A syntax teaching program (STP) circa 1970. Presented at the Conference on Innovative Treatment Programs at the University of Oregon Medical School, Portland, Ore. April 1970.

Mueller, M. W., and S. J. Weaver. 1964. Psycholinguistic abilities of institutionalized and non-institutionalized trainable mental retardates. Amer. J. Ment. Defic.,68:775-783.

Newfield, M. U., and B. B. Schlanger. 1968. The acquisition of English morphology by normals and educable mentally retarded children. J. Speech Hearing Res., 11:693-706.

O'Conner, N., and B. Hermelin. 1963. Speech and Thought in Severe Abnormality. New York, Macmillan.

Peins, Maryann. 1970. Bibliography on speech, hearing and language in relation to mental retardation, 1900-1968. Public Health Publication 2022, U. S. Department of Health, Education, and Welfare. Washington, D. C., U. S. Gov't. Printing Office.

Raymore, Sandra, and James McLean. 1970. A clinical program for articulation therapy carryover with retarded children. Presented at the Conference on Innovative Treatment Programs at the University of Oregon Medical School, Portland, Ore., April 1970.

Rosenberg, S., and B. D. Cohen. 1967. Toward a psychological analysis of verbal communication skills. In Schiefelbusch, R. L., R. J. Copeland, and J. O. Smith, Language and Mental Retardation. New York, Holt, Rinehart and Winston.

———— J. E. Spradlin, and S. Mabel. 1961. Interaction among retarded children as a function of their relative language skills. J. Abnorm. Social Psychol., 63:402-410.

Sapon, S. 1967. Operant studies in the expansion and refinement of verbal behavior in disadvantaged children. University of Rochester: Interim Report No. 3.

Schiefelbusch, R. L. 1969. Language functions of retarded children. Folia Phoniat., 21:129-144.

———— R. H. Copeland, and J. O. Smith. 1967. Language and Mental Retardation. New York, Holt, Rinehart and Winston.

Schlanger, B. B. 1961. The effects of listening training on the auditory thresholds of mentally retarded children. Cooperative Research Project, U. S. Office of Education, No. 973 (8936).

———— and R. H. Gottsleben. 1957. Clinical speech program at the training school at Vineland. Amer. J. Ment. Defic., 61:516-521.

Semmel, M. 1967. Language behavior of mentally retarded and culturally disadvantaged children. In Magary, J., and R. McIntire, eds., Distinguished Lectures in Special Education. Los Angeles, University of Southern California Press.

———— and B. Herzog. 1966. The effects of grammatical form class on the recall of Negro and Caucasian educable retarded children. Stud. Lang. Lang. Behav., 3:1966.

———— M. Lefson, and M. Sitko. 1967. Learning and transfer of paradigmatic word association by educable mentally retarded children; a preliminary report. Stud. Lang. Lang. Behav., 5:343-363.

———— L. Barritt, S. Bennett, and C. Perfetti. 1968. A grammatical analysis of word associations of educable mentally retarded and normal children. Amer. J. Ment. Defic., 72:567-576.

Siegel, G. M. 1963. Language behavior of adults and retarded children in interpersonal assemblies. J. Speech Hearing Dis. (monogr. suppl.), 10:32-53.

Sloan, W., and R. A. Cutts, 1947. Test patterns of mental defectives on the revised Stanford-Binet Scale. Amer. J. Ment. Defic., 51:394-396.

Sloane, H. N., Jr., and B. D. Macaulay. 1968. Operant procedures in remedial speech and language training. Boston, Houghton Mifflin.

Sommers, R. K. 1969. Factors in the effectiveness of articulation therapy with educable retarded children. Final report, U. S. Dept. of Health, Education, and Welfare, Project No. 7-0342, Montgomery, Ala., Public Schools, March 1969.

Spradlin, J. E. 1963. Language and communication of mental defectives. *In* Ellis, N. R., ed., Handbook of Mental Deficiency, pp. 521-555. New York, McGraw-Hill.

——— 1967. Procedures for evaluating processes associated with expressive and receptive language. *In* Schiefelbusch, R. L., R. H. Copeland, and J. O. Smith, eds., Language and Mental Retardation, Empirical and Conceptual Considerations. New York, Holt, Rinehart and Winston.

——— and J. E. McLean. 1967. Linguistics and Retardation. Parson, Kansas: Bureau of Child Research. (unpublished)

——— and S. Rosenberg. 1964. Complexity of adult verbal behavior in a dyadic situation with retarded children. J. Abnorm. Social Psychol., 68*6).

——— D. M. Baer, and Earl Butterfield. 1970. Communications Research with Retarded Children, HD 00870, to Bureau of Child Research, Lawrence, University of Kansas.

Spreen, O. 1965a. Language functions in mental retardation: a review 1. Amer. J. Ment. Defic., 69(4):482-494.

———1965b. Language functions in mental retardation: a review 2. Language in higher level performance. Amer. J. Ment. Defic., 70(3):351-362.

Staats, A. W. 1968. Learning, Language and Cognition. New York, Holt, Rinehart and Winston.

Templin, M., and F. Darley. 1960. The Templin-Darley Tests of Articulation. Iowa City, Bureau of Educational Research, State University of Iowa.

Vygotsky, L. S. 1962. Thought and Language. Cambridge, Mass., The MIT Press and New York, John Wiley & Sons.

Webb, C., S. Kinde, B. Weber, and R. Beedle. 1964. Procedures for evaluating the hearing of the mentally retarded. Cooperative research project, U. S. Office of Education, No. 1731.

Wohlwill, J. F. 1964. Piaget's theory of the development of intelligence in the concrete operations period. Paper presented at the Woods School Conference on Cognitive Models, Haddonfield, N. J. November 1964.

Zigler, E. 1964. Mental retardation: current issues and approaches. *In* Hoffman, L. W., and M. L. Hoffman, eds., Review of Child Development Research. New York, Russell Sage Foundation.

Part 3: Identification and diagnosis

9: Nonmedical diagnosis and evaluation

John V. Irwin, Jacklyn M. Moore, and Donald L. Rampp

BASES FOR COMMUNICATION

Historically, the many professions concerned with communication—both normal and abnormal—have long recognized certain prerequisites to communication. Interest in these prerequisites has reflected at least two types of motivation. In the one instance, investigators were interested in understanding normal communication. In the second instance, clinicians were interested in understanding and modifying abnormal communication. Over time, our conception of these prerequisites has, of course, varied. Relative emphases have also varied with the interest and backgrounds of particular investigators and clinicians.

The following description seeks to summarize current thinking under four headings: (1) sensory-motor, (2) cognitive, (3) emotional, (4) model and consequences.

Sensory-Motor

The successful use of language—whether oral or visual—is obviously dependent upon the ability to receive the stimuli and to produce the stimuli. Accepting the doctrine that spoken language is more basic than written language, and accepting also the doctrine that reception is basic to production, it is not surprising that interest in the precise evaluation of auditory functions and dysfunctions, and the consequences thereof to communication, has long been of scientific and clinical concern. More recently, as the importance of visual language channels in the educational process has become more generally recognized, visual and auditory dysfunctions in relationship to the reading process have been closely studied.

On the motor side, the peripheral speech mechanism has long been studied in terms of both its structure and its overt function in speaking. Recently, particularly as the impact of cybernetics has been felt, the potential importance of somatosensory input from the mechanism has been recognized. By and large, partly because of the wide tolerance for types of printing and writing, partly because of the relative motoric simplicity of writing as opposed to talking, and partly because of the availability of substitute systems such as typewriting and printing, the peripheral writing mechanism has not been studied to the extent that the peripheral speaking mechanism has been.

At the moment, we are able to generate clinically more sensory than motor data. The relative magnitude of data accumulation, however, does not necessarily reflect a complete understanding of either process.

Cognitive

The relationship of cognition to oral communication is complex. It is also ambiguous. Considerable controversy has centered about whether language makes thought possible or thinking makes language possible (Eisenson, Auer, and Irwin, 1963; Skinner, 1957: Wertheimer, 1945). Resolution of this controversy depends in part, of course, on additional data. Perhaps, even more importantly, such resolution depends upon the assumptions and definitions employed. Recently, as in the writings of Lenneberg (1967), the importance of certain types of cognitive functions as prerequisites to communication is being emphasized.

Historically, students of oral communication have been faced with two sets of data. The one set, based on man, supports the contention that intelligence as measured is related to language acquisition and usage. More precisely, a presumed general intelligence factor (as measured in conventionalized IQ type tests) can be shown to be a prerequisite for normal language development and usage. Thus, at the low extremes of intelligence, in man, language does not develop. But, at the upper extremes of intelligence, language is not necessarily more complex than in the normal ranges. This gross relationship seems to justify continued interest in general intelligence as a factor in language acquisition and usage.

But, within this gross relationship, conspicuous exceptions at the middle and upper range of intelligence have been noted. These are the children who meet the "IQ prerequisite" for language acquisition in addition to the other bases discussed in this section, and who yet do not acquire language normally. These exceptions—although always clouded by the ambiguity of testing difficulties—have long raised the possibility of some kind of language ability or function that is neurologically discrete from biological intelligence.

Data from species other than man—and particularly data from the primates—are relevant to this possibility. The chimpanzee can satisfy the "IQ prerequisite" for oral language. But he does not (and apparently cannot) acquire the oral language of man. This observation again suggests that some neurological factor other than intelligence is involved in language acquisition and usage. These data further suggest that this extra neurological factor may be species specific. Indeed, at the moment, to assume the existence of a species specific language acquisition device conveniently accounts for the rapidity of language acquisition in man, for the failures of some children to acquire language normally, and for the failure of our fellow primates to talk the way we do.

Of concern today, then, are two kinds of cognitive processes. The one—here referred to as general intelligence—continues to be of importance; the other—here referred to as a special language function—continues to acquire new stature. At the moment, both clinically and theoretically, we are able to speculate more accurately with respect to the general than to the special.

Emotional

The relationship between the emotional structure of human beings and their communicative behavior is complex. The clinical entities of stuttering and of disorders of voices have been particularly linked with emotional factors. In *hysterical* aphonia the presumed emotional basis even appears in the designation.

Many investigators have demonstrated that relationships between personality and communication can be recognized by listeners (Ball, 1958; Gilkinson and Knower, 1941; Harms, 1961). But perhaps of equal importance, the validity of these stereotypes has not been established.

Failure to communicate—or refusal to communicate readily—has been interpreted as a symptom of an individual's inner conflicts. Clinically, such behavior may be interpreted as deviant but still adaptive behavior. The experimental basis for this interpretation is still obscure.

Models and Consequences

Until recently, the role of learning in the acquisition of human language has been assumed to be relatively preeminent. Within this framework, it was convenient to recognize that French children learned to speak French; German children, German; and Japanese children, Japanese. Thus, although clinicians and linguists alike recognize the role of the model in determining the major language spoken, clinicians—and to some extent linguists—failed to recognize the possible communicative validity of variants within a language. Indeed, to the extent that dialects were recognized, with the exception of a few major geographical dialects, the recognition implied a substandard status. And, to further confound the clinical picture, many speakers of a systematic "dialect" language were not recognized as such but were regarded as nonsystematic (and therefore deviant) speakers of a standard dialect.

More bluntly, in the terminology employed by Taylor and Swinney in Chapter 2, clinicians evaluated the performance of disparate individuals against a standard competence. Traditional clinicians did not truly seek to differentiate the performance of an individual who either (1) could not learn or (2) could not successfully execute competence from the performance of an individual who was successfully executing a different competence.

The educational and social implications of this distinction are being thought—and fought—out today. Consensus has not been achieved. But the issue must be recognized even though the decision is not in.

Table 1. Traditional Classification of Organically Based Language Deficits

| | | | | Communicative functions | | | |
| | Decoding | | | | Encoding | | |
Channel	Acuity	Discrimination	Association	Central processing	Association	Motor patterns	Discrete movements
Auditory	Deafness and hearing loss	Auditory agnosias	Auditory aphasias	Categorizing Problem solving Learning	Oral aphasias	Oral apraxias	Oral paralyses
Visual	Blindness and visual loss	Visual agnosias	Visual aphasias	Storage and retrieval Language acquisition etc.	Manual aphasias	Manual apraxias	Manual paralyses

It is certainly no overstatement to suggest that some linguists and some operant psychologists have not seen eye-to-eye with respect to language acquisition. And equally certainly, this chapter is not the vehicle to attempt such reconciliation. It may be helpful, however, to note that the linguist has redrawn our attention to the importance of timing and contiguity in the development of competence even as the operant psychologist continues to insist upon the importance of the consequence.

TWO APPROACHES TO BEHAVIORAL EVALUATION

Although man has been seeking to evaluate and modify communicative behavior in both educational and medical settings for centuries, precise theories of the communicative process are relatively recent. Of these, the theory expressed by Shannon and Weaver (1964) will be emphasized, partly because its basic structure undergirds so many other theoretical formulations (Brooks, 1967), and partly because it is so applicable to disorders of communication. Nevertheless, it must be remembered that neither of the two approaches to behavioral evaluation to be emphasized in this chapter developed directly from the Shannon model.

Shannon recognized five steps in the communicative process: message source, transmitter, medium, receiver, and message destination. In human speech, the message source and the message destination are both the human brain; the transmitter, the peripheral speech mechanism with its associated tracts; the receiver, the ear with its associated tracts; and the medium, the air. It has been possible, experimentally, to clarify a great deal about the functions of the transmitter, the medium, and the receiver. But the workings of the human brain, the source and destination, remain obscure. Cognitive processing continues to defy precise evaluation.

The Traditional Clinical Approach

This description of the traditional clinical approach is exemplified in Table 1. First, noting the horizontal organization of the table, three types of activities may be recognized: decoding, central processing, and encoding. These terms reflect the basic organization of the Shannon description of communication. At the next level, the table recognizes the basic processes of acuity, discrimination, association, motor patterns, and discrete movements. Clinical terms, such as agnosia, are used in the remaining portions of the table, to specify defects in function. The vertical organization is very simple. Two channels of communication are recognized: the auditory and the visual.

The traditional speech pathologist made a sharp distinction between disorders of reception (decoding) and production (encoding). He was less certain about central processing, primarily because it is difficult to measure directly. But, for a variety of reasons, he tended to assume the existence of some type of central processing. The existence of an inner language, although not always in the sense described by Myklebust (1954), was frequently recognized.

The traditional clinician, both physician and educator, came to recognize three types of input functions and thus three types of input disorders. These steps were acuity, discrimination, and symbolic association. So far as auditory input was concerned, then, reception would break down if any one or any combination of the following events occurred: if the ear could not detect the existence of an auditory signal; if the ear could not discriminate differences in loudness, quality, and pitch (auditory agnosias); or if the semantic significance of an auditory symbol could not be established (auditory aphasia). A similar pattern existed in the visual pathway. Reading could be interfered with if the eye could not detect the existence of print on a page (blindness or visual handicap); if the eye could not discriminate form, size, color, and spatial relationships (visual agnosias); or if the semantic value of a discriminated visual stimulus could not be established (visual aphasia).

It is perhaps appropriate to expand the meaning of the clinical terms introduced above. The *agnosias* refer to the inability to discriminate in the absence of a primary acuity or detection loss; the *aphasias* refer to the inability to assign semantic values to symbols in the absence of either a loss at the acuity or discrimination level. This is a narrow definition of the term aphasia.

On the production side, the traditional language clinician again recognized three rather distinct functions and, therefore, three possible classes of disorders. These functions are the production of acoustic stimuli of precise semantic values, skilled pattern use of the peripheral speech structure or the peripheral writing structure, and the ability to perform discrete movements with the peripheral speech apparatus or the peripheral writing mechanism. Defects at the semantic level were termed expressive aphasias; defects at the motor pattern level, apraxias; and defects at the discrete movement level, paralyses. As on the input side, a hierarchy of response was recognized. Thus, ordinarily, the diagnosis of motor aphasia was made only if both pattern and discrete movements were possible; the diagnosis of apraxia was made only if discrete motions were possible; the diagnosis of discrete paralysis could, of course, stand alone.

As already stated, the details of central processing were not understood. Traditional clinicians tended to assume that basic intelligence was not necessarily impaired by either expressive or receptive interruptions up to and at the level of the aphasias themselves, although it was recognized that utilization of the intelligence would be reduced.

At issue in central processing is the question of whether the auditory and the visual channels remain separate. Recent evidence tends to support the supposition that at this level there is one symbolic mode, the auditory. If this assumption is true, then visual symbols must be interpreted ultimately in an auditory sense and must be produced ultimately from an auditory base. The possible existence of a language acquisition system at the central level also supports the notion of a single mode. Thus far, for example, acquisition curves for reading do not show the tremendous acceleration of acquisition curves for speech.

The traditional approach served two functions rather well. First, it described behavioral deficits at receptive and productive levels. Second, it provided some evidence— particularly with adults—of the clinical locus of the difficulty. Predictively, however, this approach was not particularly successful. Nor did it describe communicative behavior in linguistic terms.

Linguistic Approaches

Linguistic approaches differ from the traditional clinical approach in that they emphasize neither prerequisite behavioral functions nor locus of lesion. On the contrary, the emphasis is almost entirely upon the communicative function. As would be expected, such approaches—in contrast to the traditional clinical approach—tend to provide more detail about communication but less information about etiology. In a very real sense, these differences reflect the interest of the concerned professions. The clinician examines the process in order to change it; the linguist, in order to understand it.

Key Concepts Obviously, no one set of completely accepted linguistic postulates can be cited. But, the linguists of today, as emphasized by Tikofsky in Chapter 1, tend to concentrate their study of the communicative process around the following major functions: phonologic, syntactic, and semantic.

Phonology, as employed by linguists, embraces the sound system of oral communication. In particular, it has emphasized the phonemic structure of an oral language plus what is sometimes termed the suprasegmental features. Phonologic studies may be based on three different sets of factors: (1) physical properties, (2) production of articulation properties, and (3) perceptual properties. Physical properties include (1) the organization of the sounds, (2) insertion of sounds, (3) deletion of segments, and (4) changes in the identity of the segments. Articulation includes (1) length of sounds, (2) place and manner of articulation, and (3) which sounds begin and end words. The final division of the study of sounds is perceptual. It includes (1) length, (2) stress, (3) tone, (4) coarticulation, (5) pitch, (6) loudness, and (7) frequency. Phonological performance can be studied on either a productive or a receptive basis.

Syntax is the finite set of rules that determines the order in which the elements of a language can appear and the lawful relations among these elements. The smallest unit of syntax, the morpheme, is the minimal unit of grammatical structure that has meaning. A morpheme can be formed by a sequence of phonemes or just one phoneme. A morpheme may be a word or a stable part of a word.

Among the recognized characteristics of morphemes are the following:

1. Meaning is usually consistent.
2. Meaningless morphemes—as "to"—do exist.
3. The phonological rule may change a morpheme, as plural "s" and "z."
4. A particular sound sequence may be a morpheme at one time but not at another. Example—the "un" in unknown is a morpheme but the "un" in under is not a morpheme.
5. Morphemes may be spelled alike and pronounced differently (read and read).
6. Morphemes may be pronounced alike but spelled differently (route and root).

Three main classifications of morphemes are

1. Free vs. bound. Free morphemes can stand alone; bound morphemes cannot.
2. Full vs. empty. Full morphemes have independent meaning; empty morphemes do not.
3. Root vs. affix. A root is the core of the word of a full morpheme; affix—what is added to the root word, and in English it can be a prefix or a suffix.

The sentence is the largest unit of syntax. Although both the (1) length and (2) number of sentences in a language is theoretically infinite, sentences are generated from a finite set of symbols and in terms of a finite set of rules. At the risk of overemphasizing the separateness of morphology and syntax, it may be helpful to note that morphology is concerned with the nature and order of the word and syntax with the nature and order of the sentence.

Semantics is not always included among the prime concerns of the linguists. Increasingly, however, the psycholinguist has come to recognize that he must be concerned with the meaning of language.

Semantics, as a subsystem of language, is the study of the meaningful relationships among words, sentences, and other linguistic and nonlinguistic entities. This means that it concerns itself with the linguistic elements and the signing properties of those elements. Meaning can be evaluated productively, receptively, and in both large and small contexts.

Limitations Limitations in the linguistics approach need to be emphasized. First, many basic concepts are in a state of flux. For example, the nature of (or even the existence of) a deep structure is not unambiguous. The transformational process is not completely understood. The distinction between performance and competence, although provocative, is sometimes difficult to maintain in test situations. Norms for linguistic behavior, particularly in reception, for children, and samples not drawn from middle-class whites, are extremely limited. True longitudinal norms are virtually nonexistent for any chronological, racial, or cultural group.

The linguistic approach can describe communicative behavior. As of now, it does not automatically offer tools of modification. Nevertheless, the immediately practical implications of the linguistic approach are real. The future implications are tremendous.

LIMITATIONS IN CURRENT TESTING

It must be emphasized that, as of the present time, our ability to do complete behavioral evaluation in language disorders is at the same time both limited and spotty. Our testing is limited in the sense that we are unable to attempt certain measures. For example, direct measure of deep structure is at present beyond our clinical ability. Our testing is spotty in the sense that we can attempt certain measures with greater precision than with others. For example, the measurement of auditory perception of individual phonemes in monosyllabic environments has been well standardized; similar precision in free-running contextual units has not been achieved. Nonexistent tests and nebulous norms make both complete description and realistic production impossible. Here are some of the more serious limitations in our present evaluation procedure.

Norms

Difficulties with norms are of two types. First, and particularly true of behavioral norms but potentially true of any norm, the norm frequently reflects a particular class—such as middle-class white—rather than all possible classes. In a very real sense it is misleading, for xample, to apply the standardized norms of the Peabody Picture Vocabulary Test to an rban black population. Yet, in the absence of specialized norms, the clinician has no ther easy choice.

More obvious, but because of its very obviousness perhaps less dangerous, is the fact hat many tests are simply not standardized. Thus, Beck (1970) has developed measures f sentence complexity. These have an intuitive or face validity. But they have not been uly standardized on any definable population. The clinician, therefore, is in the dark ith respect to interpreting the performance of one child on this type of test.

mphasis on Production

s was pointed out in Chapter 2, our norms for the acquisition of language have tended) emphasize production rather than reception. This emphasis on production may stem ther from the greater identifiability of the faulty producer, from the probably greater se in testing production, or from both. In any event, although we have many studies ith respect to the age of production of a particular phoneme, we have relatively few ith respect to the age of recognition. This emphasis on production may be more true of sting at the phonological level than at other linguistic levels.

erformance versus Competence

basic assumption of behaviorism—and one which is now being brought to some critical view—is that only those data that can be independently observed are scientifically levant. Such an assumption obviously places great emphasis upon doing (which is bservable) as opposed to cognition (which is not).

The behavioristic philosophy has permeated data collection with respect to human eings. It is not surprising, therefore, that the wealth of data that we now have represents erformance in a literal sense.

But, as the distinction between performance and competence has become increas-igly clear and as the importance of the distinction has become increasingly obvious, ttention is being given to devising techniques whereby production will reveal com-etence. The work of Berko (1958), for example, is representative of this effort.

ongitudinal Data

e have remarkably few truly longitudinal studies. Most of our estimates of phoneme cquisition, for example, are based on cross-sectional rather than longitudinal approaches. lthough the cross-sectional technique yields data of great importance, findings must be iterpreted differently than from those based on longitudinal data.

igher-Level Performance

s clinicians, our attention has been on the child who does not acquire language or who cquires limited language with great difficulty. The language behavior methods that we have developed, therefore, emphasize minimal acquisition as opposed to full-scale usage. The traditional clinical diagnostic process emphasized presence or absence rather than *degree* of occurrence. This limitation becomes particularly important in any large-scale data collection attempts in relatively low-risk populations.

Central Processing

Finally, as has been noted previously, relatively little information is available with respect to central processing. Some very highly standardized measures of general intelligence are available. These, however, when evaluated strictly in terms of the assumptions on which they are based, yield relatively little information.

Age Factors

By definition, language disorders in children constitute a developmental problem. The crucial period is from birth through age 6 or 7. This range imposes several severe limitations on testing. First, and obviously, cooperation becomes a major problem. This factor complicates not only securing behavior but evaluating behavior as a best or simply as an indifferent effort. Second, unlike adult language problems, no previous self-standard of performance is available against which to measure change. This is one reason that group norms become so important. Third, current theory, as developed by McNeill (1970), suggests that age and function have crucial relations. Postponement or wait-and-see makes us carry the child beyond the crucial age. Finally, because of the limited language available, if reception is involved it is difficult to evaluate production capacities independently. A final difficulty is the fact that society has yet provided no institution—such as the school—that normally accepts children at early ages. To summarize, except in catastrophic deviation, children with developmental language problems may not even be brought into an evaluation situation until time has run out.

EVALUATION PROCEDURES

Today's clinician has available a wide variety of language related tests. Typically, the clinician's concept of the communicative process will tend to influence the battery of tests actually employed. The battery of tests to be presented in this section may be viewed as theoretical in the sense that it reflects a model. But this battery must also be viewed as practical in the sense that it reflects only the existence of tests in being today. Thus, this section will suggest both (1) the factors a clinician might like to measure and (2) those factors that current tests enable him to measure.

The Model

Earlier, in Table 1 a traditional classification of organically based language deficits was developed. Figure 1 reflects the clinical emphasis of Table 1 but attempts also to relate clinical evaluation to current linguistic and behavioral concepts. The figure is basically organized around oral language, but provision is made for written language and for simple

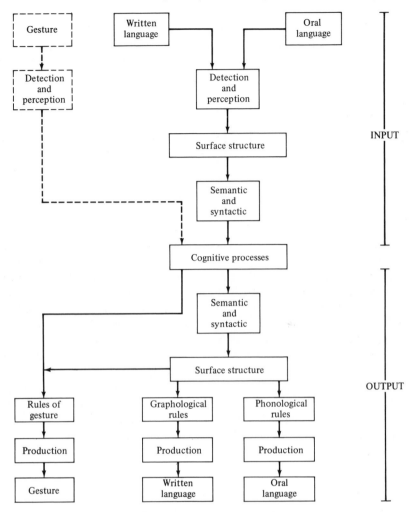

Figure 1. Proposed clinical model of communicative processes.

se of gesture. The figure may conveniently be read from top to bottom, with the input of actual oral or written language samples being shown in solid lines at the top and the output of actual written or oral samples being shown in solid lines at the bottom.

On the input level, (1) gesture and (2) detection and perception are shown with dashed lines; on the output level, the gesture function is shown in solid lines. This differentiation reflects the assumption that if gesture is the only intact input function, a true language process at either the input or output level will not develop. On the other hand, if simple gesture is the only intact output function, true language may develop as the result of oral and written input.

As of the present writing, it is not possible to evaluate each of the units diagrammed with equal precision. Even recognizing this fact, however, the model does have the advantage of both indicating the need for further test development and for providing rationale for reinterpretation of present tests. One example may make this clear. A chi whose surface structure is compatible with Standard English may produce oral sampl that deviate from standard pronunciation. The model suggests that such deviation ma result from (1) the inability to produce the sounds acceptably with his peripheral speec mechanism, (2) the faulty learning of the phonological rules of Standard English, (3) tl mastery of the phonological rules of a different (but not necessarily defective) dialect, (4) a combination of these. Thus, the model provides both for cultural and for individu differences. The traditional model emphasized individual differences.

Definition   It will be remembered that the model is basically organized around or language. Nevertheless, because of clinical and educational significance, provision is mad for an evaluation of written language. Basic definitions follow.

Written and oral language. An oral language is a set of phonological, syntactic, an semantic rules that enable humans to speak with each other about topics of mutu concern. A written language represents these rules by orthographic features.

Detection and perception. Detection is defined as the ability to react to the presenc or absence of either an auditory or visual stimulus. Perception is the ability to organiz the sensory response in terms of (1) physiological correlates and (2) learned or triggere rules. Detection is a prerequisite to but not a guarantee of perception. Although both th ear and the eye are peripheral sense organs, both detection and perception involve cortic function. Breakdowns in detection result primarily from physical factors, althoug emotional factors may be involved. Breakdowns in perception, on the other hand, ma relate primarily to learning experiences.

Surface structure: input. The term surface structure is more applicable to or language than to written language. As used here, the surface structure is a string c phonemes. As such, it represents a highly organized perceptual process. In writte reception, the surface structure may still be viewed as a string of phonemes, although i this instance the string has been interpreted from visual rather than from auditory stimul

Semantic and syntactic: input. The perceived surface structure can function a language input only if the listener or reader is able to apply rules of association and orde to the surface structure. Thus, the individual who does not know the symbolic associatio of a word or the principles of order in a sentence would be unable to interpret surfac structure. Both of these processes are dependent upon experience with a language; the may also be affected by other cultural, behavioral, and/or biological factors.

Cognitive processes. The term cognitive processes, as defined here, assumes tha language is dependent upon, rather than basic to, functioning intelligence. As indicate earlier, no definitive definition of the cognitive processes can be stated today. Appa ently, however, these processes would include such functions as categorizing, probler solving, learning, and storage and retrieval.

Semantic and syntactic: output. The basic concept generated in the cognitive proces can be transformed to surface structure only by application of semantic and syntacti principles. These principles provide for an orderly relationship between the cognitiv process and the surface structure.

Surface structure: output. Again, surface structure is primarily relevant to oral language. Surface structure may be conveived of as a strong of phonemes, not yet phonetically produced (Langacker, 1968).

Graphological and phonological rules. The string of phonemes in the surface structure can be converted either to writing or to oral speech only by the application of basic rules. For example, the rule tells the English speaker to aspirate the /p/ of *pin* but not the /p/ of *spin.*

Production. Production is the physical execution of the phonological and graphological rules for actual surface structures. Production, in the sense used here, is primarily dependent upon an intact physiological mechanism. Thus, a sharp distinction is being drawn between the rules, on the one hand, and the ability to execute the rules, on the other.

Written and oral language. These are the final outputs, either in an auditory or a visual medium.

Gesture. This term is employed in this model in a very limited sense. The term refers primarily to pointing or other spatial indicating functions. It expressly does not apply to such possible activities as fingerspelling or other symbolic applications. As defined, gesture does have validity in certain test situations as a measure of input and cognitive processing. Such gesture, however, cannot substitute for intact oral and written input channels.

An Outline of Current Tests

An outline of tests currently available is now presented. The outline follows the general organization of the proposed model and includes under each functional unit any relevant tests. It should be recognized that the location of a particular test is sometimes arbitrary in that a single test may cross several functions. Following the presentation of the outline, a systematic abstract of each of the designated tests is offered.

I. Input
    A. Detection
        1. Auditory:
            Pure-tone screening and threshold
        2. Visual:
            Ophthalmologist
    B. Perception
        1. Auditory:
            a. Word:
                Speech reception threshold
                Audiometric speech discrimination
            b. Phoneme:
                Goldman-Fristoe-Woodcock Test of Auditory Discrimination
                Wepman's Auditory Discrimination Test

    2. Visual
        a. Form:
            Bender-Gestalt Test for Young Children
            Frostig Developmental Test of Visual Perception
            Meeting Street School Screening Test
        b. Symbolic (letter and number):
            Doren Diagnostic Reading Test of Word Recognition Skills
            ITPA-Visual Reception and Visual Closure Subtests
            Peabody Individual Achievement Test
            Meeting Street School Screening Test

C. Semantic
    Full-Range Picture Vocabulary Test
    ITPA-Auditory Reception, Auditory Vocal Association, and
      Visual Motor Association Subtests
    Peabody Picture Vocabulary Test
    Picture Articulation and Language Screening Test (visual)

D. Syntactic
    1. Word:
        Doren Diagnostic Reading Test of Word Recognition Skills
        Durrell Analysis of Reading Difficulty
        Michigan Picture Language Inventory
    2. Sentence:
        Doren Diagnostic Reading Test of Word Recognition Skills
        Durrell Analysis of Reading Difficulty

II. Cognitive processes
    Goodenough-Harris Drawing Test
    Illinois Test of Psycholinguistic Abilities (ITPA)
    Meeting Street School Screening Test
    Peabody Individual Achievement Test (PIAT)
    Stanford-Binet Intelligence Scale
    Wechsler Intelligence Scale for Children

III. Output
    A. Semantic
        Basic Concept Inventory
        ITPA—Verbal Expression, Manual Expression, and Auditory Vocal
          Association Subtests
        Meeting Street School Screening Test
        PIAT—General Information Subtest
    B. Syntactic
        1. Word
            Berko Test of Exploratory Grammar
            ITPA—Grammatical Closure Subtest
            Measures of Verbal Output

2. Sentence
   Measures of Verbal Output
   Meeting Street School Screening Test
   Northwestern Syntax Screening Test

C. Overt Response
  1. Rules
     a. Phonological
        Berko Test of Exploratory Grammar
        ITPA–Grammatic Closure Subtest (with examiner
          interpretation)
     b. Graphological
        Doreen Diagnostic Reading Test of Word Recognition Skills
        Durrell Analysis of Reading Difficulty
  2. Production
     a. Oral
        (1) Word
            Goldman-Fristoe Test of Articulation–
              Sounds-in-Words Subtest
            Picture Articulation and Language Screening Test
            Predictive Screening Test of Articulation
            Templin-Darley Tests of Articulation
        (2) Co-articulation
            Goldman-Fristoe Test of Articulation–
              Sounds-in-Sentences Subtest
            McDonald Deep Screening Test of Articulation
            Templin-Darley Tests of Articulation
     b. Gesture
        Full-Range Picture Vocabulary Test
        Goldman-Fristoe-Woodcock Test of Auditory Discrimination
        ITPA–Manual Expression Subtest
        PIAT–Reading Recognition, Mathematics, Reading Comprehension
          and Spelling Subtests
        Peabody Picture Vocabulary Test

IV. Broad-comprehensive
    Communication Evaluation Charts
    Houston Test for Language Development
    Utah Test of Language Development
    Verbal Language Development Scale

ACUITY MEASURES

Category: Input-Detection-Auditory-Pure Tone

So far as the development of oral language is concerned, auditory acuity is of prime importance. Pure-tone testing of the hearing of infants and young children is now practicable. Such testing, however, should be attempted only by an experienced audiologist using proper equipment. If such personnel and equipment are not available, behavioral observations as described by the Ewings (1961) and by Myklebust (1954) may be cautiously substituted. With older children, pure-tone testing becomes simpler and more reliable. But the importance of early testing has already been emphasized.

Tests utilized in the evaluation of the peripheral hearing mechanism can be divided into two categories, that is, pure-tone and speech reception audiometry. The two categories are not mutually exclusive and the results from one category can be useful when evaluated in conjunction with results from the other category. Auditory acuity measurements involve an external auditory stimulus to which the child must respond appropriately. Observation of the response pattern gives information regarding the hearing status of the child.

Pure-tone tests are designed to indicate the faintest sounds to which a person can respond. The stimulus is a pure tone of a specific frequency. Several frequencies are employed to obtain a graphic configuration of the person's hearing acuity across the range of audible frequencies. The intensity, in decibels, of each frequency is varied systematically to ascertain the lowest intensity level that the person can hear. Pure-tone air- and bone-conduction testing is necessary when precise acuity thresholds are needed. These tests ideally would be done in a sound-treated acoustic room with the patient under earphones.

Screening procedures can be utilized with pure-tone testing. Pure-tone audiometric screening is a popular technique when large numbers of persons must be tested. The purpose of such screening techniques is to establish if a hearing loss exists. It is not designed to reveal the nature or extent of the hearing loss. The most frequently used method of pure-tone audiometric screening is the sweep-frequency technique. In this procedure the examiner sets the intensity dial of the audiometer at a specific intensity level above the environmental noise present in the testing situation. This level is usually 10 to 15 decibels ISO. If a large group is being tested the amount of available rechecking time may be a factor in the selection of the intensity level to be utilized. With a greater intensity, there will be fewer subjects to fail the screening procedures. Both ears should be tested at 500 Hz, 1,000 Hz, and 2,000 Hz; these are the so-called speech frequencies that is, the frequencies where the majority of speech sounds occur. The subject should respond to all frequencies. Failure occurs when the subject does not respond to any one frequency in either ear. Some examiners feel that if the subject fails the sweep screening procedure, he should be screened utilizing the same procedure a second time. If he fails the second screening procedure, he should be referred for a complete audiologic workup. Other examiners prefer to have all subjects who fail the first test evaluated for specific thresholds.

Carhart and Jerger (1959) advocate the Hughson-Westlake technique for determining pure-tone thresholds. The pure-tone stimulus should have a duration of 1 or 2 seconds and the first tonal presentation is presented at an intensity level well above the subject's probable threshold. After the subject responds, the intensity is reduced in 10- to 15-decibel steps until an inaudibility level is reached. At that point, intensity is increased in 5-decibel steps until the subject responds again. Intensity is then reduced another 10 to 15 decibels and another ascent in 5-decibel steps is begun. As long as the subject does not respond, each presentation is made 5 decibels stronger than its predecessor. The examiner records the levels at which the responses occur. Practically, three responses at a single intensity may be accepted as threshold for that particular frequency. The frequency range to be tested is 125, 250, 500, 1,000, 2,000, 4,000, and 8,000 Hz. The Hughson-Westlake method is applicable for both air and bone conduction testing. The only restrictions in bone conduction are those imposed by the reduced hearing levels which are testable on audiometers.

The use of masking noise is an integral part of audiometric evaluations. The air-conducted tone at approximately 60 decibels HL is capable of vibrating the bones of the skull, causing stimulation of the cochlea in the nontest ear. This must be considered when the subject's threshold indicates an asymmetrical loss, that is, if one ear is considerably worse than the other.

When air- and bone-conduction scores are approximately equivalent at each frequency, the hearing loss is considered to be sensory-neural in nature. When bone-conduction thresholds are better than air-conduction thresholds, the hearing loss is considered conductive in nature. Conductive losses are most likely to be amenable to medical treatment by otologists; ironically, these are also the losses that are most benefited by amplification. The presence or absence of an air-bone gap is a diagnostic feature of the audiometric configuration.

SPEECH RECEPTION AUDIOMETRY

Category: Input-Perception-Auditory-Word

The reception of oral language is the prime function of the peripheral hearing mechanism. It follows, then, that some of the most pertinent audiometric tests utilize the spoken word. The ability to perceive speech is not always predictable from pure-tone thresholds.

One test that audiologists find valuable is the speech reception threshold, the purpose of which is to ascertain the lowest intensity level at which a person can understand spoken words. The speech material can be administered either by live voice or recorded word lists. The two-syllable words utilized are common words in which equal emphasis is placed on each syllable; these are known as spondaic words or spondees.

The person being tested should be familiar with the words of the test, and they should be presented one at a time at a level adequately loud for the person to hear and repeat them. When the person repeats the first three words the intensity is reduced 10 decibels. If the next three words are repeated correctly, the intensity level is again reduced by 10 decibels. This procedure is continued until the person starts missing some of the words. The intensity should continue to be reduced until the person misses four consecutive words. At this point, intensity is then increased in 2-decibel steps with test words being presented at each level. After two ascending runs, the level at which the person repeats three of six words presented is considered the speech reception threshold.

AUDIOMETRIC SPEECH DISCRIMINATION

Category: Input-Perception-Auditory-Word

Once a speech reception threshold (SRT) has been attained, discrimination testing is initiated to ascertain how well the subject can understand the spoken word. The materials for this test vary from monosyllabic words to sentences. Usually, a group of 50 one-syllable words representative of the occurrence of speech sounds in English, phonetically balanced (PB) words, are presented well above the speech reception threshold. The subject repeats each word and his test score is the percentage of test words repeated correctly.

Because of the intensity/discrimination relationship, the intensity level of 40 decibels above the subject's SRT should be sufficiently loud for him to achieve a 100 percent score. If the 40-decibel sensation level is too intense for the subject, the intensity may be reduced and noted in the interpretation of results.

Loss of the ability to discriminate may be indicative of a sensory-neural type of hearing loss, whereas no loss of discrimination ability is usually apparent in conductive hearing impairments. Generally, the results of the tests indicate how socially adequate the hearing acuity of the subject is and whether or not he is a candidate or would benefit from amplification with a hearing aid.

THE BASIC CONCEPT INVENTORY

Category: Output-Semantic

Description   The Basic Concept Inventory was developed by Siegfried E. Engelmann. The purpose of the inventory is to evaluate what concepts of learning a child has acquired. The author refers to this as a criterion-referenced measure as defined by Robert Gaser (1963) in comparison to a norm-referenced test. The inventory allows one to establish a basal level of function in various conceptual areas, thus enabling objectives of training to be formulated.

The test is recommended for preschool children through grade 3. However, it can be used with children 10 years of age. Some of the basic concepts covered include concepts of *not*, *more than*, *and*, *on*, and *big*. The test is divided into three parts. Part One is Basic Concepts, Part Two is Statement Repetition and Comprehension, and Part Three is Pattern Awareness.

The test is administered on an individual basis; however, group interpretation may be made for classroom work.

The inventory materials consist of a set of nine picture cards, response booklet, and manual. The manual contains administration procedures, case studies, discussion of interpretation, general information, and technical data.

Source and Price
   Follett Educational Corporation

Department DM
P. O. Box 5705
1010 West Washington Blvd.
Chicago, Illinois 60607

Complete set	$19.32
Manual	2.16
Picture cards	2.58
Basic concept inventory,	
15 per package	2.97

Discussion Currently the Basic Concept Inventory has only been published in an experimental edition. Validity and reliability studies are forthcoming. There are no age norms available for the experimental edition; the author does not feel this is critical for a criterion-referenced measure.

Interpretation of the inventory must go beyond saying a particular concept was failed; one must ask why. The "why" should be discovered through systematic work with the child from guidelines suggested by his performance on the inventory.

THE BENDER GESTALT TEST FOR YOUNG CHILDREN (KOPPITZ NORMS)

Category: Input-Perception-Visual-Form

Description The rationale for this test, according to its author, Lauretta Bender, is based on findings that maturity in visual-motor-perception is largely a function of age and intelligence. It is a drawing test to be used with children of 5 to 10 years or retarded adults that fall in that mental-age range. The intention of this procedure is to estimate visual perception through a motor response. It is helpful as a tool to aid in the determination or presence of brain damage. This test may also be used as a reference of intellectual functioning. The test requires individual administration.

Test administration requires the subject to draw a series of nine model designs. A design is shown to the subject and not removed until the subject has completed his drawing. The subject draws with a pencil on a sheet of plain white paper. The designs are sequenced, moving from simple to complicated designs. Drawing ability does not influence test results and hearing is not a part of the test.

The test is scored by means of a checklist provided for each item regarding rotation integration, direction, or perseveration. Scoring is relatively objective and based on deviations of the drawings. E. M. Koppitz (1964) provided norms with information concerning administration and scoring.

Source and Price

The Psychological Corp.
304 East 45th St.
New York, New York 10017

Examiner's set includes
monograph, design cards,
and directions $7.00

Discussion This test was standardized utilizing 1,104 school children between the ages of 5 and 10 in eastern and midwestern states. The Bender correlated with IQ scores at 0.50, with the best reliability as a test of intelligence between the ages of 5 and 7. It is a good predictor of school achievement in grades 1 to 3. Emotional disturbances are evaluated in six deviant categories. Greatest value in identifying brain damage is in repeated testing for the presence of progressive lesion or regression. Scorer reliability correlations ranged from 0.88 to 0.96 with test/retest correlations significant at the 0.001 level. Koppitz tested 165 first and second graders to establish validity, and eliminated those items which did not differentiate good and poor students.

The primary restriction of this test is in the interpretation of results. The test is easy to administer and score, but, according to Bender (1965) ". . . requires informed, interested, and experienced workers, as does any other scientific method." It is a very popular tool that is frequently used with a retarded population.

BERKO EXPLORATORY TEST OF GRAMMAR

Category: Output-Syntactic-Word
Output-Overt Response-Rules-Phonological

Description The Berko test was originally designed as a study to explore children's ability to apply basic morphological rules to new words. Thus, it provided information regarding the procedures and patterns of grammar and additional knowledge of the systems utilized in the acquistion of language. This study analyzed the vocabulary used by children and the morphological rules they employed. It was found that all English inflectional morphemes were present in children 4 through 7 years of age.

The specific areas investigated by this test are plurals, possessives, verb tenses, derivations, and compound words. Pronouns were omitted due primarily to irregularity of form and difficulty devising appropriate new pronouns. Nonsense words and several actual words are used in the examination. The nonsense words which represent the names of animals or depict individuals performing actions are illustrated in such a way as to prevent the child from associating these with real animals or people. There are 28 test items and 27 items employing pictures. The pictures are drawn in color representing words. Test administration takes approximately 15 minutes.

Source and Price Unpublished.

Discussion The Berko Exploratory Test of Grammar is not a standardized instrument. The subjects of this study included both adults and children. The adult responses were considered accurate and used as a base to judge the answers of the children. Several questions which were answered from this study show that children do extend and operate with morphological rules. The results of the test indicated that there was no significant sex differences employing a chi-square criterion with Yates's correction applied. There were some significant differences in performance between preschool and first-grade children. Reportedly, they were refining what knowledge they possessed.

Tables are available from this study that illustrate distribution of children at each age level for comparison of the sexes, age differences on inflectional items, percentages of children supplying correct plural forms, percentages of children supplying correct verb forms, and percentages of children supplying correct possessive forms. Many investigators are now devising tests employing Berko's technique to study language acquisition. Children enjoy this type of test because of the uniqueness of the nonsense pictures and words. Motivation of the subject is usually good, administration is simple. It is a good screening device in the areas of morphology and syntax.

COMMUNICATION EVALUATION CHARTS

Category: Broad-Comprehensive

Description This chart can be utilized as a quick appraisal of a child's abilities in language and performance. This scale was constructed to assess a child's comprehension abilities or disabilities in language. The communication evaluation chart (CEC) is composed of two groups of items in language and performance areas. It can be administered by various professional disciplines. The prime function of the chart is to determine if a child is functioning within normal limits or if he needs to be referred for more extensive evaluation.

Source and Price

Educators Publishing Service, Inc.
75 Moulton St.
Cambridge, Massachusetts 02138

20¢ each

Discussion The items were taken from various standardized sources such as Gesell and Cattell. Therefore, the authors did not restandardize the items utilized in the scale. The CEC is a beneficial tool especially useful for unskilled examiners. Results may be quickly surveyed and compared to a child's chronological age to determine if the child is functioning below average limits. It contains the same disadvantages that any such screening device exhibits.

The CEC chart includes directions and blanks for scoring. A plus (+) sign is used to indicate an item is present. A minus (−) sign is used to indicate that a function is not present and a plus and minus (±) sign indicates that the item fluctuates.

The chart is divided into nine age levels. The age levels are 3 months, 6 months, 9 months, 1 year, 1.5 years, 2 years, 3 years, 4 years, and 5 years.

Information for the chart may be obtained through an interview technique or direct observation.

DOREN DIAGNOSTIC READING TEST OF WORD RECOGNITION SKILLS

Category: Input-Syntactic-Word
   And Various Subtests in Other Categories

Description The Doren Diagnostic Reading Test of Word Recognition Skills was developed by Margaret Doren for the purpose of analyzing a child's basic skills of word recognition. Administration of the test is intended for primary and intermediate grades. Group testing is usual; however, it can be administered individually.

There are 390 test items, which form 11 divisions called units. The units are Unit I, Letter Recognition; Unit II, Beginning Sounds; Unit III, Whole Word Recognition; Unit IV, Words within Words; Unit V, Speech Consonants; Unit VI, Ending Sounds; Unit VII, Blending; Unit VIII, Rhyming; Unit IX, Vowels; Unit X, Sight Words; and Unit XI, Discrimination Guessing.

Test instructions are suggested but may be modified to meet a child's specific needs. The number of accurate responses are recorded on the score sheet. The number of inaccurate responses may be plotted on a profile that allows interpretation of areas which need special attention. The materials needed are test booklets, score sheets, and manual of instructions.

Source and Price

American Guidance Service, Inc.
Publisher's Building
Circle Pines, Minnesota 55014

Tests, per package of 25	$4.85
Manual	1.75
Complete set special translucent overlay keys	1.50
Specimen set, with manual (without special keys)	2.00

Discussion Validity and reliability studies are few in number. However, a 0.90 correlation of Reading Achievement with the Coordinated Scales of Attainment was reported. Reliability studies indicate a 0.53 for Letter Recognition and an 0.88 for Blending.

The instruction manual contains suggestions for designing programs of study. This diagnostic instrument is designed to provide an educator valuable guidance with class grouping and curriculum selection. Thus, the practical utility of this test and curriculum guidelines appear good.

DURRELL ANALYSIS OF READING DIFFICULTY

Category: Input-Syntactic-Sentence
      And Various Subtests in Other Categories

Description The Durrell Analysis of Reading Difficulty was developed by Donald D. Durrell for the purpose of detecting reading problems which are amendable through adjustments of educational procedures. The test is designed for administration from a nonreader level to an intermediate (sixth-grade) level. The test assumes no physical disabilities. It is composed for three reading levels: nonreader, or preprimer, level; primary-grade reading level; and intermediate-grade reading level. The test is divided into specific parts: Oral Reading Tests, Silent Reading Tests, Listening Comprehension Tests, Supplementary Paragraphs, Word Recognition and Word Analysis, Visual Memory of Word Forms, Auditory Analysis of Word Elements, and Spelling and Handwriting. Suggestions for supplementary tests and observations are also presented.

Materials required are a manual of directions, reading paragraph booklet, tachisto-scope, individual record booklets, and stopwatch. The time required to administer the Analysis is from 30 to 90 minutes. It should only be administered by experienced teachers or diagnosticians.

Testing procedures are explained for each part of the analysis. Norms are given for most parts of the test. On the front of each record booklet a profile chart is provided for recording grade, age, and norms in oral reading, silent reading, listening comprehension, word recognition, word analysis, and spelling and handwriting.

Source and Price

   Harcourt Brace Jovanovich
   Test Department
   757 Third Ave.
   New York, New York 10017

   Examiner's kit $6.90

Discussion The majority of the tests included in the analysis have been standardized on, minimally, 1,000 children. Test results have been compared to other tests and are reported to correlate well.

The Durrell is a comprehensive instrument. The checklists are the most important feature of the test. The items on the checklists are those of highest frequency and significance in remedial work. The items failed indicate what areas need remediation, which is the basic purpose of the analysis.

The Analysis is an individual test and not designed for group administration. Other instruments would be employed for screening. Low performance on screening tests would indicate the need of this type of analysis.

THE FROSTIG DEVELOPMENTAL TEST OF VISUAL PERCEPTION

Category: Input-Perception-Visual-Form

Description The Frostig Developmental Test of Visual Perception was constructed to measure and identify disabilities of specific visual perceptual functions. It is not a prognostic tool of reading ability. The functions viewed are in five different areas, each of which is a separate subtest. The five subtests are eye-hand coordination, figure-ground perception, form constancy, position in space and spatial relationships. Norms are given for ages 4 through 8, but it may be used with other children.

The test battery is composed of a 35-page test booklet which includes a scoring sheet, a set of 11 demonstration cards, 3 transparent scoring tissues, 4 colored pencils, a regular pencil, an administration and scoring manual, and a 1963 standardization manual. Instructions are given for each test item in the administration manual. This test is verbal but alternative instructions may be used for subjects who have special limitations, such as a hearing handicap.

Test administration may be on a group or individual basis. The approximate testing time for an individual is 45 minutes. Grading of the test may be completed in about 7 minutes. Objective grading procedures are given in the administration manual.

Scale scores may be transmuted to a perceptual age equivalent or perceptual quotient. The perceptual age equivalent is the average age of achievement and is given for each subtest. The perceptual quotient is reported to be more reliable as a prognostic indicator than the perceptual age. Individual scores are not a satisfactory index when viewed in isolation.

Source and Price

Consulting Psychologists Press
577 College Ave.
Palo Alto, California 94306

Manual	$ 3.00
Specimen set	5.00
Test booklets, 25	11.00 (or $0.50 each)
Examiner's kit	10.50

Discussion This test is not well-standardized. A population of 2,116 was utilized, with 88 for each group of norms. The population was from a rather restricted area and no reliable information regarding socioeconomic class was available. The test-retest reliability ranged from 0.69 to 0.98 and split-half correlations for the 4-year intervals from 0.74 to 0.89. Product moment and chi-square correlations with classroom teacher ratings were 0.441.

Studies completed with the Frostig indicate that development of perceptual abilities is greatest between 4 and 7 years of age. The visual perceptual activities are reported to develop in a definite progression. The manual purports that the items of each subtest were chosen and formed to maximize a pure test avoiding pollution of the specified ability.

The Frostig is utilized frequently in clinical settings. Educators have become aware of the role of visual perception in learning and behavior, thus rapidly increasing its use in educational settings. A common pitfall is that unskilled examiners attempt to administer, interpret, and recommend therapeutic programs, thus confounding the child's problems by using the results of a test whose validity is questionable.

Since the standardization is weak, this test should not be used as a criterion. It may be most useful as a test-retest to monitor improvement following a specific program. It is the only test of its kind available and Frostig has designed a series of worksheets for remedial help that accompany the test. Another restriction is that it is a time-consuming test to administer and is relatively expensive.

THE FULL-RANGE PICTURE VOCABULARY TEST

Category: Input-Semantic
   Output-Overt Response-Production-Gesture

Description   This test was developed by Robert B. Ammons and Helen S. Ammons. The Full-Range Picture Vocabulary Test is a measurement of verbal comprehension of single words, not unlike the Peabody Picture Vocabulary Test. The age range for the Full-Range Picture Vocabulary Test (FRPVT) is from 2 years through adult levels.

Test materials are composed of 16 picture plates with each plate containing 4 cartoon-like black-and-white line drawings. There are from 1 to 11 test words for each plate. There are two forms, A and B, each having 85 test words listed according to chronological age. One additional plate includes the administration and scoring procedures. Answer sheets for each test form contain space for recording of the score obtained on each plate.

Test administration involves an examiner speaking a test word with the subject directed to point to the picture which indicates what the word means. If the subject is unable to point to the picture the examiner can point and have the subject indicate a yes/no response. The FRPVT does require adequate vision but can be adapted for administration to motorically involved or hearing-handicapped persons if they are able to read. The instructions suggest a checkmark to indicate a correct response and a circle to indicate a wrong response marked next to the test word. It is suggested that the order of presentation of test words be varied to maintain interest.

A basal and ceiling are determined for each test plate by passing or failing three consecutive point levels. Norms are given on the reverse side of the word-list form. The total raw score transmutes into a mental age or adult percentile rating if over 16.5 years. Interpolation is necessary for some scores.

Source and Price

Psychological Test Specialists
Box 1441
Missoula, Montana 59801

Test kit with set of plates, instructions,
   norms, and sample answer sheets $7.50
Set of forms A or B, 100 per package   4.00

Discussion   The Full-Range Picture Vocabulary Test is a standardized test. Norms were determined by a sampling of 589 cases of the general population from 2 years of age through adult levels. Reliability is 0.93, and validity is reportedly high. Correlation with the Stanford-Binet vocabulary subtest resulted in high reliability and validity. There are separate norms for white farm children, Spanish-American children, and Negro children and adults.

The Full-Range Picture Vocabulary test is easy to administer but not as easily scored as some other available one-word vocabulary tests of word usage. The drawings in this test contain artifacts that may be confusing to the child taking the test. Many of the drawings are also very dated, and modern children are unable to recognize some of the items.

GOLDMAN-FRISTOE TEST OF ARTICULATION

Category: Output-Production-Oral-Word
Output-Production-Oral-Co-articulation

Description   The Goldman-Fristoe Test of Articulation was developed by Ronald Goldman and Macalyne Fristoe. The purpose of the Goldman-Fristoe test is to provide a systematic means of assessing an individual's articulation of consonant sounds. It has three subtests: (1) the Sounds-in-Word Subtest, which was designed to sample all but one of the consonants that appear in spoken English; (2) the Sounds-in-Sentences Subtest, which samples a smaller number of phonemes, that is, those most likely to be misarticulated; and (3) the Stimulability Subtest, which samples a smaller number of phonemes, that is, those most likely to be misarticulated. It tests articulation at two levels, including judgments for the presence of an error and judgments as to the type of error. Testing and scoring time is approximately 10 minutes. There are 44 picture cards in a spiral-bound folder. Age range is 2 years and above. Thirty-six of the pictures are of familiar objects for elicitation of spontaneous speech of a single-word level. This is assumed to measure the general production of the sound, not just the sound production in a specific word. Twenty-three consonant phonemes in English are measured plus 12 consonantal blends. For examination of connected speech there are two story sets. The stories are first read by the examiner and then the child is asked to retell the story as he is shown the pictures. An alternative method of test presentation is offered. There is also a filmstrip version of 60 full-color frames which is optional. Recording of responses is completed on a color-coded form which reflects the child's articulatory profile.

Source and Price

American Guidance Service, Inc.
Publishers Building
Circle Pines, Minnesota 55014

Complete G-F easel-kit $19.00
(includes 44 spiral-bound
pictures, 50 response forms,
and manual)

Response forms, per package of 50	3.50
Manual	1.50
G-F filmstrip, 60 full-color frames	7.50

Discussion   Test-retest reliability in Sounds-in-Words Subtest, median agreement, for the presence or absence of error and for type of error, was 0.95 and 0.89, respectively. The Sound-in-Sentences subtest was 0.94 and 0.85, respectively. Interrater reliability for Sounds-in-Words subtest was 0.92 and 0.88, respectively, and intrarater reliability for Sounds-in-Words was 0.91 for both presence or absence of error and for type of error. This test does not allow for any specific comparison of its results to that of others. Results of the test are often compared to normative studies of articulation, usually those of Mildred Templin (1957), to see what the defective sounds are in relation to the age at which children often master the sounds. Test materials are designed for ease in administration. The pictures are colorful and realistic. Also, the pictures have the advantage of not being dated. This test does not offer any predictive information except for stimulability results.

GOLDMAN-FRISTOE-WOODCOCK TEST OF AUDITORY DISCRIMINATION

Category: Input-Perception-Phoneme
         Output-Overt response-Production-Gesture

Description   The Goldman-Fristoe-Woodcock Test of Auditory Discrimination was developed by Ronald Goldman, Macalyne Fristoe, and Richard W. Woodcock. The primary purpose of the Goldman-Fristoe-Woodcock test is to detect those whose auditory discrimination abilities are below age level. The design of this test includes such features as (1) a set of training plates for the purpose of teaching the child the vocabulary utilized on the test plates prior to administration of the test; (2) a minimum requirement of auditory memory since only one word is spoken per plate; (3) avoiding a same-different concept because no verbal response on the part of the child is required; and (4) providing a recorded test under controlled acoustic conditions, thus avoiding the confounding variable of different examiners' oral presentation. It is a test of the ability to discriminate speech sounds in one-syllable words in the presence of controlled noise and in quiet conditions. It is designed for administration to subjects 4 years old and above. There are three subtests: Training Procedure, Auditory Discrimination-Quiet Subtest, and Auditory Discrimination-Noise Subtest. The noise subtest was developed in an attempt to assimilate a natural situation in which a child makes discriminations in a listening environment confused by background noises. The background of the noise subtest was recorded in a school cafeteria.

The two subtests recorded on the audio tape contain instructions and the stimulus items. The child is asked to point to the line drawing of the stimulus word which is one of four pictures on a given plate. There are 79 such plates, each of which has four pictures of words which are alike with the exception of one phoneme. This different phoneme is always in the same word position on a single plate. The test is done with the child wearing earphones.

The response form is divided into three sections for separate scoring of the three subtests. The Quiet and Noise Subtests sections allow for sound-error analysis. Norms are given for each subtest. The norms are in percentiles by age level.

Source and Price

> American Guidance Service, Inc.
> Publishers Building
> Circle Pines, Minnesota 55014

> Complete G-F-W easel-kit $19.50
> 50 response forms   3.00
> Prerecorded test tape   5.00

Discussion The Goldman-Fristoe-Woodcock Test of Auditory Discrimination was standardized on 745 subjects, 3 to 84 years of age, without regard to the presence or absence of auditory-discrimination problems. Age and sex differences were found. Females were superior in auditory discrimination in the age range 4 to 12 years, but the authors felt that the significance was not sufficient to construct a separate test for males. Results of the quiet subtest indicated an improvement in performance until age 10 and a gradual decrease beginning at age 34. The results of the noise subtest indicated improvement in performance until age 13, gradually decreasing around the age of 25.

This test was administered to 242 subjects with various communicative disorders, and the reliability coefficients were low when compared to other psychological instruments. The authors, however, felt this test to be useful as a clinical and research tool. For validity, the training procedure is used to ensure prior knowledge of each picture. The words selected were supposedly highly meaningful to children, but some cultural bias is apparent. The scores of both subtests on subjects with disabilities, as might be expected, was low when compared to the general population.

Although the background in the noise subtest is controlled acoustically, the choice of a school cafeteria as exemplary may have been unrealistic considering the other choices possible. This test has, however, attempted to minimize many of the poorer features of other similar meaningful word tests, such as auditory memory, test procedures, materials, and so forth.

THE GOODENOUGH-HARRIS DRAWING TEST

Category: Cognitive Processes

Description The Goodenough-Harris Drawing Test is a revision and extension of the Goodenough Draw-A-Man Test by Dale B. Harris. The changes that were incorporated include (1) extension of the test to an older age group; (2) the addition of the drawing of a woman and the self; (3) restandardization to derive a more defensible quantitative expression of the child's performance; and (4) the establishment of a more convenient approximation to full-scale scoring. It is used primarily as a measurement of intelligence, although several modifications of this test have been introduced as "projective tests." It was developed to be administered to preschool and school-age children either individually or in a group situation.

Materials needed for administration and scoring are the manual, a pencil, and a test booklet. The task is to have the subject draw three pictures, one of a man, one of a woman, and one of the subject. No assistance or cues should be given the subject. The examiner should score carefully following the detailed directions of the manual. Rules dictate whether items of a drawing are passed or failed. No partial credit is given. The test booklet provides space for scoring and a summary of the test results. Two scales are available for scoring, one is a point scale and the other is a quality scale. The Point Scale allows a point for each item scored as passed. The sum of points equals the raw score and converts to a Standard Score.

The Quality Scale is available for a quick estimate of the drawing of the man and woman; however, this scale is not as accurate as the Point Scale. The Quality Scale scores may be converted into a Standard Score. Standard Scores may be converted into percentile ranks.

Source and Price

Harcourt Brace Jovanovich
Test Department Office
372 Peachtree St. N.E.
Atlanta, Georgia 30309

Examiner's test kit $5.00

Discussion   The Goodenough-Harris Drawing Test is a quick measure of intellectual functioning. It is necessary for the child to understand spoken language, but he does not have to respond verbally. The test does not require artistic ability and the points are given for the amount of detail present in the drawings.

The test can be scored by any person capable of following instructions faithfully. Very careful study of the manual is imperative if the results are to be of any value. Because subjective judgment is required to score some items, reliability between two scorings may be poor. This test is widely used by a variety of professional disciplines.

THE HOUSTON TEST FOR LANGUAGE DEVELOPMENT

Category: Broad-Comprehensive

Description   The Houston Test for Language Development was authored by Margaret Crabtree to assess language functioning in children. The Houston Test is divided into two parts. Part I is a language scale for children 6 months of age through 3 years of age, and

Part II is an extension of the language scale through age 6. Part I is primarily observation of behavior of the young child by a teacher-observer team. The categories of language included are gesture, articulation, and melody of speech. Part II assesses self-identity, vocabulary, syntactical complexity, and communicative behavior.

Test materials include a manual of instructions, a set of 20 vocabulary cards for Part I, a set of 20 vocabulary cards for Part II, miniature objects, paper, crayons, and a score sheet. It takes approximately 30 minutes to administer this test.

Test instructions are printed in the manual. Response guidelines for scoring are illustrated on the score sheet. A score for each age level is obtained by counting the failures and subtracting it from the total possible points. A Basal Age is determined by the lowest age level where all items are correctly completed, and the Upper Age is the highest age any item is correctly completed. The total points convert into a Language Age.

Source and Price

The Houston Test Company
P. O. Box 35152
Houston, Texas 77035

Part I:

Complete kit	$ 9.50
Manual of instructions	3.50
Set of 25 score sheets	3.00
Set of vocabulary cards (20)	3.00

Part II:

Complete kit	$20.00
Manual of instructions	4.00
Set of 20 score sheets	3.50
Set of vocabulary cards (38)	4.50
Miniature objects	8.00
Parts I and II in same order	$27.00

Discussion Part I of the test was standardized on 113 and Part II was standardized on 1,102 white children in Metropolitan Houston. They were equated as to age and sex. Handicapped children were avoided in the standardization procedures. The items were scored on a percentage basis and rearranged by difficulty. A correlation coefficient of 0.84 was found between observations for Part I. No data on reliability for Part II are available.

The Houston Test is a relatively popular one, primarily with persons unsophisticated with the language development of young children. It does provide developmental-language-age levels that many clinicians need for explanation to parents.

ILLINOIS TEST OF PSYCHOLINGUISTIC ABILITIES

**Category: Cognitive Processing (General)
And Various Subtests in Other Categories**

Description The experimental edition of the Illinois Test of Psycholinguistic Abilities became available in 1961 (McCarthy and Kirk), and a revised edition was initiated in 1965, in an attempt to improve each of the subtests and to add subtests which were not originally included. A complete description of the administration and scoring of the ITPA can be obtained in the Examiner's Manual of the ITPA (revised edition) by Samuel A. Kirk, James J. McCarthy, and Winifred D. Kirk. This is a comprehensive test of psycholinguistic abilities in children. This test is designed to provide a framework within which tests of educational and discrete abilities have been generated, and to provide a base for developing an instructional program for children. Thus, this diagnostic teaching tool serves as a model for evaluating psycholinguistic disorders as well as a tool for selecting and programming remedial procedures.

There are 10 basic subtests: Auditory Reception, Visual Reception, Auditory Association, Visual Association, Verbal Expression, Manual Expression, Grammatic Closure, Visual Closure, Auditory Closure, and Sound Blending. Each subtest has its own administration, scoring procedures, and norms. In addition, two supplementary subtests provide additional clinical information. These supplementary tests are Auditory Closure and Sound Blending.

The starting points for each subtest are specified according to ability levels. A basal and ceiling are established for each subtest. Testing examples are provided. The prescribed order of presentation must be followed for each of the subtests. The record form includes a summary sheet.

Source and Price

Illinois Test of Psycholinguistic Abilities
University of Illinois Press
Urbana, Illinois 61801

Complete kit	$ 43.50
Examiner's manual only	5.75
Package of record forms and visual closure picture strips (25 12-page record forms and 25 each of 5 picture strips for the new Visual Closure Test)	7.75
Four packages	$ 27.90
Filmed demonstration of the ITPA	$360.00

Discussion This is a standardized test. The norms for the ITPA were derived from the responses of approximately 1,000 children between 2 and 10 years of age. This sample of children was selected as being of average performance on measures of intelligence, school achievement, and socioeconomic status and of intact motor development.

Four types of scores can be obtained from the ITPA: (1) raw scores, which are obtained directly from each of the subtests and are not really open to interpretation (2) psycholinguistic age (PLA), which is derived from each subtest, which can be similarly derived from the raw score; (3) scaled scores (SS), which are transformations of the raw scores such that at each age and for each of the 12 subtests the mean performance of the referral group is equal to a score of 36 with a standard deviation of 6; and (4) an estimated Stanford-Binet mental age and IQ, which are gross indices of a child's intellectual development.

A description of the 10 subtests and the 2 supplementary tests is listed below. Although each subtest is dependent upon cognitive function, various combinations of input and output functions are emphasized in the tests.

1. *Auditory Reception.* This assesses the ability of a child to derive meaning from verbally presented material. The receptive rather than the expressive process is being sampled; therefore, the response is kept at the simple level of "yes" or "no" or a shake of the head. The vocabulary becomes more difficult as the test proceeds, but the response remains at a two-year level. The automatic function of determining meaning from syntax has been minimized by retaining only one sentence form. Semantic input (auditory).

2. *Visual Reception.* This measures the child's ability to gain meaning from visual symbols. The child is shown the stimulus picture on one page and must choose a similar picture on the second page which consists of four response pictures. The credited choice is the object or situation that is conceptually similar to the stimulus. Perception (visual).

3. *Auditory-Vocal Association.* This test assesses the child's ability to relate concepts presented orally, or the ability to relate words meaningfully. The organizing process of manipulating linguistic symbols in a meaningful way is tested by verbal analogies of increasing difficulty. It taps verbal concepts of a more automatic sort than Verbal Expression. Semantic input (auditory) and semantic output (oral).

4. *Visual-Motor Association.* This test provides a picture association with which to assess the child's ability to relate concepts presented visually. The child is presented with a single stimulus picture surrounded by four optional pictures, one of which is associated with the stimulus. The child must choose the picture which is most closely related to the stimulus picture. This test assesses the ability of the child to comprehend relationships through visual stimuli. Semantic input (visual).

5. *Verbal Expression.* This test taps verbal fluency and the number of concepts the child can employ. It tests his ability to express his own concepts orally when presented with a concrete object and asked "Tell me about this." Semantic output (oral).

6. *Manual Expression.* This tests the child's ability to express ideas through movement and gesture or to express ideas manually. The child is shown a picture of various common objects (one at a time) and asked to "Show me what we do with a _____." The child must then pantomime the appropriate action. Semantic output (manual).

7. *Grammatic Closure.* This assesses the child's ability to make use of the redundancies of oral language in acquiring automatic habits for handling syntax and grammatic inflections. It tests his ability to speak grammatically. It is considered automatic because the child is not taught formally, but learns through imitation. Syntactic output (oral).

8. *Visual Closure.* This assesses the child's ability to identify a particular common object from an incomplete visual presentation. The object is seen in varying degrees of concealment and the child must point out all the examples of the object within a certain time limit. Perception (visual).

9. *Auditory-Sequential Memory.* This assesses the child's ability to reproduce sequences of digits from memory. The digits increase in length from two to eight digits. Input (auditory) and output (oral).

10. *Visual-Sequential Memory.* This assesses the child's ability to reproduce from memory sequences of nonmeaningful figures. The visual figures increase in length from two to eight figures. Input (visual and manual) and Output (visual and manual).

Supplementary Test 1–Auditory Closure. This assesses the child's ability to fill in missing parts of a word (which were omitted in the auditory presentation) and the child must produce the complete word. For example, the child will hear "bo / le" and he must respond "bottle." Morphologic competence as represented in the auditory mode.

Supplementary Test 2–Sound Blending. This provides another means of assessing the organizing process in the auditory-vocal channel. The child hears the sounds of a word and he has to synthesize the separate parts of the word and produce an integrated whole word. Phonologic competence again as represented in the auditory mode.

THE MCDONALD SCREENING DEEP TEST OF ARTICULATION

Category: Output-Overt Response-Production-Oral-Co-articulation

Description The Screening Deep Test of Articulation is designed for children. It is an assessment of nine frequently misarticulated consonant sounds. These sounds are /s/, /l/, /r/, /t/, /θ/, /ʃ/, /k/, /f/, and /t/. Multiple elicitations of each sound in possible contexts are completed. The sounds are tested by presentation of picture pairs. It is necessary that the monosyllables that each picture represents be combined into a bisyllable. There are several example cards and 31 test cards which have two pictures on each card. The examiner records the results on a record sheet. For each response the examiner must judge several sounds. The examiner has the freedom to design his own system of recording errors. The results are transferred to blank spaces to indicate the number of correct responses for each sound. These results may be plotted on a phonetic profile provided on the record sheet. The manual gives a table and profile for interpretation of the results. A separate form is also available for reporting the test results to teachers.

Source and Price
Stanwix House, Inc.
3020 Chartiers Ave.
Pittsburgh, Pennsylvania 15204

Screening Deep Test of Articulation	$8.50
Individual record sheet	7.00
Individual screening sheets per pad	.50
Teacher report form screening per pad	.30

Discussion Validity and reliability considerations of the McDonald Deep Screening Test are discussed in the administration booklet; however, it is not a standardized test. The aspects of validity and reliability are assumed as with other phonetic proficiency measures. McDonald feels that the traditional viewing of sounds by initial, medial, and final groupings is erroneous. His philosophy reflects the idea that speech is dynamic, thus, the syllable should be used as the basic physiologic and acoustic unit—not isolated sounds. Speech is made up of a series of sounds and in reality there are few initial and final sounds. Sounds are observed to be influenced by their blending effects, or release and arrest.

The trend popular with most therapists is to view the individual sound in initial, medial, and final positions as the basic unit for testing purposes. The McDonald Deep Screening Test is considered to be good in a therapeutic situation for evaluation of the consistency of error sounds in various contexts. The consistency of sound errors might also be utilized as a prognostic tool. If the sound occurs in many of the contexts as an error, this may indicate that special assistance is required for its acquisition.

MEASURES OF OUTPUT VERBALIZATIONS

Category: Output-Syntactic-Word
Output-Syntactic-Sentence

Description Measures of verbalizations are frequently subjective examiner ratings of the child's output. These ratings often judge such factors as the amount of verbalization appropriateness, structure, length of response, and so forth.

There have been a number of studies concerned with verbal output, but there are few standardized, commercial measures available. McCarthy (1954) made extensive studies of the language of children and introduced a technique of gathering verbal output data. Some current linguistic studies are challenging the validity of these types of measures however, the techniques to follow are still accepted and utilized by many examiners.

The general technique of obtaining verbal output for analysis is to elicit a language sample from the child by means of stimulation with toys, pictures, or other materials. Usually following the first 10 utterances of the child, the next 50 spontaneous verbalizations (not necessarily consecutive utterances) are recorded. With this basic language sample, certain basic measures of verbal output are available.

Mean length of response. McCarthy used this measure as her primary estimate of children's linguistic achievement. This method was earlier advocated by Nice (1925) and Smith (1926). McCarthy (1954) stated that the utilization of the MLR measure has not been superceded by any other measure as to reliability, ease of determination, objectivity, and most easily understood measure of linguistic maturity.

Procedurally, the method consists of counting the number of words in each separate verbal response, totaling these numbers, and dividing by 50. If less than 50 verbalizations were achieved, division is made employing the total number of verbalizations recorded. The results can be compared with norms for mean length of response derived by Templin (1957). Certain standards as to the determination of how words should be counted are available from McCarthy's (1954) original work, and amplification of the counting procedure may be found in Davis (1937) and Winitz (1959).

Mean of five longest responses. Davis (1937) was the first to indicate that another good procedure for obtaining the child's maximum linguistic skill in a given situation would be the mean of the child's five longest responses. The same language sample previously discussed is utilized in this method. M5L may be achieved by calculating the total words the child used in his five longest responses and dividing by five. Templin (1957) also has norms available for this data.

Number of one-word responses. A decreasing number of one-word responses by children is usually thought of as an indication of increasing language maturity. The number of one-word responses from the original language sample of a particular child may also be compared to normative data provided by Templin. These norms represent the median number of one-word responses made by children in her study (1957).

Discussion. Mean Length of Response, Mean Length of the Five Longest Responses, and the Number of One-Word Responses as measurements of the verbal output of children are infrequently employed by examiners. The primary reason for their lack of use is probably related to the amount of time required in the analysis of the child's verbal output. Nevertheless, these measures are practical in that they provide basic information about the linguistic nature of a child's language.

THE MEETING STREET SCHOOL SCREENING TEST

Category: Cognitive Processing (General) and
Various Subtests in Other Categories

Description The purpose of this test is the early identification of children with learning disabilities. The Meeting Street School Screening Test (MSSST) can be employed either for screening large numbers of children or as a part of a diagnostic evaluation of an individual child. For screening purposes, classroom observation and previous test results are incorporated with the results of the MSSST. When used as an individual test, it surveys gross motor, visual-perceptual-motor, and language skills of kindergarten and first-grade children.

Utilization of the MSSST provides a determination of how effectively a child is processing information through the three subtest modalities. Five normative tables are available in the manual that span the age range 5.0 to 7.5 years. The MSSST raw scores, scaled scores, and ratings on a behavior rating scale may be used to identify children with learning disabilities. How these scores and ratings are employed in combination with other information depends on whether the purpose is group screening or that of understanding the skills of a learning disabled child.

Each of the three modalities evaluated by the MSSST has five test areas. A brief description of each follows:

I. Motor Patterning Subtest. Samples a variety of sequential movement patterns and awareness of the body in space. The areas within this subtest, except Follow Directions I, are completed with the child imitating the examiner's demonstration.

A. Gait Patterns. Samples the child's ability to execute unilateral and bilateral body movement patterns consisting of hopping, skipping, and dancing.

B. Clap Hands. Evaluates the child's ability to see, remember, and reproduce unlearned, sequential movement patterns in appropriate spatial relationships.

C. Hand Patterns. Similar to clap hands, but child imitates hand patterns demonstrated by the examiner.

D. Follow Direction I. Tests the child's ability to comprehend and remember verbal directions concerning spatial concepts and to perform the requested tasks.

E. Touch Fingers. Tests the child's ability to coordinate his hands and fingers in rapid bilateral patterned movements.

II. Visual-Perceptual-Motor Subtest. Samples the child's visual discrimination, visual memory, reproduction of geometric and letter forms in correct spatial orientation and sequence, and the understanding of spatial and directional concepts on a piece of paper. The five areas of evaluation included are:

A. Block Tapping. Measures the child's memory for place sequences by reproducing the tapping patterns of the examiner.

B. Visual Matching. Samples visual-perceptual discrimination of form constancy by visually matching one geometric design with another like it in a series of similarly shaped designs.

C. Visual Memory. Measures the child's short-term memory for geometric designs and letter forms.

D. Copy Forms. Evaluates the child's ability to coordinate hand and eye in reproducing geometric and letter forms in the correct shape, orientation, and spacing.

E. Follow Directions II. Tests the child's understanding of spatial and directional concepts when drawing on a piece of paper. Child attempts to do what the examiner instructs him to do.

III. Language Subtest. Evaluates the child's ability to listen, remember, sequence, and formulate language. The five areas constituting this subtest include:

A. Repeat Words. Assesses the child's ability to listen to and repeat familiar and unknown speech sound sequences in their correct form, order, and rhythm.

B. Repeated Sentences. Tests the child's ability to listen and repeat language material that is more complex, both in length and grammatical form, than found in the above.

C. Counting. Evaluates the child's ability to sequence numbers in automatically learned and in interrupted sequences.

D. Tell a Story. Samples the child's ability to formulate and express his thoughts about an abstract picture in meaningful language.

E. Language Sequencing. Measures the ability of the child to sequence time concepts and to understand the order and meaning of time units.

The manual for the MSSST contains a discussion of early identification programs, administering and scoring directions for the test, stimulation materials, uses of the MSSST (including general meaning and validity studies), and an information-processing view of childrens' behavior. The appendixes provide scoring rationale and examples of the copying of forms, and tables for converting raw scores to scaled score equivalents.

Source and Price

> Meeting Street School
> 333 Grotto Ave.
> Providence, Rhode Island 02906

> Manual and
> > test record forms $10.00

Discussion   The MSSST is designed to permit administration by nonprofessional, as well as professionally trained, examiners. Scaled scores obtained from raw scores allow an individual child's performance to be compared with that expected for his chronological age. Time necessary for this test approximates 15 to 20 minutes per child.

The total and subtest MSSST correlated with the ITPA and the Frostig Developmental Tests of Visual Perception at a level indicating the MSSST can be used to survey the skills tapped in the test. A control group's ($N = 20$) composite score on the ITPA correlated significantly with the total MSSST ($r = 0.77$) and with the language subtest ($r = 0.71$). The MSSST motor patterning and visual-perceptual-motor subtests correlated positively with the visual-motor sequencing of the ITPA ($r = 0.62$ and 0.41).

High-risk children (low scores on the MSSST) showed significantly poorer performance than the control group on the ITPA ($t = 4.21, p = 0.01$), Frostig ($t = 3.63, p = 0.01$), and a school achievement test ($t = 3.65, p = 0.01$). The MSSST has also been found to have predictive validity for identifying children with learning disabilities; these predictions have been based solely on intelligence scores of 220 kindergarten and 274 first-grade children. The MSSST has been used in large-scale screening programs and found to be a good predictor of children who will encounter academic difficulty. Further information concerning the reliability and validity of both the individual and screening tests may be found in the manual.

Although not widely used, the MSSST holds promise for the early identification of children with learning disabilities.

THE MICHIGAN PICTURE LANGUAGE INVENTORY

Category: Input-Syntax-Word

Description   The test was originally designed by Lerea (1958) to develop a standardized procedure which would measure the normal and the language-retarded child's ability to express and comprehend vocabulary and language functioning. It is divided into two linguistic components, including lexical and structural relationships, and consists of a picture vocabulary inventory including 35 items, 5 each at each of seven age levels, ages 3 to 9 years. Two scores are derived from this section of the test and are in the areas of vocabulary expression and vocabulary comprehension. A second section of the test consists of a picture language structure inventory designed to indicate the child's structure or grasp of the syntax of English. The examiner first describes to the child each of 50 cards broken into classes of function words, generally resembling nouns, adjectives, verbs, and adverbs. Subsequently, the examiner attempts to elicit an oral response from the child to key items on the cards. The number of correct responses determines the language structure expression score. The pictures are shown to the child a third time to derive a measure of language structure comprehension of singular and plural, present and past tense, comparative and superlative forms of adjectives, possessive and demonstrative pronouns, and relative terms such as prepositions.

Source and Price

Speech Clinic
1111 East Catherine St.
Ann Arbor, Michigan 48168

$5.00 per set

Discussion Initial standardization suggested that this test possessed validity as a diagnostic tool because the results yielded scores of increasing magnitude at successive levels and demonstrated differences in performance between groups of children known to vary markedly in their language skills. Lerea's study (1958) reported the coefficients for vocabulary comprehension, vocabulary expression, structural comprehension, and structural expression to be 0.93, 0.90, 0.94, and 0.95, respectively. This has not been a widely used test. Its most useful application appears to be as a guideline for the initiation of remediation. It may also be useful for assessing language development and defining language retardation in some children.

NORTHWESTERN SYNTAX SCREENING TEST

Category: Output-Syntactic-Sentence

Description The purpose of this test is to screen children delayed in syntactic development. The test measures receptive and expressive use of syntactic forms, using identical linguistic structures in both parts of the test. The NSST consists of 20 paired sentences to be identified receptively by selection of a picture in response to stimulus pictures. Administration time is approximately 15 minutes. Age range is three through eight years.

Source and Price

Northwestern University Press
1735 Benson Ave.
Evanston, Illinois 60020

$10.00 for the set
  2.50 for additional packages of 50 record forms

Discussion   Two hundred forty-two children were utilized to establish the norms for this test. Its greatest utility appears to be as a reliable screening instrument for children exhibiting receptive or expressive syntactic delay.

THE PEABODY INDIVIDUAL ACHIEVEMENT TEST

**Category: Cognitive Processes (General)
      And Various Subtests in Other Categories**

Description   The Peabody Individual Achievement Test was developed by Lloyd M. Dunn and Frederick C. Markwardt, Jr. This is a wide-range screening test of achievement in the areas of mathematics, spelling, reading, and general information. This instrument gives information of scholastic accomplishment. The PIAT is designed for use with kindergarten-age children through adult levels.

There are five subtests: Mathematics, Reading Recognition, Reading Comprehension, Spelling, and General Information. Each subtest has its own administration procedures. The items of each subtest are arranged in progressive order of difficulty. A basal and ceiling are established and the number of correct responses equals a raw score for each subtest. The raw score can be changed by the use of norm tables into Grade Equivalents, Age Equivalents, Percentile Ranks, and Standard Scores. An overall achievement level may be derived from the Total Score and test results plotted on a profile provided on the response booklet. This is an untimed instrument which is administered on an individual basis. The usual testing session is approximately 35 minutes in duration.

Test stimulation materials come in two hard-bound, easel-style volumes. A convenient manual contains general information, administration procedures, technical data, and norm tables. A response booklet allows easy scoring of test results and analysis of achievement.

Source and Price

Complete test kit, including PIAT easel-kit Volume I, PIAT easel-kit Volume II, 25 individual record booklets, and manual	$24.00
PIAT easel-kit Volume I (Mathematics, Reading Recognition), if ordered separately	$10.00
PIAT easel-kit Volume II (Reading Comprehension, Spelling, and General Information), if ordered separately	11.00
Individual record booklets, 25 per page	3.00
Manual, if ordered separately	2.25
Training tape (optional) (not included in complete test kit)	4.00

Discussion   The PIAT has been standardized. Reliability studies were completed o[n] each subtest and for the total test. Six levels were sampled: kindergarten, grades 1, 3, [5,] 8, and 12. Median values obtained for each of the areas are as follows: Readin[g] Recognition 0.89, Reading Comprehension 0.64, Spelling 0.65, Mathematics 0.7[4,] General Information 0.76, and an 0.89 for the total test. These results indicate reliabilit[y] would be greatest in the total test and Reading Recognition and lowest in Readin[g] Comprehension and Spelling.

Validity studies were concerned with content and item validity and concurre[nt] validity. Content was chosen that was not biased by methods or types of material but wa[s] rather material of a general nature. Concurrent validity studies have been complete[d] correlating the PIAT with the Peabody Picture Vocabulary Test and the Wide Ran[ge] Achievement Test. A detailed discussion of reliability and validity studies is present i[n] the PIAT manual. Further studies of this instrument are needed.

The PIAT is an easy test to administer. The examiner should be very familiar with t[he] test but does not have to be a sophisticated examiner to administer this test. T[he] administration procedures are explicit, easy for the examiner to present, and easy for t[he] subject to follow. Picture stimulus is good and is not ambiguous, dated, or regionalize[d.] This is a relatively new test which may become very popular.

PEABODY PICTURE VOCABULARY TEST

Category: Input-Semantic
    Output-Overt Response-Production-Gesture

Description   The Peabody Picture Vocabulary Test was developed by Lloyd [M.] Dunn. The purpose of this test is to measure single-word receptive vocabulary. The a[ge] range of the Peabody Picture Vocabulary Test is 2 years 3 months to 18 years 5 mont[hs.]

Test materials consist of a spiral-bound booklet which contains 3 example plates a[nd] 150 test plates. The test plates are arranged in order of increasing difficulty. There a[re] four black-and-white pictures on each plate. A manual contains administration a[nd] scoring procedures; general information; and age, standard score, percentile equivalen[ts,] and intelligence quotients.

Administration of the test is a simple procedure. A test word is spoken by t[he] examiner, and the child indicates which picture best represents the word. The testee c[an] indicate his response by pointing to the picture, saying the number of the picture, or ev[en] by blinking his eye for a yes/no response. There are two forms of the Peabody Pict[ure] Vocabulary Test. Each form has its own set of norm tables. A base and ceiling [are] established and the number of correct responses equals the raw score. The recording [of] the responses is completed by the examiner writing the number of the picture indicat[ed] by the testee as his response. The scores can be converted into mental age, IQ, standa[rd] score equivalent, and percentile equivalent. Administration and scoring time is appro[xi-]mately 15 minutes.

Source and Price
    American Guidance Service, Inc.
    Publishers Buildings
    Circle Pines, Minnesota 55014

Complete test kit $17.00
Individual test records
Form A or B, package of 50   3.25

Discussion The Peabody Picture Vocabulary Test is a standardized test with a minimum of 11 studies attesting to its reliability. These studies are reported in the manual that accompanies the test. It is a reliable instrument for both handicapped and average children. The Peabody Picture Vocabulary Test and Stanford-Binet correlated at 0.71, while the Peabody Picture Vocabulary Test and the Wechsler correlated at 0.61.

This is a most popular instrument and is included as a basic item in many test batteries. One of the criticisms of this test currently is its popularity. For example, handicapped children who are often evaluated by several different agencies may have been given the Peabody Picture Vocabulary Test by each agency and perhaps by even two different departments within the same agency. The ease and speed of administration and scoring have increased its popularity. Also, it has had much attention brought to it because of many validity and reliability studies. In addition, it has been used as an instrument for many other types of research studies, especially in academic settings. One hazard that many professionals fail to avoid is that the Peabody Picture Vocabulary Test is not an intelligence test, but a test of a child's one-word receptive vocabulary. It should not be considered an intelligence test. Another limiting factor is that the Peabody Picture Vocabulary Test is a culturally biased test.

THE PICTURE ARTICULATION AND LANGUAGE SCREENING TEST

Category: Input-Semantic
         Output-Overt Response-Production-Oral-Word

Description The Picture Articulation and Language Screening Test was developed by William C. Rodgers. This test is a quick articulation and language screening instrument primarily designed for use in a school situation. The test is constructed for children on a first-grade level. The time required for its administration is less than 2 minutes.

This test is comprised of three parts: Initial Screening, Sound Evaluation, and Stimulus Materials. The first part, the Initial Screening section, elicits sentence responses from picture stimulation for language and articulation performance. If the first part is successfully completed, the next two sections are not administered. The Sound Evaluation part presents 13 pictures to elicit spontaneous speech with sounds in initial and final positions on the word level. The Stimulus Materials part consists of three stimulus pictures to elicit three phonemes produced in isolation to reportedly aid in case selection. A simple score sheet is provided for recording test results.

Source and Price
  Word Making Productions
  P O. Box 305
  Salt Lake City, Utah 84110

PALST Articulation Screening Test
with one (1) pad of score sheets $16.00
Additional grading pads (25 pages
per pad; each pad records 7
children)   1.00

Discussion This test was compared to the Templin-Darley Articulation Test and t
Riley Articulation and Language Test and a level of confidence was achieved beyo
0.001 using a chi-square comparison. The test appears to be most efficient in identify
those children in need of detailed evaluations. Also, it may be utilized to select child
for the public school clinician's case load. A distinct disadvantage of this test is
screening nature. It is not an objective measuring instrument and its validity a
reliability are certainly open to question.

THE PREDICTIVE SCREENING TEST OF ARTICULATION

Category: Output-Overt Response-Production-Oral-Word

Description The Predictive Screening Test of Articulation was designed by Char
Van Riper and Robert L. Erickson. The revised edition was printed in July 1970. T
purpose of this test is to separate children who have an articulation disorder into tv
categories: (1) those children who will correct their misarticulations and not requ
speech therapy, and (2) those children who probably will not correct their misarticu
tions and will require speech therapy. The test is most appropriate for first-gra
students.

The Predictive Screening Test of Articulation is divided into nine parts. There is
total of 47 test items. All instructions are given orally and 45 items require a verl
response. No visual materials are used. A response sheet provides scoring by circling a o
(1) for correctly completing an item or a zero (0) if the item was incorrect. A total sco
is computed by counting the number of responses which received a 1 point score. T
total score is recorded on the front of the response record sheet. The test and scori
time is typically 7 or 8 minutes. Tables listed in the manual reflect cutoff scores f
comparison to the norm samples. The selection of a cutoff score should be completed l
the therapist according to the appropriateness for that particular program and populatic

Source and Price
Continuing Education Office
Western Michigan University
Kalamazoo, Michigan 49001

Available at current printing cost

Discussion The test manual presents a discussion of the predictive validity a
reliability of the Predictive Screening Test of Articulation. A reliability of 0.89 w

estimated by use of the Spearman-Brown Formula. The interexaminer reliability correlation mean was 0.97. Validity of cross-validation groups was high.

This is a quick test that is often utilized by public school speech therapists. However, therapists often do not properly analyze the results of their particular population for establishment of appropriate cutoff scores in selection of case loads. Perhaps this is due in part to their difficulty in understanding the test construction and the techniques utilized to establish cutoff scores.

In addition, time is often of essence to the public school therapist due to the large population he serves. But, omission of the interpretation aspect of the test results defeats the purpose of the Predictive Screening Test of Articulation, which is to predict those who have misarticulations but will probably not need speech therapy.

THE STANFORD-BINET INTELLIGENCE SCALE

Category: Cognitive Processing

Description The Stanford-Binet Intelligence Scale originally consisted of a 30-item scale in 1905. It has undergone many revisions and improvements. In 1937 major revisions were made and two forms were developed. In 1960 the most recent revision resulted in the combination of the two forms, L and M, into one form, the L-M. In the 1960 revision no new test items were added.

The 1960 revision is grouped, as was the 1937 revision, into 20 age groups from 2 years through superior adult levels. Through year level five there are half-year groupings. Above the 14-year level, grouping is divided into Average-Adult and Superior-Adult Levels I, II, and III. Most of the levels contain six tests with content varying considerably from level to level. Alternative tests on each level are also available. The lower-age level tasks consist primarily of sensorimotor activities and simple verbalizations. At the upper level, tasks are more abstract and are very verbal.

The test is comprised of a variety of tasks, including object manipulation and eye-hand coordination, perceptual discrimination, identification and observation of common objects, practical judgment or common sense, memory tests, spatial orientation, numerical tests, and verbal tests. The test materials consist of standard toys, printed-card sets, a manual, and a 16-page response booklet or 6-page record form.

A basal level of performance is established and testing is continued until a terminal age is reached. Terminal age is the point where all test items at one age level are failed. Results may be converted into a deviation IQ as an extension of mental age and chronological age factors.

Source and Price

Houghton and Mifflin Co.
3108 Piedmont Road, N. E.
Atlanta, Georgia 30305

Revised Stanford-Binet Intelligence Scale,
   3rd edition: examiner's kit, Form L-M $39.00

Discussion Extensive reliability and validity studies were conducted in the 1937 revision and results showed that IQs were essentially stable. The use of the deviation IQ in the 1960 revision appears to be more reliable. Validity studies are strong and indicate that predictive value of the Stanford-Binet is good. There is a positive correlation of the Stanford-Binet with school performance.

The Stanford-Binet has been recognized as a good measure of intellectual functioning and is probably the most widely used age scale. Test results appear to be stable. This test does require a skilled and experienced examiner for administration, scoring, and interpretation. It is especially valuable due to the wide range of age levels. However, because of the arrangement of test items in age levels, repetition of instructions is necessary, requiring additional administration time and examiner talent for smooth testing.

The Stanford-Binet is extremely useful with children or adults suspected of being mentally retarded, but is impractical for use with speech, language, or visually impaired individuals. It is verbally loaded at the young age levels.

THE TEMPLIN-DARLEY TESTS OF ARTICULATION

Category: Output-Overt Response-Production-Oral-Word-Co-articulation

Description The Templin-Darley Tests of Articulation were written by M. C. Templin and F. L. Darley as a measure of the production of specific phonetic elements of children. The test was designed so that it may be used as a 141-item diagnostic test. The screening test is used to identify children having unsatisfactory articulation patterns. The 141-item test is diagnostic in nature, permits a detailed description and evaluation of the child's articulation, and is used more frequently with children already identified as having articulatory problems to aid in prescribing the nature of the speech-therapy program. The diagnostic portion includes nine areas, of which 43 of the 141 items compose the Iowa Pressure Articulation Test, 42 items test intial- and final-consonant singles, 31 items test two- and three-phoneme /r/ clusters, 18 items test two- and three-phoneme /l/ clusters, 17 items test two- and three-phoneme /s/ clusters. In addition, 9 miscellaneous items test two-phoneme clusters, 11 vowels, and 6 diphthong and combination items. This screening and diagnostic test has 57 cards with 2, 3, or 4 pictures to a plate to evoke the single-word responses. The stimulus pictures are available in color. The test set consists of a booklet which contains an introduction, test instructions, norms, and overlays for ease in scoring. A list of test words and sentences is available for older subjects.

The responses are recorded in a test form as follows: To indicate a correct sound, a checkmark is used to indicate substitutions and the sound substituted is recorded; to indicate an omission, a dash is used; for a distorted sound, an X is used; and no response is recorded as (NR). Page 3 of the form is an analysis sheet, thus allowing the responses to be compared with the test norms.

Source and Price
Bureau of Educational Research & Service
Extension Division C-20 East Hall

The University of Iowa
Iowa City, Iowa 52240

Manual	$4.50 each
Articulation test form	.06 each
Overlays (set of 9)	.50 each

Discussion The Templin-Darley is one of the few articulation tests which has norms. Templin used 480 subjects divided into groups. The norms give the percentage of sounds correctly produced at eight age levels between 3 and 8 years, divided by socioeconomic, sex, and age factors. Reliability coefficients for the screening test ranged from 0.93 to 0.99 on single-age groups between 2 and 5 years. Validity of the diagnostic test was 0.78 using a Pearson r. It does not provide a developmental level of sound production.

THE UTAH TEST OF LANGUAGE DEVELOPMENT

Category: Broad-Comprehensive

Description The Utah Test of Language Development, authored by M. J. Mecham, J. R. Jex, and J. D. Jones, is a comprehensive screening test of receptive and expressive language functions. The underlying purpose is to determine if a child is delayed in language functions, and if so, the language processes involved. This is an extension of the Verbal Language Development Scale in a test form. The test may be administered to children from age 1 to 15 years. The test items were taken from several standardized behavioral developmental scales and tests. The items were chosen on the theory that there are four basic language processes: semantic decoding and encoding, grammatical or sequential decoding and encoding. Test items in these areas are sampled and arranged in developmental age levels. There are 51 test items and administration time is approximately 35 minutes.

The test consists of a manual with specific instructions and guides for scoring each item on the test. Testing materials are in a separate booklet. A convenient response form is available. A base and ceiling are obtained and the number of correct responses can be converted into a language quotient. Standard scores and percentile equivalents are not available at this time but are forthcoming.

Source and Price

Communication Research Associated, Inc.
P. O. Box 11012
Salt Lake City, Utah 84111

Test kit	$15.00
Score sheets—per package	1.00

Discussion The validity of this test in relationship to the Verbal Language Development Scale was 0.967 ($N = 117$). The norms for each of the test items vary.

However, the norm sample size is approximately 1,880 and represents most regions of th
United States. Therapists who have used this tool feel that it is basically a good screenin
instrument which covers a wide range of items. The test is still being revised an
improvement of the test stimulation materials is felt by many examiners to be necessary

One basic criticism of the test is that certain pictures illustrated as answer choices ar
ambiguous, especially the items of receptive language measures. Another criticism of th
current test is the picture size and style. Also, the design of the test is viewed as tim
consuming, and requires jumping from one task to another and then back to the fir
task. This procedure increases administration time in repeating the instructions, an
interrupts the flow of the test. Data are still being collected on this test and revisions ma
be forthcoming.

VERBAL LANGUAGE DEVELOPMENT SCALE

Category: Broad-Comprehensive

Description The Verbal Language Development Scale by M. J. Mecham is a
extension of the communication portion of the Vineland Social Maturity Scale by Edg
A. Doll. The informant-interview method is utilized to provide a description of the child
communication behavior in the areas of listening, speaking, reading, and writin
Questions are asked of the informant so that the information obtained is not biased. Th
age range of the scale is from 1 month to 15 years.

A score sheet provides for quick recording of the information obtained. There are 5
items and each item is worth a full point if it is, or has been, routinely or habitual
performed by the child. One-half point credit is given for items which are in a transition
or emergent state. No credit is received for items that are absent or cursory. The poin
earned are totaled and transmuted to a language age equivalent.

Source and Price

American Guidance Service, Inc.
Publishers Building
Circle Pines, Minnesota 55014

Specimen set	$0.65
Score sheets, per package of 25	1.70
Manual, per copy	0.50

Discussion Item calibration and tentative norm scores for the VLDS were deriv
from a sample of 120 "normal"-speaking children randomly selected from a sample fro
urban and rural areas, five boys and five girls at each of the 12 age levels. Reliabili
testing yielded a correlation coefficient of 0.989. No validation information is y
available.

This scale is a useful clinical tool. It assists in collecting data on the child who
difficult to test. Also, if the child is testable it gives comparative performance data a

indications of how the informant views and evaluates the child's performance. Information can be biased by the examiner if questions are not properly presented or if the examiner is not familiar with the item definitions of the scale. The competence of the examiner is most important in utilization of this scale.

THE WECHSLER INTELLIGENCE SCALE FOR CHILDREN

Category: Cognitive Processes

Description   The Wechsler Intelligence Scale for Children was developed by David Wechsler. The age range is from 5 years through 15 years. The Wechsler Intelligence Scale for Children is composed of 12 subtests. Of the 12 subtests, 2 may be used as supplementary or alternative tests. The subtests are classified as verbal or performance. The verbal portion includes the subtests of General Information, General Comprehension, Arithmetic, Similarities, Vocabulary, and an alternative subtest, Digit Span. The performance portion includes the subtests of Picture Completion, Picture Arrangement, Block Design, Object Assemble, Coding, and an alternative subtest of Mazes.

In contrast to a mental age obtained on a Stanford-Binet, the WISC provides a point scale. Raw scores are obtained for each subtest, and are converted into normalized standard scores according to the testee's age level. Standard scores of the various subtests are added and changed into a deviation IQ with a mean of 100 and a standard deviation of 15. A Verbal, Performance, or a Full Scale IQ can be obtained. The manual discusses the criteria for scoring in detail.

Source and Price

Psychological Corporation
304 East 45th St.
New York, New York 10017

$25.00 complete

Discussion   The Wechsler Intelligence Scale for Children is a standardized test of intelligence and the procedures used are considered to be very good. It was standardized on 2,200 subjects. Reliability for the subtests individually is not considered to be stable. However, stability of the Verbal and Performance IQs is reported to be between 0.80 and 0.90 by Wechsler, according to split-half reliabilities. Validity studies indicate that there is a higher correlation between the Verbal Scale than the Performance Scale and the Stanford-Binet Intelligence Test.

The WISC is a versatile instrument for test result interpretation. It yields a great deal of information and is felt to be more diagnostic than the Stanford-Binet. The WISC may even be assistive for psychodiagnostic purposes. But, as with any test, some examiners find that it is not a useful tool for young children because of the nature of its construction. This test does have limited use with moderate or severe sensory-motor handicaps. Many examiners ordinarily do not administer this test to subjects under 7 years. For ages 16 and above, the Wechsler Adult Intelligence Scale is available.

WEPMAN'S AUDITORY DISCRIMINATION TEST

Category: Input-Perception-Phoneme

Description Wepman's Auditory Discrimination Test was designed by Joseph M. Wepman. The intent of this test is to detect those who have difficulty with auditory discrimination of phonemes. There are no visual cues. Although the test was written primarily for children of the early elementary level, it is often used with older children. There are two equated forms of the test. The test consists of 40 word pairs. Thirty word pairs are similar phonemically and in length but with one single phoneme different in each pair; 10 word pairs are the same. The phonemes compared consist of 13 initial consonants, 13 final consonants, and 4 medial vowels. Word pairs were selected to meet three criteria: (1) all word pairs had to be of the same syllable length; (2) each word of a pair had to appear with the same frequency in the language of children as the other word of the pair, and (3) the phoneme or vowel to be compared had to be in the same position in each word pair and each comparison was required to be in the same phonetic category. The test administration is not complicated. The child is presented a pair of words and asked to listen and indicate if the words spoken were the same words or two different words.

Test instructions are given but do not have to be followed rigidly. The important thing is that the child understand the task. Example word pairs are presented to the child until the examiner feels confident of the child's understanding of the procedure. The child's back is then turned to the examiner to eliminate visual cues and the test is administered. The test forms are easily scored. A plus (+) is used for appropriate answers and a minus (−) for inappropriate answers. The final scores can then be compared to a chart which lists the minimum score considered adequate, according to age level for discrimination maturation. Also, cutoff points are given to indicate if the test was valid.

Source and Price

Language Research Association
300 N. State St.
Chicago, Illinois 60610

One set $6.00

Discussion The Wepman is a standardized auditory discrimination test if the cutoff points listed in the test are used. This test can be useful in identifying young children with auditory discrimination problems which may be related to speech, language, and reading disturbances. This test has been rather popular among clinicians, primarily because its administration is easy and only takes approximately five minutes. A disadvantage of this type of assessment is that it requires an understanding of the same-different concept which is frequently difficult for young children. Also, because linguistic units are the stimuli to be discriminated, the child's language functioning may be a crucial feature in his judgments. Auditory memory may also be impaired, and invalidate the test's meaningfulness. Variation is possible in test-word presentation of an individual examiner and between different examiners. Variations may occur because of rate of presentation and emphasis of word pairs may affect the results. Therefore, interpretation should only be made with an overview of the examiner's competence, environment of the test situation in relation to the child's articulatory pattern, behavior, intelligence, attention, motivation, the child's performance on other tests in related areas, and so forth. An additional factor which might be considered in interpretation of results is the vocabulary of the test.

REFERENCES

Ball, J. 1958. The relationship between the ability to speak efficiently and the primary mental abilities, verbal comprehension and general reasoning. Speech Monogr., 25:285-290.

Beck, R. N. 1970. Syntactic abilities of normal and mentally retarded children of similar mental age. Ph.D. Dissertation, Lawrence, University of Kansas.

Berko, Jean. 1958. The child's learning of English morphology. Word, 14:150-177.

Brooks, Keith. 1967. The Communicative Arts and Sciences of Speech. Columbus, Ohio, Charles E. Merrill Books.

Carhart, R., and J. Jerger. 1959. Preferred method of clinical determination of pure tone thresholds. J. Speech Hearing Dis., 24:330-345.

Davis, E. A. 1937. The development of linguistic skill in twins, singletons with siblings, and only children from age five to ten years. Child Welfare Monographs, No. 14. Minneapolis, University of Minnesota Press.

Deese, J. 1970. Psycholinguistics. Boston, Allyn and Bacon.

Eisenson, J., J. J. Auer, and J. V. Irwin. 1963. The Psychology of Communication. New York, Appleton-Century-Crofts.

Ewing, I. R., and A. W. G. Ewing. 1961. New Opportunities for Deaf Children. London, University of London Press.

Gaser, Robert. 1963. Instructional technology and the measurement of learning outcomes: some questions. Amer. Psychol., 18:519-521.

Gilkinson, H., and F. H. Knower. 1941. A study of personality traits and skill in speech. J. Educ. Psychol., 32:161-175.

Harms, S. L. 1961. Listener judgments of status clues in speech. Quart. J. Speech, 47:164-169.

Koppitz, E. M. 1964. The Bender Gestalt Test for Young Children. New York, Grune & Stratton.

Langacker, R. W. 1968 Language and Its Structure. New York, Harcourt Brace Jovanovich.

Lenneberg, E. H. 1967. Biological Foundations of Language. New York, John Wiley & Sons.

Lerea, Louis. 1958. Assessing Language Development. J. Speech Hearing Res., 1:75-85.

McCarthy, D. 1954. Language Development in Children. In Carmichael, L., ed., Manual of Child Psychology. New York, John Wiley & Sons.

McNeill, D. 1970. The Acquisition of Language. New York, Harper & Row.

Myklebust, H. R. 1954. Auditory Disorders in Children. New York, Grune & Stratton.

Nice, M. N. 1925. Length of sentences as a criterion of child's progress in speech. J. Educ. Psychol., 16:370-379.

Shannon, C. E., and W. Weaver. 1964. The Mathematical Theory of Communication. Urbana, Ill., University of Illinois Press.

Skinner, B. F. 1957. Verbal Behavior. New York, Appleton-Century-Crofts.

Smith, M. E. 1926. An investigation of the development of the sentence and the extent of vocabulary in young children. Univ. Iowa Stud. Child Welfare, 3.

Templin, M. C. 1957. Certain language skills in children; their development and interrelationships. Child Welfare Monographs, No. 26. Minneapolis, University of Minnesota Press.

Wertheimer, M. 1945. Productive Thinking. New York, Harper & Row.

Winitz, H. 1959. Language skills of male and female kindergarten children. J. Speech Hearing Res., 2:377-386.

10: Medical diagnosis and evaluation of language disabilities

Sylvia Onesti Richardson

The term language disabilities, as used in this chapter, refers to the inability or limited ability of a child to use symbols for purposes of communication and may be characterized by speech, reading, and/or writing difficulties. Dysphasia is concerned exclusively with an inability to receive and/or express spoken symbols. Dyslexia indicates a problem in the reception of written symbols. Dysgraphia refers to a problem in the expression of written symbols. Thus, developmental dysphasia, dyslexia, and dysgraphia[1] all represent disturbances in the development of particular language functions. They are closely related conditions and often are found together in the same patient or in members of the same family. There are many points of similarity in their etiology and clinical pictures. In each, the process of symbolization is impaired. Yet there is a tendency to regard them as separate clinical entities, and particularly to explain dyslexia and dysgraphia in terms of "lateralizing confusion" or to attribute them to "mixed hand and eye dominance." The fact is too often ignored that specific developmental dyslexia and dysgraphia, like developmental dysphasia, are disorders of language.

At present, there is a strong consensus that language disorders in children are caused by dysfunction of the central nervous system, presumably due to cerebral immaturity or damage, and associated with perceptual impairment. They are sometimes classified under neuropsychiatric (or psychoneurological) learning disorders. These children may show behavior problems, which are sometimes referred to as "organic behavior disorders." Dysphasia, dyslexia, and dysgraphia have also been gathered into the cumbersome portmanteau of "minimal brain dysfunction," of which the signs and symptoms most commonly reported can be grouped into disorders of (1) neuromotor coordination,

[1] The terms aphasia, alexia, and agraphia may also be used. The difference in prefix is arbitrary. Originally the argument was held that the prefix, a-, refers to loss of a function and is, therefore, inappropriate for children who never have developed that function.

287

(2) attention, (3) perception, and (4) language (Clements, 1966). Many educators, however, prefer the label "specific learning disability," since it does not connote a medical diagnosis and does differentiate the learning problem from intellectual subnormality.

Good treatment is dependent on an accurate diagnosis and an understanding of the pathogenesis. An all-encompassing label that covers a multitude of disabilities, instead of describing a particular child's specific problems, is not helpful in planning appropriate educational procedures and management. Classification based on description of the language disorder and related clinical and environmental findings is safer, more useful, and may eventually lead to a sounder classification of language, speech, and hearing disorders.

The purposes of medical evaluation and diagnosis are to demonstrate the presence or absence of a language disorder and to determine the existence of any etiological factors such as disease or injury. Medical diagnosis, however, is only one part of the total evaluation required for the child with a language disability. No less important is the assessment of the child by representatives of other disciplines, including speech clinician, audiologist, psychologist, educator, social worker, and others as indicated. A period of observation and diagnostic therapy in a classroom setting may be required before a precise diagnosis can be reached.

DIAGNOSIS

In the very young child the major manifestation of dysphasia is retarded development of speech. Symptoms may include failure of speech development, failure of auditory comprehension, and possibly clues with regard to central nervous system involvement. These, along with an abnormal birth and/or neonatal history, may add to a presumptive diagnosis of dysphasia and would be particularly significant if there was relatively normal development in other areas. In assessing the child's speech and language, one must consider whether the primary problem is one of reception (understanding speech), expression (expressing himself with speech), or, most commonly, a combination of these two. Certainly the large majority of children with developmental dysphasia demonstrate auditory imperception or receptive problems, and, of course, expression cannot help but be affected. The differential diagnosis of dysphasia must include other disorders which cause significant retardation of speech development, such as severe hearing loss, deafness, intellectual subnormality, and severe psychiatric disorders. Neurological or structural abnormalities affecting the articulatory organs, and gross uncomplicated environmental deprivation, rarely cause serious retardation of speech development, and when they are severe enough to do so, they are usually obvious.

It may be extremely difficult to distinguish hypoacusis, or reduced auditory acuity, from dysacusis, or central auditory imperception, or receptive aphasia. Young children with either tend to rely on gesture and to lipread. Fortunately, by the time children suffering from dysacusis reach the speech clinic, appreciation of sounds other than those of speech may be apparent. A significant number of dysphasic children may also have a sensorineural loss, which must not be overlooked. A positive family history of retarded speech development, reading and writing difficulties, delayed establishment of cerebral dominance, or ambidexterity, without abnormalities of hearing, may be helpful clues. Definitive diagnosis must depend on detailed clinical and audiological examination.

Children who are intellectually subnormal may present clinical manifestations similar to those of dysphasia. Patients with either condition may show inattention to the spoken word, relatively normal motor milestones, and grossly retarded speech development. It is not uncommon for mental retardation and developmental dysphasia to be associated in the same patient. Although a history of uniform retardation in motor, adaptive, language, and social aspects of development is in favor of the diagnosis of intellectual subnormality, many retarded children will show remarkably normal motor development, and their parents may fail to recognize or to report slowness in adaptive and social behavior.

Gross psychiatric disorders are rare in very young children, but autistic children may be quite late in speaking; their inattention to speech and other environmental sounds may suggest deafness or intellectual subnormality. However, it is more common for children with severe dysphasia and secondary behavior reactions to be diagnosed as demonstrating "autistic traits" than for autistic children to be diagnosed as dysphasic. The dysphasic child usually does not react to internal stimuli in the manner of a psychotic child. Although he may seem disturbed and will sometimes react violently because he is unable to cope with his environment, his emotionality will be relatively superficial and quite distinguishable from the phobias, the compulsivity, and the countless expressions of anxiety seen in psychoneurotic children. The dysphasic's deviant emotionality is mainly due to his inability to understand his environment.

Similar problems to those found in the diagnosis of dysphasia in childhood occur with dyslexia and dysgraphia. However, these disorders in symbolization are usually not apparent until the child is of school age, and are frequently overlooked or underestimated by the schools until he is in approximately the third grade. Mental retardation, visual defects, environmental problems, severe psychiatric disturbances, or psychogenic stress may all interfere with the processes of learning to read and write. Detailed history-taking and careful, complete physical and psychological examinations usually will clarify the diagnosis. The family history of school achievement is essential, since specific developmental dyslexia can be familial and uncomplicated by neurological or environmental handicap (Critchley, 1964). A thorough evaluation of the child's reading skills is imperative.

In any of these conditions the case history may indicate encephalopathy as the possible cause of the disability. In other cases no such history is found and the disability may be due to developmental neurological deficit or immaturity. Other possible causes of reading, writing, and spelling difficulties include psychological, educational, and/or environmental factors, all to be considered in the differential diagnosis.

In general, when teachers or parents report that a child is "immature," that he is "lazy," a "daydreamer," or an "underachiever"; when he has particular problems with verbal, reading, or number tasks; when he has difficulty retaining visual or auditory information; when he is very verbal but does not communicate meaningfully and there is an absence of conventional grammar; when there is a marked discrepancy between apparent capacity and actual achievement, it is advisable to consider the possibility of a language disorder.

EVALUATION

The essentials for medical evaluation of a child with a language disability include (1) the case history, and (2) comprehensive general and special physical examinations, including a complete battery of laboratory examinations.

Case History

Family Whenever possible, both parents should be interviewed as well as the child. The family history should include detailed information regarding the family constellation, educational and employment status of the parents, growth and development data on the siblings, and the family history of disease. Particular attention should be given to the history of other language disorders in the family.

In interviews with the parents and child, one must attempt to determine the specific interpersonal dynamics, especially the emotional stresses and strains, that exist in the family.

It is particularly important to get an educational history of every member of the family of a dyslexic child, since this condition can be familial in nature.

Birth This includes prenatal and postnatal information as well as the birth history itself. When possible, the child's birth record should be obtained from the hospital where he was born. It is also useful to have the mother describe the child's personality as an infant, or his characteristic type of reaction pattern.

Developmental Details of motor, language, adaptive, and social development are obtained. Of particular interest is the feeding history, the development and status of handedness, gross and fine motor coordination, the child's responses to sound as well as to speech, and the efficiency of communication by means other than speech. In assessing the child's social development, it is important to note the "sociability" of the environment in which he must function. One must determine whether the problem involves a normal child in an abnormal environment, or an abnormal child in a normal environment.

School This can be one of the most valuable portions of the case history. Whenever possible, reports should be secured from the child's teachers. Much information of value can be derived from the preschool and kindergarten teacher's observations of language development, gross and fine motor coordination, and social maturity.

Medical This is essentially the child's history of illness, including a complete review of all systems. It is important to note the age of the child at the time of an illness, the symptoms, severity, treatment, and the course of the illness. If the child has been hospitalized, these records can be obtained.

Physical Examination

The general physical examination is not simply a "checkup," although the general physical examination of a child includes evaluation of eyes, ears, nose, and throat, as well as of the nervous system. Children with language disorders should also be referred to specialists in the fields of ophthalmology, otolaryngology, and pediatric neurology. These specialists must be skilled in examining children and in the interpretation of their findings within the framework of developmental medicine.

The special points of focus in the physical examination of the child with language disabilities include these listed below (Richardson and Normanly, 1965):

Motor Abilities Gross motor function is evaluated by observing the gait, heel-and-toe walking, hopping on a single foot, skipping, rapid alternating movements, and finger-to-nose maneuvers. Fine motor coordination (and praxis) is evaluated by watching the child button and unbutton, tie laces, and so forth, and by paper-and-pencil tests. How the child grasps, points, and grips a pencil can be observed while he is drawing. He may be asked to demonstrate with his fingers how he would use scissors, brush his teeth, comb his hair, and so on. Similar evaluation of praxis, skilled performance of certain learned or consciously planned acts, is commonly tested by the psychologist, utilizing such tests as the Bender for copying, or the Graham-Kendell to evaluate reproduction from memory, or utilizing the Koh's blocks in the assembly of designs, and so on.

Speech is a motor function of special interest. One looks for any structural defect of the speech apparatus, such as a submucous cleft palate or severe dental malocclusion; special note is made of the child's ability to manipulate the tongue voluntarily and also of the diadochokinesis of the articulatory muscles. If there is any suspicion of dysarthria, additional tests, probably with the aid of an ENT specialist and a speech clinician, may be necessary.

Abnormal postural reflexes are noted; for example, when the child extends his arms with eyes closed, it is abnormal to have wide divergence or convergence of the arms, or variation in the levels at which the arms are held. Abnormal hand postures and fine tremor or choreiform movements must be noted. Not uncommonly, this may be seen in the so-called fidgety child, the one who literally cannot sit still. Throughout the examination, the examiner will look for possible tremor, mild choreoathetosis, or nonspecific general clumsiness. Tests for cerebellar signs include observations for ataxia on tandem walking, poor balance standing on one foot, poor diadochokinesis, and tremor.

Associated movements, known also as synkinesia or mirror movements, often accompany voluntary or involuntary movements in young children, generally in contralateral parts of the body. They decrease with age and their disappearance is considered to be a sign of the functional maturation of the nervous system.

Visual Functions The physician checks visual acuity, visual fields, and will also do funduscopic examination. It is particularly important to note the movement of the eyes in following an object and also to command, since oculomotor incoordination or strabismus is unusually frequent among children with organic neurological problems, and since lack of fusion or nonparallel vision can affect the formation of three-dimensional concepts. Because color coding is used in some educational approaches, color vision should be tested. It must be remembered that the child's visual acuity at 16 to 18 inches distance is almost more important than his visual acuity at 20 feet, since most of his school day will be spent in reading and also in shifting focus between book and blackboard.

Hearing Evaluation   Hearing is screened grossly during the general physical examination. Audiologic evaluation (and otologic evaluation if indicated) should be scheduled to determine the presence of hypacusis or dysacusis. One can be misled by seemingly normal responses on cursory examination. A bright child with hearing loss often receives enough visual cues to communicate appropriately. One must also remember that audiograms are notoriously inconsistent from one trial to another in dysphasic children. The inability to obtain a consistent audiogram and also a history that the child seems to hear at times and does not seem to hear at other times, or that he ignores even the loudest sounds, all are suggestive diagnostic signs. Comprehensive and thorough audiologic evaluation will be one of the most important steps in the total assessment of the child.

Psychomotor Abilities   The preferred hand, eye, and foot is recorded since "mixed or crossed dominance" is a frequent observation among these children, even though it is difficult to integrate this finding in a specific diagnosis, and its significance is not quite clear. If there is a difference in visual acuity between the two eyes, the child will probably use the better eye, so that eye dominance cannot always be determined with accuracy unless the visual acuity is essentially the same in both eyes.

Right-left confusion is to be noted. Normally, by the age of 6 to 7 years the child knows his own right and left sides. To differentiate this on another person standing opposite him requires an additional 2 years of maturity (Benton and Kemble, 1960). Tests of right-left discrimination and finger recognition or localization involve, in addition to perception, at least a concept of body image and extracorporeal space.

Examination of the Reflexes   This is, of course, a traditional part of neurological assessment and the examiner checks for the threshold of tendon reflexes as well as intensity of reflexes.

The physician who is experienced in evaluating children with language and learning problems may incorporate within the physical examination the use of adaptation of some tests which overlap the fields of neurology and psychology. In this way he will be able to utilize, chiefly for purposes of screening, tests of perception, some tests of memory, and some tests of praxis. For example, he will ask the child to copy forms and to draw a person. He may test for auditory digit span and may include a similar test using nonsense syllables. As mentioned, he will probably do tests of right-left discrimination and finger gnosia, and may check for unilateral tactile inattention to simultaneous stimulation. As part of the sensory examination he will usually check for atereognosis and graphesthesia. When a formal psychological evaluation is planned, the physician should not borrow from it items which will provide the child with advance experience, but some of these items do serve a useful function of screening when the physician is trying to determine how far he needs to go in ordering additional tests or consultations.

The assessment of vision, hearing, and speech needs specialized techniques, and specialists for these functions must be consulted if they are indicated.

The physician can do some rough screening for developmental dyslexia and dysgraphia, as well as dyscalculia. There are graded Durrell cards available which are useful, as well as the Gray Oral Reading Paragraphs. The physician may devise his own word-recognition test, may administer a brief spelling test, and may ask the youngster to do some calculation involving the four functions of number: addition, subtraction, multiplication, and division.

The child's behavioral characteristics are under continued observation throughout the entire evaluation. Routine psychiatric evaluation is rarely available. However, through the social and family histories and observation of parental attitudes, it is possible to assess the more obvious psychodynamic factors. It must be determined whether the child's emotional overlay is severe enough to require psychiatric referral. Actually, the psychotherapeutic value of a proper diagnosis and appropriate educational therapy can be dramatic in its impact on the child and on the parents and may, itself, provide a turning point in the child's emotional development and school adjustment.

Laboratory Tests

Routine laboratory tests include serology, hematology, and urinalysis, with routine test for phenylketonuria. Some physicians routinely obtain metabolic studies, such as blood cholesterol or protein-bound iodine. Others may include galactose, lipid, and calcium studies in order to complete their differential diagnosis. When available, urine chromatography may be done for screening amino acids and other abnormal metabolites. X-rays of the skull, long bones, and wrists may be ordered. If genetic assessment seems indicated, the physician can order a chromosome analysis. An electroencephalogram may be ordered, including wake, sleep, and serial tracings. However, it should be emphasized that, except where seizures are suspected, the electroencephalogram usually contributes little of practical value in the diagnosis or management of children with language disorders. If the child has focal brain dysrhythmia or a frank convulsive disorder, this will easily be detected on the electroencephalogram; but, if there is any damage subcortically, below the cortex of the brain, it may not be recorded on the electroencephalogram. Therefore, a positive electroencephalogram may confirm the diagnosis, but a normal electroencephalogram does not necessarily exclude neurological dysfunction. It is well to remember, also, that many children with grossly abnormal electroencephalograms and overt epilepsy have no particular language disorder, and many children with language disorders have normal electroencephalograms. Parenthetically, it should be mentioned that children with developmental dysphasia almost never show electroencephalographic abnormality over specific areas conventionally associated with language functions, such as Broca's area or Wernicke's area.

As stated earlier, the purpose of medical evaluation is to demonstrate the presence or absence of a language disorder and to determine the existence of any disease or injury. This is only the first step in the complete diagnostic evaluation of the child. Complete language and behavioral assessments are necessary. These involve evaluation by specialists in speech, language and audiology, a psychologist, the child's teacher, an educational diagnostician, and others as indicated. Ideally, the physicians who have participated in the evaluation of the child should confer together and with these other specialists in order to arrive at a diagnosis that will provide the basis for appropriate recommendations, management, and educational planning.

In the case of a child with a language disorder, the initial evaluation may not result in a definitive diagnosis that is as simple and clear-cut as, for example, right lower lobe pneumonia. The diagnostic impressions may be mostly descriptive and etiology may be obscure. However, this is the first step, the baseline for subsequent observations and re-assessments. Recommendations for management or treatment must be evaluated for their effectiveness and revised as indicated on a continuing basis. For these children there is no cut and dried diagnosis and treatment.

REFERENCES

Benton, A. A., and J. D. Kemble. 1960. Right-left orientation and reading disability. Psychiat. Neurol., 139:49-60.

Clements, S. D. 1966. Minimal Brain Dysfunctions in Children—Terminology and Identification. Co-sponsored by The Easter Seal Research Foundation of the National Society for Crippled Children and National Institute of Neurological Disease and Blindness, U. S. Department of Health, Education and Welfare.

Critchley, M. 1964. Developmental Dyslexia. Springfield, Ill., Charles C. Thomas.

Davidoff, R. A., and L. C. Johnson. 1964. Paroxysmal EEG activity and cognitive-motor performance. Electroenceph. Clin. Neurophysiol., 16:343.

Drew, A. L. 1955. Familial reading disability. Univ. Michigan Med. Bull., 21:245.

Eisenson, J. 1968. Developmental aphasia—a speculative view with therapeutic implications. J. Speech Hearing Dis., 33:3-13.

Ingram, T. T. S. 1963. Delayed development of speech with special reference to dyslexia. Proc. Roy. Soc. Med., 56:199.

Keenan, J. S. 1968. The nature of receptive and expressive impairments in aphasia. J. Speech Hearing Dis., 33:20-25.

MacKeith, R., and M. Bax. 1963. Minimal brain damage—a concept discarded. *In* Bax, M., and R. MacKeith, eds., Little Club Clinics in Developmental Medicine, No. 10: Minimal Cerebral Dysfunction. London, The National Spastics Society and Heinemann Medical Books.

Morrell, F. 1962. Electrophysiological contributions to the neural basis of learning. Physiol. Rev., 41:443.

Orton, S. 1937. Reading, Writing, and Speech Problems in Children. New York, W. W. Norton.

Paine, R. S. 1962. Minimal chronic brain syndromes in children. Develop. Med. Child Neurol., 4:21.

Richardson, S. O. 1968. Voice and speech disorders of mental and emotional origin. *In* Gibbs, S. S., and B. M. Kagan, eds., Current Pediatric Therapy. Philadelphia, Saunders.

——— and J. Normanly. 1965. Incidence of pseudoretardation in a clinic population. Amer. J. Dis. Child., 109:432-435.

Touwen, B. C. L., and H. Prechtl. 1970. The neurological examination of the child with minor nervous dysfunction. Philadelphia, Lippincott.

Part 4: Management and corrective education

11: The general problem of management and corrective education

Michael Marge

Once the language-handicapped child has been identified and has received a careful diagnostic examination, many problems concerned with the provision of essential clinical and educational services must be faced. Decisions must be made about the goals of the language training program for each child; the personnel providing the language training; the time appropriate for initiating the program; the type of program, which includes considerations of the frequency and length of training, individual versus group sessions, and the content of the instruction; and the ancillary services necessary for the program (e.g., medicine, psychology, and school work). The purpose of this chapter is to provide an overview of these problems and their implications for the development of an effective management and corrective education program for children with language disabilities.

THE MANAGEMENT PROCESS

The process of managing any program which provides services and special training to the handicapped may be evaluated by determining if each of three criteria is met. These are

1. *Comprehensiveness of services*—every effort should be made to provide the handicapped individual with all the services and training necessary to attend to his specific needs.

2. *Continuity of services*—from the time the handicapped individual is entered into a program of services and training to the time he is successfully released, he should be provided with a consistently effective program.

The author wishes to express his appreciation to Laura Lee (Northwestern University), Donald Harrington (Childrens Bureau, Washington, D. C.), James J. Gallagher (University of North Carolina), and Philip J. Schmitt (Gallaudet College)—all of whom reviewed the manuscript for this chapter and offered many valuable suggestions.

3. *Coordination of services*—related to the points 1 and 2, there should be a mechanism for assuring that the individual benefits from the combined efforts of all pertinent agencies and persons in a given community throughout the period of his program of services and training.

What implications do these factors have for the best management practices for children with language disabilities? First, it is proposed that language disabilities are best managed by the responsible professional person or agency which has available and frequently utilizes a team of specialists throughout the entire program of training. For example, in the case of diagnosis of the language problem, it is not enough to use a comprehensive approach with a team of consultants just for the initial examination (Wood, 1964). It is untenable to believe that an initial examination alone provides all the necessary information for the development of an effective training program. The diagnostic process, which should continue throughout the program of intervention, often resulting in essential modifications of techniques and direction, requires the continual use of a team of consultants to provide the managing professional with a dimension of comprehensiveness of approach.

Another implication is that one agency or professional person should accept the responsibility not only for initiating the program but also for managing it from its inception to its termination. The fact that some children are not managed by a single professional resource in the community may be a function of the belief that the responsibility is that of the parents and not the professional. The practice of receiving a diagnosis in one agency and language training in another is a common problem in the current provision of services for atypical children which has resulted in serious complications for specialists as well as for the child and his family. Some of these complications include confusion of goals and practices resulting from differences in professional definitions and philosophies, difficulty in providing a smooth transition for the family from one agency to another, and duplication of effort when the diagnostic procedures have to be repeated. Also, lack of coordinated management often leads to "agency shopping" by the family, in which case the child shifts from one service agency to another during the critical stages of the child's language development, with long periods of interruption or reduction in intensity of programming. Among the most serious repercussions of this practice may be the loss of the child's motivation for and cooperation with the language training program.

And finally, to ensure the provision of the best possible services throughout the training period by drawing together all necessary elements, one person or agency should function as liaison with various professionals in the community, with the schools, and with the family. In the management of atypical children, one often finds serious gaps in the communication among diverse groups of specialists interested in the child, not only at specific times during the management process but throughout the entire process. The coordination of these diverse efforts increases the probability of successful management of the child.

GENERAL AND SPECIFIC GOALS FOR CHILDREN WITH LANGUAGE DISABILITIES

The primary goal of management and corrective education for all children with language disabilities is to help each child develop effective language ability as soon as possible. *Effective* is the key term in the statement of the primary goal. This term refers to the development of a language function, especially oral language, appropriate for the child's age and maturational level, which allows him to listen, understand, and communicate his thoughts and feelings in a meaningful and understandable manner to peers and adults. Secondary goals that identify specific skills and behaviors for all children which should result from the language training program include

1. Development of facile expression of thoughts and feelings.

2. Development of "linguistic shifting behavior"—i.e., a skill which allows a speaker to readily adjust from one communicative situation, with its inherent requirements, to another, by adapting to the appropriate oral language needs of the situation, e.g., the ability to communicate with adults as well as with peers.

3. Expansion of the linguistic repertoire of words and concepts.

4. By the use of readiness activities, provision of a linguistic foundation for the further development of language skills, such as reading and writing.

5. Assistance to the child, family, and the school in accepting the language disability without emotional overreaction and with a greater degree of objectivity.

In Chapter 3 it was stated that there are commonalities of need among all children with language disabilities as well as individual needs which must be considered in the management process. Though there is an acceptance of this position, there appears to be a tendency to develop training programs on the basis of broad categories of need often related to etiological classification schemes. For example, Wood (1964) discusses the needs of children classified according to these categories: brain injury, aphasia, dysarthria, mental retardation, hearing loss, emotional disturbance, and immaturity. In a similar vein, Lenneberg (1964) reviews the needs among children in the various categories listed by Wood but adds the categories of congenital inarticulation, congenital receptive disorder, structural abnormalities in the oropharyngeal cavity, and minor articulatory deficits. Both authors present generalizations about each category, indicating what differences in training approaches may be necessary. They caution, however, that generalizations are subject to many exceptions and that individual needs must be identified and met by the training program. In our view, if each child is perceived as a functioning or potentially functioning linguistic system, the training program should be based in large part on his current and potential linguistic capacity rather than on the limitations which are implied by the etiological category into which he has been placed. Therefore, the description of his linguistic ability and disability and not the etiology of his disability should determine the form of the management process.

Some attempts have been made to develop diagnostic tests which analyze language behavior and avoid etiological classifications. One of the most promising and perhaps the most comprehensive test is the Illinois Test of Psycholinguistic Abilities (McCarthy and Kirk, 1961). The ITPA has been useful in describing a child's language status, revealing his linguistic strengths and weaknesses, and suggesting the most appropriate ways to provide a remedial program. Based on the theoretical model of language by Osgood (1957a, b), the test appraises linguistic abilities on (1) two levels of language usage—representational and automatic-sequential; (2) three main psycholinguistic processes—decoding, encoding, and association; (3) certain channels of communication—auditory or visual and motor or vocal. McCarthy and Kirk (1961) believe that a remedial program can be more easily programmed from learning theory than from neurological speculations. For this reason, the ITPA relies on operationally defined functions based primarily on behavioral, not neurological, theory.

In developing a specific course of action for an appropriate program of assistance and utilizing all the available data obtained from the diagnostic process, answers to the following questions should be sought:

1. When should the language training program begin?
2. What are the specific goals for the child based on the current status of his language ability?
3. Should the child be seen individually or in a group?
4. How frequently should the child be seen?
5. What ancillary services must be provided?

Let us consider now some of the issues raised by each question.

When Should Language Training Begin?

In previous chapters, the importance of early identification and diagnosis of language disabilities was stressed. Most scholars agree that it is equally important to apply interventional techniques as early as possible, though there is some disagreement about the type and intensity of training required to meet the primary goal of assisting the child in his development of language skills as adequately and as soon as possible (Webster et al., 1966; Wood, 1964; Bangs, J., 1957; Bangs, T., 1968; Frostig and Maslow, 1968; Schlanger, 1959; Lowell, 1968). The arguments in favor of early intervention arise from the evidence supporting the preventive nature of such programs and the observation that the programs of intervention at early ages (preschool) present fewer problems and are considerably less complicated than training provided at later age levels (school-age).

It should be noted that Lenneberg (1966) argues for a postponement of language training for the young child since he feels there is very little which can be done to modify language behavior during the period of language acquisition. He observes that maturation plays the single most significant role in the development of early language behavior. Environmental stimulation and intensive training, therefore, will not noticeably result in higher stages of language development when the young child has not matured to a period of readiness for specific linguistic behaviors. Further, it is suggested that since almost all children, even the most dramatically atypical, eventually attain meaningful language ability according to their own rate of development, we should wait until the process of language maturation is completed. Then, if adequate language function has not been attained as a result of the "natural" process of maturation, special training may be needed and, contrary to the views of the early interventionalists, the training effort is less difficult because the child is more linguistically mature, has had more social experience, and is capable of understanding the purpose and details of the instruction. The observation that the postponement of training will lead to a cumulative deficit in language learning and a greater tendency toward emotional problems is obviously not accepted by those who support later intervention for language disabilities. Most educators would find this approach unacceptable. The research and clinical evidence, moreover, is noticeably in favor of the efficacy of early intervention for all linguistically handicapped children. The "wait-and-see policy" invariably has led to many unnecessary complications which enlarge the problem of providing an effective training program.

What Are the Specific Goals for the Child Based on the Current Status of His Language Ability?

It has been stated that the primary goal of management and corrective education for the language-handicapped child is to help each child develop effective language ability as soon as possible. There are at least three broad approaches to language teaching which identify specific goals for the child—phonetic, development of perceptual skills and concept formation, and grammatical. Each will be considered in a later section. For the present discussion, let us review the specific goals of the grammatical approach.

In determining the level of a child's linguistic ability, the grammatical approach, emanating from modern linguistic theory and research in child language acquisition, appears to hold great promise. This approach suggests that children with language disabilities should be evaluated according to their phonological, morphological, syntactic, and semantic functioning. Using developmental sentence types, such as those suggested by Lee (1966) which draw upon the observations and studies of McNeill (1966) and Chomsky (1957), the level of development in the progression from simple to complex structures (i.e., from one-word sentences to complex sentences) can be described in a manner meaningful for the language training program. Specific goals on a day-to-day and week-to-week basis could be identified by following the principle of presenting linguistic forms (1) in the developmental sequence in which a child may be expected to acquire grammatical structure and (2) at the time when he is ready to relate the new linguistic form to his inner organization of experience and concepts. The assumption underlying this approach is as follows: Most children spontaneously abstract from the adult models in their environment those semantic, syntactic, and morphological features for which they have developed, or are ready to develop, a meaningful counterpart in experience, observation, and cognitive growth (Lee, 1969). Therefore, oral language ability increases in relation to internal mechanisms of competence, sometimes referred to as the "deep structure" of meaningful content. This explanation of language acquisition implies that the child induces for himself the linguistic structures of his native language from the stimulation of speech models without direct teaching by the adult. The child acquires adult rules of syntax, for example, in a series of steps which are cumulative, each higher level depending upon the success at earlier stages (Lee, 1966).

Should the Child Be Seen Individually or in a Group?

This question has been the subject of many debates about the provision of effective special educational services to language-handicapped children. The arguments for and against either arrangement concern what is best for the child. On the one hand, some authorities hold that individual training sessions allow for greater depth and intensity of programming, resulting in a more effective effort which will take less time to reach a successful termination when compared with group sessions. On the other hand, some feel that group sessions, especially if the groups are small, provide communicative experiences among the peer members which enhance the training and cannot be offered by individual sessions. It is further argued that since children do learn from one another as readily as they do from adults, and since peer-group communications are an important function in a child's life, group sessions are not only useful but also essential.

In deciding which approach will be chosen, other considerations must be explored. If a child has a severe language disability, is easily distracted in group situations or noticeably aware and upset about his disability, individual attention may be the most desirable choice. Another factor concerns whether or not the specialist or agency providing services can afford to train children in individual sessions. Limitations in staff, equipment, and facilities may prohibit the use of individual training.

A recommended course of action is to deal with young children first on an individual basis with the intention of gradually placing them in groups as they become more accustomed to the management process.

How Frequently Should the Child Be Seen?

The severity of the disability, the age of the child, the cooperation of the parents, and the limitations in staff and facilities of the agency determine how often and how long the child should be seen. The recommended range of frequency of sessions for any effectiveness in training is two to five times weekly with sessions from ½ hour to 1 hour in duration. The general rule is that the more severe the disability, the more frequent and longer the sessions. In addition to the specific language training sessions in the agency, the management of the child's language disabilities should be extended to as many of his other daily activities as possible. It is essential that the parents and the child are carefully prepared for the program by identifying weekly or monthly objectives for the child and by specifying days and hours for sessions on a scheduled basis. As Wood (1964) points out, a routine must be established which is planned and organized in such a way that a learning climate is created to which the child could attach meaning.

What Ancillary Services Must Be Provided?

The management process should entail not only the provision of an appropriate training program to modify and improve the child's language behavior and a mechanism for continual evaluation of progress in training, but also the services of specialists from various disciplines to attend to any other of the child's problems which are concurrent with his language disability. Once the training program is initiated, the child's entire complex of needs should be met by the management program either by provision of necessary services through the agency or in collaboration with other agencies. For example, in the case of a language-handicapped child with a hearing loss, provision should be made for periodic otological and audiological examinations to assess the status of his impairment and his prosthesis (if a hearing aid is prescribed). The major ancillary services which should be provided are periodic medical, psychological, and educational evaluations.

SPECIALISTS OF LANGUAGE DISABILITIES

The type and nature of the management process is primarily determined by the language limitations and assets currently possessed by the child. Other influential factors include the availability of ancillary professional personnel, limitations of current evalution and interventional techniques, and the skills of the language specialist. The success of the management program is primarily dependent upon the professional who is responsible for the child. Ideally, he should be the "manager of the language program" and should have the skill to handle all types of severities of language disability. Furthermore, he should have a grasp of the current knowledge about language and its related disabilities, including theory and training in child psychology, speech pathology and audiology, descriptive linguistics, psycholinguistics (especially child language acquisition), and teaching English as a second language, in addition to a substantial background in early childhood and primary-grade education. This idealized specialist should be capable of managing the diagnostic process and training program for any child with language problems. He should possess a working knowledge of necessary diagnostic tests and procedures, of the contributions of other professionals who may be involved in the diagnostic process, and the various types of interventional techniques available for meeting the individual needs of children. Also, he should have the professional skill to coordinate the various resources to provide the child with necessary services, even to the extent that he may actively engage in both the diagnosis and training program. With regard to his role in implementing the training program, if he does not actually perform the training, but transfers this responsibility to one of a number of specialists, he should retain a supervisory and resource role in the program. Unfortunately, specialists with these requisites are few in number and cannot represent a national resource for the language-handicapped child. Instead, services must be sought from professionals representing no fewer than six disciplines:

1. Speech pathologists (and audiologists)
2. Teachers of English as a second language
3. Applied linguists
4. Clinical child psychologists
5. Language-arts teachers (including speech-improvement teachers)
6. Special educators (including learning-disability teachers and teachers of the deaf and hard-of-hearing)

In Chapter 3 a discussion of the skills generally offered by each of these specialists indicated that the concept of a manager of language disabilities is not found in the training of those who provide services to children with various types of disabilities. Speech pathologists are found to provide services in diagnosis and training for types I, II, and III.[1] Some clinical child psychologists and most teachers of learning disabilities have the skills to engage in diagnostic activity and in training programs for types II and III. Some teachers of the deaf and hard-of-hearing can provide training services for children with types I and II disabilities. Though they cannot be expected to assist types I, II, and III disabilities, most teachers of English as a second language and language-arts teachers can apply their skills to implement training programs for children who speak dialects and become handicapped in their school programs. Finally, few, if any, applied linguists have the training to assist children either in the dialect-speaking category or with language disabilities. Though some speech pathologists possess the capability of determining language deviations (types I, II, and III) among speakers of dialect, they are in the minority because of their inability to differentiate a bona fide disability from the dialect pattern presented by the child. This is especially true of children who may possess what appears to be an articulation disorder or delayed syntactic development. The diagnostician must know the linguistic characteristics of the standard dialect pattern before an evaluation of disability within the dialect can be made.

Let us consider the role of the parents in the management process. For a number of reasons, parents should be incorporated as an integral part of the program of training for the child. First, the motivation and cooperation of the child for the program are, in large part, dependent upon the attitudes of the parents. Second, the program becomes more meaningful and effective if some of the activities conducted in the agency are continued at home by the child's parents (Wood, 1964). Of course, it should be fully realized that the parents cannot substitute for a language specialist, and therefore the goals for linguistic activities for the home should be considerably less ambitious than those for the formal training sessions. At best the parents can assist in reinforcing certain learned language behaviors. And third, with limited training, parents are able to assist the specialist in evaluating the progress of the child in the language program. Again, clinical objectivity in the assessment of their child is an unreasonable demand to place upon the

---

[1] Type I. *Failure to acquire any language.* Children who by age 4 years have not shown any sign of acquiring the language of their speech community, which is that set of people who communicate with each other, directly or indirectly, via a common language.

Type II. *Delayed Language Acquisition.* Children whose language acquisition is below levels attained by their age peers in their speech community. The delay may occur in all, one, or some combination of the phonological, semantic, and syntactic components of the language of their speech community.

Type III. *Acquired language disabilities.* Members of a speech community who had at some point in their developmental history acquired the language of their speech community, who subsequent to such adequate language acquisition suffered a complete loss or reduction of their capacity to use the language common to their speech community.

parents. But, since the parents are able to observe the child in many situ
elicit spontaneous linguistic utterances, they can be of assistance in providin.
evaluation of progress.

If the community program for management of language disabilities in children is to
be effective, therefore, some one individual or agency, other than the parents, should
assume the responsibility for the provision of *comprehensive*, *continuous*, and *coordinated* services.

APPROACHES TO LANGUAGE TRAINING

The rapidly expanding literature on language disabilities in children is rich with
descriptions of various programs of training. Broadly speaking, if primary consideration is
given to the inception and chief focus of the language program, there appear to be at least
three general approaches to language training. They are phonetic, development of
perceptual skills and concept formation, and grammatical approaches. Each may be
discussed according to general strategy, specific training techniques, and recommended
grouping. Table 1 summarizes each approach.

Phonetic Approach

The general strategy recommended by the phonetic approach (Berry and Eisenson, 1956;
Wood, 1964; Kohl, 1966; Clements et al., 1964) is to begin with the correct formation of
speech sounds. Regardless of the etiology, the specialist focuses upon the discrimination
and production of sounds, gradually progressing to syllables, words, phrases, and
sentences. The rationale for this strategy is based on two assumptions: (1) language
development naturally follows the sequence from sound formation to words and
sentences, and (2) sounds are the building blocks with which all other language forms are
created. Specific teaching techniques include auditory-discrimination training, development of articulatory flexibility, imitation of the specialist's speech, phonetic placement
(for older children), drillwork, practice of the speech sounds in increasingly more
complex linguistic forms, and practice in use of correct sounds in conversational speech
and in oral reading. These are generally applied in a semistructured program of
instruction. Once the child learns the correct sound formations, it is expected that with
little drillwork on vocabulary and sentence formation, he will eventually realize language
skills comparable to those of his peers.

It is recommended that the training be conducted with small groups of children
primarily for the socialization which will result and most likely accelerate the acquisition
of complex language forms. However, if a child is having difficulty in adjusting to groups,
he should be seen individually.

The phonetic approach represents the traditional program of training used by a large
proportion of speech pathologists, teachers of the deaf and hard-of-hearing, and teachers
of aphasic children.

Table 1. Summary of Major Approaches to Language Training

Approach	General strategy	Specific training techniques	Recommended grouping
Phonetic	Focus on correct speech sound formulation; progress to words and sentences	Imitation of teacher or specialist; auditory discrimination training; drillwork; strengthening visual and kinesthetic cues; phonetic placement and sound analysis (for older children); vocabulary building	Small groups are recommended unless child cannot tolerate groups, then should be seen individually
Development of perceptual skills and concept formation	Focus on auditory and visual perceptual skills development and concept formation; concept development leads to words and sentences	Use of special materials in carefully ordered, highly structured lessons; imitation of verbal labels of events and experiences; speech sounds are taught in relation to alphabet	Small groups of children who interact with the teacher or specialist on a one-to-one basis
Grammatical	Stress on instruction of grammatical development; begins at child's level of grammar on a continuum of language development and progresses to more complex and adult levels	Teach kernel sentences and transformations; drillwork; limited imitation of instructor; use of expansions and interpretations; teach concepts, then word or appropriate grammatical form	No consensus, but proponents tend to suggest individual management unless children are grouped according to comparable levels of language comprehension and production

Development of Perceptual Skills and Concept Formation Approach

The major proponents of the developmental approach (Richardson, 1963; Schechter, 1966) are teachers and specialists who utilize the Montessori methodologies and materials in training language-handicapped children. The major focus of the program of instruction is to enrich the experiences of the child in a carefully prescribed sequence of activities with the goal of improving perceptual skills and developing a rich organization of oncepts. Essentially, it is assumed that if the child realizes the meaning of an experience or event (i.e., understands it in relation to other experiences) and builds a hierarchy of meanings, language skills will readily develop. Therefore, comprehension of experiences precedes production of language forms. Specific training techniques include providing the verbal label to an experience or event which the child appears to understand, practice in recalling labels of experiences and events, limited imitation for correct sound formation, and learning the alphabet as it relates to speech sounds. Practice in oral language is encouraged during structured sessions when the child is taught concepts.

Though children are grouped, each child is treated as an individual who is allowed to progress at his own rate.

Grammatical Approach

The general strategy of this approach (Lee, 1966, 1970; Monsees, 1967; Stark, 1968; Brown, 1966) is to improve the grammatical development of the child's language production. Instead of emphasizing sounds or concept formation, this approach focuses upon teaching grammar, which is thought to be the most significant aspect of language development. Based on the theories and postulates of Chomsky (1957), it is believed that language consists of a small number of elementary sentence types and that all the meaningful and grammatical utterances of the language can be produced from these sentences by certain operational processes called transformations. Language teaching, then, becomes a matter of learning and practicing these basic patterns (Monsees, 1967). The child is taught basic types of patterns which represent the next step in the developmental sequence above his current grammatical production. For example, if a child is still using a single noun as a noun phrase, omitting any modifiers (as in the case of saying *car* instead of *Daddy's car* or *my little car*), the language program would attempt to teach the noun phrase as a grammatical unit.

Specific training techniques include practice and drill in the basic sentence patterns and transformations of these patterns, repeating the child's utterances in longer and more complex sentences (called "expansions"), responding to the child's utterances by more complex statements or interpretation, and engaging in development of concepts and verbal labeling of experiences and events.

Because of the amount of material to cover, lessons are generally well structured, with some time for spontaneous activity. There appears to be no consensus about the most desirable grouping.

In addition to these major approaches to language training, one finds many eclectic developments. As an example, let us consider a typical eclectic program of language training which may be found in a university setting. Children with language disabilities are evaluated according to the following functions: (1) sensory acuity, (2) attention and retention spans, (3) perceptual skills, (4) concept-formation ability, (5) receptive language level, and (6) expressive language skills (i.e., phonemic, morphemic, syntactic, and semantic abilities). The battery of tests which are administered to assess these functions may include audiological evaluation, the Wepman Auditory Discrimination Test, the Rosewell-Chall Auditory Blending Test, Frostig Test of Visual Perceptual Abilities,

Peabody Picture Vocabulary Test, Berko Test of Grammatical Ability, Illinois Test of Psycholinguistic Ability, and others as needed.

Language training incorporates the development of auditory and visual perceptual skills and proper sentence structure. With regard to the latter, the specialist will structure the lessons so that grammar is taught in the developmental sequence suggested by Lee (1969) and Stark (1968). In addition to practice with kernel sentences and transformations of these sentences, a multisensory approach will be utilized so that the child may match word cards to appropriate pictures, select a picture or word card after hearing the auditory command, or produce the sentences after seeing the pictures or the word cards in sequential order.

Unfortunately, there is no reported evidence on the effectiveness of any approach in current use. The literature reveals discussions of individual cases of successful results with language disabilities in children, but one finds it difficult to generalize because of the multiplicity of factors which may individually or in combination lead to failure or success in managing language handicaps.

MANAGEMENT SETTINGS

The problem of limitations in the manpower resources available to language-handicapped children is compounded by the limitations in the settings where services are offered. The quantity and quality of services in each setting is dependent upon many factors, some of which are training and expertise of professional personnel, type and number of personnel, priorities for managing handicapped children, physical facilities and equipment, and community need and demands for services.

The settings in which management services are provided include regular day-school programs, preschool education programs, college and university speech and hearing centers, hospital and community speech and hearing centers, and private practice. To determine the effectiveness of the services provided, it is suggested that each setting be evaluated by the critiera of *comprehensiveness, continuity,* and *coordination* of services (see pages 297-298 for a description of these criteria).

Regular Day-School Programs

Though the exact number of public and nonpublic regular day-school systems which offer special services to children with language disabilities is not currently known, it has been estimated that 59.1 percent of the nation's elementary schools and 40.7 percent of the secondary schools have available the service of an estimated 9,000 speech clinicians (NEA, 1967) who, in many cases, can provide appropriate management of the language-handicapped child. In addition, there are teachers of the deaf and hard-of-hearing, an estimated 6,050, who manage day-school programs, and teachers of specific learning disabilities, who are estimated at 9,400. Few school programs offer a full range of management services for all types of language disabilities, except for type II, and not all can be expected to meet the needs of these children. Further, the other criteria of good management are met by few school systems. Most educational programs in the chools list the development of speech and language skills as one of their major objectives, nd instruction in these skills for the typical child is interwoven throughout the urriculum. However, though there has been a steady growth in the schools in the rovision of language services for the atypical child, his needs are far from being met.

It would appear that the ideal setting for the provision of a full range of language raining is the schools because (1) they are geographically accessible; (2) they occupy a ubstantial part of the child's day and therefore make him available for extensive and ntensive intervention; (3) they allow for the specific training program to function within he meaningful context of the educational curriculum; and (4) they are best suited for naintaining continuity of programming throughout the child's elementary and secondary ducational career.

Preschool Education Programs

Early intervention in language training for children with language disabilities is the desirable course of action. In many instances, it is noted that speech and language skills or typical children are taught as part of the regular preschool curriculum. Unfortunately, widespread and comprehensive services for preschool language-handicapped children are elatively unavailable through preschool educational programs. Except deaf children, dequate specific services for children with language disabilities as part of the preschool program have not realized substantial growth.

In the past 5 years, there have been some major developments in preschool education which have stepped up national interest in language training. Several federal programs— Project Head Start; Parent and Child Centers; Follow-Through; Education of the Disadvantaged through Title I of the Elementary and Secondary Education Act of 1965, and Education of the Handicapped through Title VI of the Elementary and Secondary Education Act Amendments of 1967—have prompted the planning and development of comprehensive preschool programs which include, as one of their necessary components, services for all children with language disabilities. The rapid initiation and expansion of these programs, which attend to the needs of all children, is anticipated.

With the realization that early educational intervention is a significant factor in the later academic achievement of children, public school programs are rapidly establishing preschool classes and services. It is predicted that these programs may eventually reach children as young as 1 year of age. Concern for language acquisition in young children will lead to the incorporation of special language training to prevent the development of communicative difficulties and/or to accelerate the growth and development of language skills.

College and University Speech and Hearing Centers

All colleges and universities with training programs in speech pathology and audiology maintain a clinical center which offers services to one or more of the various types of language disabilities. At present, there are 271 institutions (J. Fricke, personal communication, 1968) with a professional working force of an estimated 1,900

professionals broadly distributed throughout the United States. Almost all can b
expected to provide services to types II and III language disabilities and many serve type
but few have programs for speakers of dialect. Some centers may focus upon th
provision of services for all children with language disabilities, regardless of etiology
while another may restrict its program to children whose language problems appea
related to certain etiologies. Services differ in quality and quantity from institution t
institution and may be related to whether the center exists as a community-oriented
agency or chiefly as a training ground for the institution's students. Since these purpose
are not necessarily mutually exclusive and both may be served at the same time, there i
little apparent justification for some institutions to argue that they find it necessary t
sacrifice one for the other.

One of the major advantages in the development of language training programs i
colleges and universities is that in many circumstances the program generally reflects th
most recent advances in language training and is modified accordingly to the benefit o
the children under management. In an estimated 64 centers located in university-affiliate
hospitals (J. Fricke, personal communication, 1968), all necessary ancillary services ar
provided. There are, however, several disadvantages of this setting which should b
considered. First, by the nature of their limited facilities and professional manpower
college and university programs cannot be expected to serve the entire community o
preschool and school-age children with language disabilities. Second, these programs fac
the difficulty of maintaining comprehensiveness and continuity of services. Lines o
communication between the institutions of higher education and other institutions in th
community—especially the public schools—generally are not well established, resulting i
isolated management of children. And third, the turnover of students-in-training assigne
to the children renders the overall training program less effective.

As public school and preschool educational programs for language-handicappe
children realize greater expansion, colleges and universities eventually may limit thei
programs to private school children for whom language training may not be available an
to children referred by other agencies for an additional opinion about appropriate
management.

Hospital and Community Speech and Hearing Centers

These represent an estimated 575 nonuniversity hospital and community centers (J
Fricke, personal communication, 1968) with a professional manpower resource estimated
at 2,700, which deal primarily with types I, II, and III cases of language disability. Again,
it is observed that only a few provide necessary services for children who speak dialects.
Of all the available agencies, the hospital centers usually provide all the ancillary services
necessary for the appropriate management of the children. Though continuity and
coordination of services may be somewhat better than those found in other agencies
hospital and community centers still function relatively autonomous of the other
significant resources in the community. A common complaint by the public schools, for
example, is that these centers not only have little or no understanding of the child's
educational needs but also do not really communicate with the schools about the child's

inguistic problems. As a result, the child is not carefully managed as he shuffles back and orth between the two settings or from one setting to the other.

Private Practice

To realistically assess the clinical management effectiveness of the category of private practice, it is necessary to make a distinction between those who are in serious full-time practice and those who engage in practice on a part-time basis (less than 20 hours per week) in addition to a full-time position in another setting.

Berlinsky et al. (1971) state that because of his relatively independent and isolated working situation and his ready availability to members of the general public, the private

Table 2. Estimates of Availability of Management Services for Children with Language Disabilities by Setting

Criteria for evaluating management	No. regular day-school programs[a]	No. preschool educational programs	No. college and university speech and hearing centers	No. hospital and community speech and hearing centers	No. full-time private practices
A. Comprehensiveness of services					
1. Diagnostic and training services					
a. Type I	Few	Few	Many	Many	Few
b. Type II	Many	Few	All	All	Many
c. Type III	Few	Few	All	All	Many
d. Dialect	Few	Few	Few	Few	Few
e. All types	Few	Few	Few	Few	Few
2. Availability of ancillary services	Few	Few	Many	All	Many
B. Continuity of services	Few	Few	Few	Few	Few
C. Coordination of services	Few	Few	Few	Few	Few

[a]Excludes special residential schools for the deaf, mentally retarded, and emotionally disturbed.

practicioner assumes a responsibility for patient care greater and more hazardous than that of clinicians in other settings. With this caution in mind, the American Academy of Private Practice in Speech Pathology and Audiology has recommended standards for training and experience of clinicians in private practice which exceed those required for clinical certification by the American Speech and Hearing Association. Full-time practicioners who meet these standards are generally sensitive to the need for providing comprehensiveness and continuity of services for their patients.

Although most part-time private practicioners dealing with language disabilities have some relationship, formal or informal, with other professional consultants whose services are pertinent to the problems of the children, it has been observed that they have greater difficulty than full-time practicioners in providing necessary ancillary services on an effective basis. Even during the language-training phase of the service program, when a team approach is not as critical as it is during the diagnostic phase, the private practicioner functions at a disadvantage without the consultation of other professional specialists on a readily available basis.

In all the above settings, there are common limitations which add to the problem of providing adequate services to children with language disabilities. These limitations may be summarized as follows:

1. Few programs meet the needs of all types of language disabilities.

2. Limited available resources for the number of children in need of services.

3. Service programs which are not geographically accessible to all language handicapped children.

4. Limited concern for the communication problems of children who speak a dialect

5. Few programs which provide comprehensiveness and continuity of services.

The ideal setting for providing necessary services to the child with language disabilities appears to be in the public schools, if language training programs are designed to meet the individual needs of the child and if the school program demonstrates a concern for the *comprehensiveness, continuity*, and *coordination* of services.

Table 2 summarizes the current availability of management services by agency according to the three major criteria. Since exact data and careful documentation about current services are not available, the information in Table 2 represents estimates based on the author's experience and observations. These judgments, therefore, should be used with caution and with the qualification that they are tentative.

REFERENCES

Bangs, J. 1957. Preschool language education for the brain-damaged child. Volta Rev. 69:17-19.

Bangs, Tina 1968. Language and Learning Disorders of the Pre-Academic Child. New York, Appleton-Century-Crofts.

Berlinsky et al. 1971. Preparation for private practice: academic, clinical, experiential Asha, 13:599-600.

Berry, M., and J. Eisenson. 1956. Speech Disorders. New York, Appleton-Century-Crofts

Brown, R. 1966. From codability to coding ability. *In* Bruner, J., ed., Learning about Learning, A Conference Report (Cooperative Research Monograph No. 15). Washington, D. C., Office of Education.

Chomsky, N. 1957. Syntactic Structures. The Hague, Mouton and Co.

Clements, S., L. Lehtinen, and J. Lukens. 1964. Children with Minimal Brain Injury. Chicago, National Society for Crippled Children and Adults.

Frostig, M., and P. Maslow. 1968. Language training: a form of ability training. J. Learning Dis., 1:105-115.

Kohl, H. 1966. Language and Education of the Deaf. New York, Center for Urban Education.

Lee, L. 1966. Developmental sentence types: a method for comparing normal and deviant syntactic development. J. Speech Hearing Dis., 31:311-330.

————1969. Recent studies in language acquisition. ASHA, 11:272-274.

————1970. A screening test for syntax development. Speech Hearing Dis., 35:103-112.

Lenneberg, E. 1964. Language disorders in children. Harvard Educ. Rev., 34:152-177.

————1966. The natural history of language. In Smith, F., and G. Miller, eds., The Genesis of Language. Cambridge, Mass., The MIT Press.

Lowell, E. 1968. John Tracy Clinic Correspondence Course for Parents of Preschool Deaf Children. Los Angeles, John Tracy Clinic.

McCarthy, J. J., and S. A. Kirk. 1961. Illinois Test of Psycholinguistic Abilities: Examiner's Manual. Urbana, Ill., University of Illinois Institute for Research on Exceptional Children.

McNeill, D. 1966. Developmental psycholinguistics. In Smith, F., and G. Miller, eds., The Genesis of Language. Cambridge, Mass., The MIT Press.

Monsees, E. 1967. Language curriculum for teachers of language-deficient children. Proc. Int. Conference on the Oral Education of the Deaf. Washington, D. C., Alexander Graham Bell Association for the Deaf.

National Education Association. 1967. Public school programs and practices. N.E.A. Research Bulletin, December:105-116.

Osgood, C. E. 1957a. A behavioristic analysis. In Contemporary Approaches to Cognition: A Symposium held at the University of Colorado. Cambridge, Mass., Harvard University Press.

————1957b. Motivational dynamics of language behavior. In Nebraska Symposium on Motivation. Lincoln, Neb., University of Nebraska Press.

Richardson, S. 1963. Language training for the mentally retarded. In Schiefelbusch, R., and J. Smith, eds., Research in Speech and Hearing for Mentally Retarded Children. Lawrence, University of Kansas.

Schechter, M. 1966. Montessori and the child's natural development (Part II). Children's House, November/December:31-33.

Schlanger, B. 1959. A longitudinal study of speech and language development of brain damaged retarded children. J. Speech Hearing Dis., 24:354-360.

Stark, J. 1968. Programmed Instruction for Perceptually Handicapped Children with Language Difficulties. Final report, U. S. Office of Education Grant No. 6-8527. Palo Alto, Calif., Stanford University.

Webster, E., W. Perkins, H. Bloomer, and W. Pronovost. 1966. Case selection in the schools. J. Speech Hearing Dis., 31:352-358.

Wood, N. 1964. Delayed Speech and Language Development. Englewood Cliffs, N. J., Prentice-Hall.

12: Educational management of speaking and listening

D. D. Kluppel

Speaking and listening are integral aspects of a human communication system. The history, traditions, and cultures of man have been perpetuated by communication from one generation to the next. The infant is born into a society which demands that he learn to function as an independent, contributing member of his society. In order to do that, the child must learn to communicate. In most instances speaking and listening are the primary means of communication. Thus the skills involved in speaking and listening prepare and aid the child in assuming his role in society.

When there is interaction within a social group, some kind of communication has taken place (Ruesch, 1959). This communication may be verbal or nonverbal (i.e., written, spoken, or gestured) or a combination. Communication, or interactions, may occur between countries, between friends, or between parent and child, to name a few, but it is in childhood when the skills of communication are usually developed. Essentially, the child must be capable of behaving appropriately in various interactions, and it is the educator's delegated responsibility to make certain that the child has the ability to do so.

The most frequent and obvious components of the oral communicative act are those of speaking and listening (i.e., the comprehension and production of the oral symbols which form the language). This implies neural processing, storage, retrieval, and memory. If the sequential ordering and manipulation of input and output is not accomplished, for whatever reason, there would be only sounds produced without referents and comprehension would not occur because the sounds would be meaningless. The listening situation is usually a covert type of activity with active processing of information.

The theories proposed to account for the acquisition of oral language by children are quite varied (McNeill, 1966; Bijou and Baer, 1965). The process does not seem to be accounted for by a conventional learning paradigm, but perhaps by a different or special kind of learning. Nevertheless, the assumption has to be made that the acquisition of oral language is a sufficiently flexible process that can be altered by learning.

CHILDREN WITH ORAL LANGUAGE PROBLEMS

The traditional classification of children with communicative handicaps has involved use of a medical model. Consequently, children have been labeled according to their medical etiology, or suspected etiology (e.g. minimally brain damaged, emotionally disturbed, and so forth). The labeling has the accompanying implication that the communicative handicap is unique to the etiological classification and hence its treatment is etiology-bound. It has become more apparent in recent years that there are very few "pure" cases of any of these causes. Currently, it seems more appropriate to organize treatment programs according to the educational needs and areas of deficit rather than the medical etiology of the child. The communicative deficits seem to distribute themselves across all medical etiological types. Furthermore, in the practical sense of working with a child, the teacher must take him from where he is, with whatever deficiencies he demonstrates, and help him to strengthen these areas of weakness. With few exceptions knowledge of the medical classification is relatively unhelpful in the educational management of the child (Hardy, 1965). Obviously, if the child has a hearing impairment and amplification will help, the teacher would be foolish to ignore the use of an aid, but the child would still need remedial education for the specific deficits he displays.

When children are evaluated for the development of an educational program it is necessary to obtain quite a bit of information concerning the child's abilities and disabilities. In this instance, it is not sufficient to be aware of general behavior, but rather it is necessary to have specific information about the child. A first requisite of the evaluation would be a complete description of the child's oral language behavior, or lack of it. Next, some determination must be made of the child's comprehension of oral language. This may be measured by various tests or by asking for responses from the child which indicate his comprehension of the auditory signal. These descriptions should be representative of his typical responding. A comparison of his oral language behavior can now be made against the normative data for his age group. Once it is determined that the child is performing below what should be expected, specific assessment must be made of a number of factors which could influence his behavior. Awareness of his perceptual, motor, verbal, and cognitive abilities and disabilities not only provides clues about why there is a problem in oral language, but indicates the appropriate areas of concern in planning a remediation program.

The specific information required includes the child's sensory and perceptual abilities: Is sensory acuity and discrimination normal, does sensory input have meaning for him? Next, an evaluation must be made of the child's response modes: What is his gross and fine motor behavior like, does he have sufficient motor control to produce the sound symbols of the language, does he rely on gesture to communicate? Whether with standardized tests or observational techniques, assessment of the verbal level at which the child is functioning should be determined: Does the child demonstrate the ability to use the phonology, morphology, and/or syntax of the oral language? What is his knowledge of phonology, morphology, and syntax?

Finally, it is necessary to evaluate the more complex cognitive functions, such as memory, concept formation, and problem solving. Recognizing that these cognitive functions are in part dependent on the sensory input to the child, independent assessment of short- and long-term memory, abstraction of qualities, concept formation and categorization, and problem solving should be determined for each sensory input (i.e., auditory, visual, and tactile).

Additional information concerning the child's interests, his activity level, and his distractibility aids in designing the educational program for the child because it answers questions about how to structure motivation, attention, and appropriate reinforcement. The child's performance earlier in the evaluation will help to determine the kind of stimulus input, the difficulty of the stimulus materials, how they are sequenced, and the kind of response to be expected or worked toward.

With the above information obtained, the educator is now in the position of selecting an appropriate educational program under which he can group the children for maximum benefit. Individual programming for differences among the children is possible because of the base-line assessment.

CRITERIA FOR PLANNING OPTIMAL LEARNING

Traditional learning theories have focused their analyses of the learning process in a variety of ways. Depending upon the explanation they wish to offer to account for the change in behavior of the organism, they have chosen to look at various aspects which are common from one learning situation to another. Almost all theories (Guthrie, 1952; Skinner, 1953; Hull, 1951) indicate that they have to see evidence that learning has taken place (the *appropriate response*); many of them (Tolman, 1932; Guthrie, 1952; Hull, 1951; Skinner, 1953) insist that what takes place must be a response to something (the *stimulus*) that has been attended to (*attention*); most of them (Hull, 1951; Tolman, 1932) are concerned about why the response takes place (*motivation*); and several of them (Hull, 1951; Skinner, 1953) note that the feedback to the organism (*reinforcement*) is essential for optimal learning to take place. The impact of any of these factors varies from theory to theory, depending upon the explanatory value it holds within the theory. Many current theories of learning present only more highly specified formulas to account for the behavior observed. There is, in addition, a vast literature of empirical support for the role of these various factors in learning.

Considering the number of learning theories that find these factors useful in their explanatory power, and considering the differences in meaning these factors take on as one employs one theory after another, it seems reasonable to accept that they, in a very general sense, provide a set of criteria for evaluating an educational process. The argument is that to date no theory of learning is sufficient to account for the available data and that the general concepts of these five criteria as they relate to an explanation of the learning process are what are important and not their definitions according to a specific set of words or symbols.

When these five criteria (motivation, attention, stimulus control, response appropriateness, and reinforcement) are taken together, they should describe an optimal learning experience. This is not to say that there have not been demonstrations of learning when one or the other of these criteria was not obviously present or accounted for, but that to ensure the optimum conditions for learning to take place, each criterion should be known and be able to be specified independently for each individual.

At the pragmatic level of teaching children speaking and listening skills, the application of the five criteria is relatively straightforward. It is necessary for the child to be interested (motivated) in what he is doing. Next, if he is going to be able to do anything at all with the stimuli, he must be able to attend. The stimulus conditions (environment for attention) must be regulated so as to fit adequately into the level at which the child is performing. Responses must be chosen that are in the child's behavioral repertoire (or that can be shaped). And finally, some kind of feedback (reinforcement) must be given the child so that he can assess the consequences of his behavior.

While there are times when it may seem unnecessary to specify all five criteria, attention to each one will assure an optimum learning opportunity for each child. This is not to be viewed as a sterile approach to learning simply because it specifies what the relevant variables are. Rather, it provides a very rich opportunity to program for the learning of all sorts of specific behavior, as well as concept formation, the development of abstract ideas, meaning, and problem solving. The unique advantage of this approach is that it not only allows for designing educational programs for children with individual differences, but makes it mandatory.

The following discussion of the five critera should provide a general awareness of each and some indication of the use of the criteria and how they interact in the learning process.

Motivation

Motivation has been described by many psychologists (Bruner, 1966; Kendler, 1963) as the "energizer" of behavior. It propels the person along a particular path of behavior and generally with a particular goal in mind. Motivation is a criterion which interacts with almost all the other criteria. The child must be motivated to attend, motivated to remember, motivated to respond, and so forth. Teachers in preparing their materials should not only evaluate them as to the information they contain, but also for the interest they provide for children.

When motivation is deficient or absent, the educator must create a need within the child. This need could be for information, for a pleasant smile, for a piece of candy, or for a hug. Thus, the relationship between motivation and reinforcement is a very close one. Adequate motivation increases the chances that the desired response will be made, and reinforcement maintains and strengthens the response (Bijou and Baer, 1961, 1965; Staats, 1968).

The child will have a desire for speaking and listening if he has been reinforced for communication. If not, it is the teacher's job to instill in him a need for speaking and for listening. The child must understand why communication is a "good thing." The attitude toward communication of children with speaking and listening problems is quite frequently bad. The child may have been punished for, or ignored in, his oral communication. He may not see the value of it, and therefore, may have to be encouraged to use oral language to convey his needs and ideas. The association of unpleasant consequences with his attempts at oral language must be erased. Once the need for speaking and listening is developed, it is much easier to help the child make appropriate oral responses or analyze what he has heard.

Attention

Attention is a primary concern for educators (Haring, 1968). The child must select from numerous stimulus events the particular one or ones to which he must attend. At first glance, attention seems to be more relevant to the listening process. Certainly it is an important element, since the child does not experience sensorily and perceptively any auditory stimulus to which he is attending if other stimuli conflict with it and distract him. Equally important is the use of attention in speaking. The child must be able to produce an utterance while keeping track of where he is and what is to follow. Sequential abilities are, therefore, dependent upon attention. It cannot be stressed enough that attending and length of attention are major factors in speaking and listening and should be pursued as a "skill development" (Haring, 1968).

Lack of attention in a child may coexist with unresponsiveness or hyperactivity and/or lack of an appropriate response. Attention must be built up on the basis of stimulation of interest (motivaton) in the child, and the reinforcement of "attending responses." The "attending responses" are those by which the child isolates some particular aspect of the environment to observe. There are two dimensions which determine the difficulty of the stimulus: length and complexity. Training the child to attend to either of these aspects involves moving from a simple, long presentation to a short, complex presentation. The two aspects can be varied independently of one another and in most cases should be. Thus, the relationship among "attending responses," motivation, and selection of stimuli is an intertwined one.

The necessity of attending is important, not only for the educational situation, but also for the child's home and play environments. The child must attend to get information and to follow instructions in the classroom and at home, and also he must attend in order to play games with his peers. His basic interactions with people in his environment, therefore, depend upon his attending and responding appropriately.

The Stimulus Environment

Arranging for the appropriate environment is a critical variable in optimal learning. It must reflect prior planning on the part of the teacher. The physical environment should be stimulating but not distracting. The psychological environment should be warm and comfortable. The number and kinds of potential stimuli vary with the type of sensory input and the complexity of the stimuli. The choice of teaching to strengths or weaknesses has been debated by many educators (Johnson and Myklebust, 1967;

McGinnis, 1963; Bangs, 1968) with varying opinions. Whatever the choice, the end product must be the child's successful utilization of incoming stimulation. Care in choosing stimulus materials must be exercised so that it is appropriate to the child's interest and level of functioning. In addition, the stimuli must be sequenced so that there is a logical change or progression for the child to follow. Initially, it may be necessary to proceed in a repetitive fashion, moving to a new condition only after mastery of the preceding one. This allows for the building up of logical thinking on the part of the child; that is, he can learn a specific concept as well as its relationship to other concepts.

Response Appropriateness

In general, any measurement of learning is made directly on the responses of the individual to the stimuli presented. Those responses must be appropriate to the situation. Frequently, however, the response which is desired cannot be produced by the child. In those instances, the teacher must determine what kind of response the child can make and start from there. Since the ultimate goal is to help the child achieve proficiency in speaking and listening, the procedure is to work from a response the child can make toward the stated objective. This allows the child to experience success (reinforcement) and may help change his attitude (motivation) toward speaking and listening activities.

At the most basic level the teacher may have to accept an eye blink, pointing, or a rudimentary vocal response. When these are produced by the child, they should be reinforced. After they occur with some regularity in the presence of the stimuli, the response can be modified into one that more closely resembles the desired behavior. Clearly, there must be many intermediate goals for the child to achieve between his initial responses and the final performance if motivation is to be maintained. The value of reinforcement may vary during the child's learning so that the nature or type of the reinforcement may have to be changed to ensure the maintenance of the response.

Reinforcement

Reinforcement is a very controversial concept in the eyes of many educators. To some, it smacks of bribery, and to others, it is the logical consequence of behavior. It has been described as anything from a tangible reward (food or candy) through social stimuli (approval or affection) to knowledge of results (feedback). Reinforcement has a role in producing behavior change which is very dramatic. If a stimulus is reinforcing, the response which it follows will be strengthened and will be more likely to occur again. The time relationship between the response and the reinforcement is critical to ensure the association between them. The child must learn the consequences of his responses.

When attempting to arrange for optimal learning by children, the choice of a reinforcer is quite crucial. The nature of reinforcement is very individual (Bijou and Baer, 1961, 1965); what may be a reward for one child may not be for another. This is not just the case for tangible rewards, but also for social reinforcement. Many children will work hard for the approval of their teachers while for others that would not be important.

Table 1. Specific Educational Programs Categorized According to the Five Criteria for Optimal Learning

Motivation	Attention	Stimulus control	Response appropriateness	Reinforcement
	Strauss and Lehtinen	Strauss and Lehtinen		
	McGinnis	McGinnis	McGinnis	
		Montesorri	Montesorri	
	Johnson and Myklebust	Johnson and Myklebust	Johnson and Myklebust	
Bangs		Bangs		
Bereiter and Engelmann	Bereiter and Engelmann	Bereiter and Engelmann	Bereiter and Engelmann	Bereiter and Engelmann
Hewett	Hewett	Hewett	Hewett	Hewett

Gradually, however, the use of social stimulation and feedback as reinforcement must be introduced to the child, so that optimum performance can be associated with it in the classroom.

SPECIFIC EDUCATIONAL PROGRAMS

Using the five criteria for optimal learning an evaluation of a number of educational programs for teaching children listening and speaking will follow. Some of the programs focus on one aspect or another of these criteria and might appropriately be used with specific types of children; indeed some of these techniques were designed for specific children. Designation of the criteria not only improves the opportunities that exist for the child's learning, but it helps the therapist or educator to analyze exactly what is happening in the remediation setting. With this knowledge the teacher will then be better able to evaluate what is being successful for the child and what is not.

In Table 1 various educational programs have been assigned to those criteria that they tend to focus on. Obviously if a child has difficulty in relationship to one or the other of these criteria, an appropriate program dealing with this factor could be chosen. However, for optimum learning, control and specification of all these criteria are necessary. Either a program which does all of these things should be selected, or components of various programs should be put together to designate each of the criteria.

Strauss and Lehtinen

Strauss and Lehtinen (1947) have proposed a theoretical and procedural basis for working with "minimally brain-damaged" children. In large measure it consists of structuring the environment and stimuli so that the hyperactive and highly distractible child can attend more easily to the materials presented, therefore, allowing the child to work on those skills which are deficient. Very simply, what is done is that the room or area in which the child works is bare of as much visual stimuli as is possible; even the teacher dresses carefully with no swinging earrings or bright print blouses. The teacher may surround the child with screens to block his view of the other children in the class. Materials are carefully chosen, in terms of their difficulty level or complexity, to be appropriate to the level on which the individual child is functioning. The child works in relative isolation where his attention can be directed to specific tasks and he is not distracted by watching other children or by the teacher's movements. The teacher attempts to control exactly what the child is attending to and supervises his study. In this procedure it is assumed that if the stimulus materials are chosen appropriately, the child will be adequately motivated. Perhaps this would be the case with an experienced teacher, but with someone less sophisticated it might be less apparent. The appropriateness of the response and its consequences are also assumed; that is, specific ordering of responses with consistent reinforcement or feedback is not focused on. If this were to be done, the teacher and the child would have a much better idea of the child's progress.

McGinnis

The Association Method of teaching language was developed by Mildred McGinnis (1963). It is so called because the technique brings in close association various processes of learning (i.e., attention, retention, and recall) in the child. The Association Method is particularly concerned with training the aphasic child. A major component of this technique is the development of attention in the child. McGinnis provides suggestions for "attention-getting exercises" which she sees as supplementary to the teaching of sounds and words. She has sequenced items to be practiced by the child in what she calls the "vertical program." This consists of "the basic language and speech curriculum, which the child will be expected to complete over a period of time" (McGinnis, 1963, p. 61). The vertical program is arranged in a hierarchy of three units of language through which the child progresses. Additionally, she has developed correlative programs to aid in such areas as attention, writing, and other activities necessary to academic success.

McGinnis specifies very carefully the sequencing of stimuli and the teacher's monitoring of the child's responses. She encourages multiple sensory input and provides for various kinds of responses (i.e., motor and verbal). The details of the curriculum can be found in her book, Aphasic Children.

McGinnis makes the assumption that motivation and attention are inextricably tied together: If the child goes through the attention-getting exercises, he will be motivated to learn. This may not necessarily be the case. Activities for a group of children may not stimulate them uniformly. In addition, the individual differences shown by children with speaking and listening problems do not lend themselves to a specific set of activities; nor do activities always motivate a child.

McGinnis is concerned about the appropriateness of the response of the child, but she does not go into detail about how the child finds out that he has responded correctly. Perhaps she assumes that a good teacher would supply that information automatically.

However, for the best possible educational experience, both the child and the teacher should know what the stimulus was, what the response was, and whether or not the response was correct.

Johnson and Myklebust

Johnson and Myklebust (1967) have proposed the technique of "clinical teaching" for the remediation of children with learning disabilities. This is a highly individualized approach taking into account a number of characteristics of the child (e.g., integrities, deficits, tolerance levels). The authors state very explicitly that "Clinical Teaching does not assume that the same methodologies are applied to every child" (*ibid.*, p. 64). Therefore, the basis for clinical teaching is an extremely comprehensive diagnostic evaluation. The treatment program is then planned taking the results of this evaluation into account. Johnson and Myklebust take note of the fact that attending behavior is necessary for learning to occur. They also specify that the stimuli must be selected at the level of functioning of the child. Responses appropriate to the stimuli and available to the child are stressed.

Johnson and Myklebust do not dwell on the necessity of motivating the child. They seem to assume that if the stimulus materials are thoughtfully chosen and if the child is capable of attending, he will be adequately motivated. Additionally they make no special mention that the child be provided with knowledge of the results of his responses, even though feedback is essential for efficient learning.

Montesorri

The Montessori method (1970) was originally developed for intellectually and environmentally deprived children. In it very selected materials are to be used by the child in a prescribed manner. Thus this technique specifies both the stimulus and the response to be made to it. The different sets of materials are graded in difficulty and the child proceeds with them at his own rate. Within this philosophical approach, it is assumed that the child provides his own motivation and that he is capable of attending. Finally, it is assumed that the completion of the response provides the child with self-reinforcement. The Montesorri directoress monitors the child's activities to be sure that he is using the materials appropriately. Of all the programs, the philosophy behind Montesorri makes it virtually impossible to manipulate motivation and reinforcement independently and still operate within its framework.

Tina Bangs

Tina Bangs (1968) has explored the idea that early preschool activities for getting the child "ready" for academic endeavors are essential for many, if not most, children. This is particularly true for those children who suffer from language and learning problems. Her thesis is to evaluate the child while he is young and before he is left behind in a regular classroom. In that way her program is preventative, but also offers many ideas for remediation should that be necessary. She has proposed a way of looking at young children to determine their abilities and disabilities in terms of their avenues of learning. She states that "It is the detailed assessment of the avenues of learning that suggests the dynamics of language disorders" (Bangs, 1968, p. 27). The avenues of learning that she specifies are sensation, perception, memory retrieval, attention, and integration. In addition, she notes that certain other social and emotional skills are necessary for the child to function well in the academic setting.

In her book she provides not only assessment techniques and evaluation forms, but an extremely complete curriculum guide. This guide is ordered in terms of difficulty from below 3 years of age to above the kindergarten level, which she calls the readiness level (the child has the basic information necessary for a successful encounter with the first grade). Contained within the curriculum guide are things to enhance motivation and particular attention is given to the ordering of the materials (stimuli) in terms of their difficulty. Bangs seems to make the assumption that if the situation is motivating, attention will almost automatically occur. In her discussion of attention as an avenue of learning she comments specifically on auditory and visual attention, but does not, either in this section or later in the guide, provide a paradigm for the learning of attending behavior by the child.

Bereiter and Engelmann

Although it has been said that Bereiter and Engelmann developed their approach (1966) without particular regard to learning theories, it is one of few that seems to take into .account all those things necessary for an optimal learning situation. After deciding that a major handicap of disadvantaged children was their poor performance in language skills and other cognitive functions, they set about to establish a curriculum and to train teachers to help the child improve his performance. They acknowledge the role of motivating the child through various ways of getting him to participate in the learning situation. Included in this is a mild degree of stress moving him to achieve competence. They are conscious of the necessity of attending behavior and underscore the requirement that all the children in the group must participate. It is the teacher's job to help the child attend to the appropriate characteristic of the stimulus.

In the developing of the curriculum, the stimulus materials are organized in such a way that differences between children and differences in abilities as the child learns are acknowledged. The ultimate goal is to give the child sufficient language ability and the concomitant conceptual behaviors that he can succeed in academic endeavors.

The responses that the children make to the stimulus materials are guided, prompted, and/or cued by the teacher. Initially, they are provided with the correct response, later they must produce it, either by rote or by logical deduction, themselves. They are immediately told that their response was correct. In the early part of training Bereiter and Engelmann allow more tangible reinforcement to be provided. Most of their responses are correct, since the learning situation is so carefully structured. This allows children, who frequently have been wrong, to experience success.

Hewett

Hewett (1968, p. 55) says that "The goal of all education is to promote children's eventual involvement with learning on . . . a self-directed basis." The developmental sequence by which the child reaches this state is thought to be a hierarchical system consisting of attention, response, order, exploration, mastery, and achievement. The educational program for each child is developed with this hierarchical sequence in mind. The basic assumption is that all children can learn; the teacher's task is to find what level is appropriate for each child and to plan his program accordingly. Since Hewett's rationale was developed with severely disturbed children in mind and there is a broad range of abilities in these children, it could be expected that the program could be used with children with a variety of abilities. The range of responding which Hewett discusses runs from absolutely no apparent response in a catatonic schizophrenic to responding at the "achievement" level.

The fundamentals on which Hewett's (1968, p. 240) "engineered classroom" operates are as follows:

1. Start where the child is and get him ready for more complex tasks through assignment of basic readiness tasks.
2. Settle for "thimblesfull" of accomplishment and resist preoccupation with a "bucket" orientation in learning.
3. Once you have established contact with a child gradually increase demands and expectations at a pace which the child can tolerate.
4. Attempt to guarantee that the child will experience continual success in the classroom.
5. Create a predictable learning environment for the child in which he is rewarded for his accomplishments, nonrewarded if he fails to meet demands which, according to everything known about him, are reasonable to expect of him.
6. Be prepared to back up, modify tasks, and reset expectations if the child fails.

The concept of an "engineered classroom" is dependent upon the teacher determining exactly what is of interest to each child and of ordering the stimulus materials and the required responses in terms of the child's abilities. Knowledge of the results, or the correctness of his response, is a crucial factor in the child's learning. Hewett discusses the role of reinforcement, or feedback, as a necessary consequence for both the child and the teacher to know how he is progressing. Thus, Hewett focuses his educational technique on all five factors that seem to be essential for optimal learning.

CONCLUSIONS

All the educational programs (Bangs, 1968; Hewett, 1968; Strauss and Lehtinen, 1947; Johnson and Myklebust, 1967; McGinnis, 1963; Montesorri, 1970; Bereiter and Engelmann, 1966) note the necessity of planning for each individual child even though the children may be grouped together in a classroom for remedial work. The choice of the specific educational program is a matter of personal preference and theoretical or philosophical orientation. It is suggested that the five criteria proposed for optimal learning (motivation, attention, stimulus control, response appropriateness, and reinforcement) can be utilized within almost all the specific educational programs previously discussed. The exception is the Montesorri program (1970), which precludes the direct control of motivation and reinforcement because of its basic tenets.

For those children with problems of oral languages the complex of behaviors required for speaking and listening (i.e., comprehending) must be taught. They may start with differing ability levels and with varying degrees of potential. They may respond to one kind of stimulus input better than another, and the responses themselves may be distributed in relevance and complexity. The function of the educational program, then, is to start where the child is, to allow him to proceed at his own rate and with his own degree of progress, to provide him with the motivation and reinforcement that makes progress possible, and ultimately to help him to realize the goal of using oral language, both speaking and listening, at a level comparable to the normative standards appropriate for him. The child in our society needs to be able to communicate. He needs to express his ideas and thoughts as well as to understand the ideas and thoughts of others. Speaking and listening are such integral parts of social exchange that any strengthening of the skills necessary for them to take place will aid the child in assuming his social role in the community.

REFERENCES

Bangs, T. E. 1968. Language and Learning Disorders of the Pre-Academic Child: with Curriculum Guide. New York, Appleton-Century-Crofts.

Bereiter, C., and S. Engelmann. 1966. Teaching Disadvantaged Children in the Preschool. Englewood Cliffs, N. J., Prentice-Hall.

Bijou, S. W., and D. M. Baer. 1961. Child Development: A Systematic and Empirical Theory, Vol. 1. New York, Appleton-Century-Crofts.

———— and D. M. Baer. 1965. Child Development II: Universal Stage of Infancy, Vol. 2. New York, Appleton-Century-Crofts.

Bruner, J. S. 1966. Toward a Theory of Instruction. Cambridge, Mass., Harvard University Press (Belknap Press).

Guthrie, E. R. 1952. The Psychology of Learning, rev. ed. New York, Harper & Row.

Hardy, W. G. 1965. On language disorders in young children: A reorganization of thinking. J. Speech Hearing Dis., 30:3-16.

Haring, N. G. 1968. Attending and Responding. San Rafael, Calif., Dimensions Publishing Co.

Hewett, F. M. 1968. The Emotionally Disturbed Child in the Classroom. Boston, Allyn and Bacon.

Hull, C. L. 1951. Essentials of Behavior. New Haven, Yale University Press.

Johnson, D. J., and H. R. Myklebust. 1967. Learning Disabilities: Educational Principles and Practices. New York, Grune & Stratton.

Kendler, H. H. 1963. Basic Psychology. New York, Appleton-Century-Crofts.

McGinnis, M. A. 1963. Aphasic Children: Identification and Education by the Association Method. Washington, D. C., Alexander Graham Bell Association for the Deaf.

McNeill, D. 1966. Developmental psycholinguistics. *In* Smith, F., and G. A. Miller, eds., The Genesis of Language. Cambridge, Mass., The MIT Press.

Montesorri, M. 1970. The Child in the Family. (Translated by Nancy Rockmore Cirillo.) New York, Avon Books.

Ruesch, J. 1959. General theory of communication in psychiatry. *In* Arieti, S., ed., American Handbook of Psychiatry. New York, Basic Books.

Skinner, B. F. 1953. Science and Human Behavior. New York, Macmillan.

Staats, A. W. 1968. Learning, Language, and Cognition. New York, Holt, Rinehart and Winston.

Strauss, A. A., and L. E. Lehtinen. 1947. Psychopathology and Education of the Brain-Injured Child. New York, Grune & Stratton.

Tolman, E. C. 1932. Purposive Behavior in Animals and Men. New York, Appleton-Century-Crofts.

13: Educational management of reading deficits

Corrine E. Kass

Reading is a complex communication act, and the inability to read is recognized as a severe problem in our society. Currently, the neurological term "dyslexia" has become the popular label for severe reading deficits. In this section, reading deficits are defined as specific integrational difficulties associated with reading as a skill or habit. The focus in these few pages will be on the automatic process of the complex act of reading (in educational terminology, this may be designated as "word calling").

A complete treatment of deviations from the normal development of reading and their educational management would, of course, make this section unwieldly and confusing. The literature is replete with descriptions of methods; the publishing market provides an array of materials. This section will present only one point of view, and the reader is referred to some recent references for more complete reviews of reading problems and remedial methods (Strang, 1964; Harris, 1968).

The point of view to be presented in this section will include a *theoretical philosophy* about the types of reading deficits commonly found in children with learning disabilities, and three steps in the *educational management* of such deficits.

It is only fair to point out at the outset that the state of present knowledge regarding specific integrational difficulties associated with reading as a skill or habit is incomplete. The theoretical basis for educational management is shaky at best. However, courage is necessary for progress to occur, and necessity dictates that the problem of educational management be faced squarely. A common question of teachers is: What can we *do* about this problem?

A THEORETICAL PHILOSOPHY

The children who display reading deficits in specific integrational or automatic processes of the reading act are often puzzling to teachers. They possess adequate intellectual ability for learning to read, they have adequate sight and hearing, but they are not reading up to their expected level. They are variously described as not recognizing letters, not having word-attack skills, not perceiving word wholes, or as not remembering words. These are children who display the characteristics found within the following definition of special learning disabilities (National Advisory Committee on Handicapped Children, 1968):

> Children with special learning disabilities exhibit a disorder in one or more of the basic psychological processes involved in understanding or in using spoken or written language. These may be manifested in disorders of listening, thinking, talking, reading, writing, spelling or arithmetic. They include conditions which have been referred to as perceptual handicaps, brain injury, minimal brain dysfunction, dyslexia, developmental aphasia, etc. They do *not* include learning problems which are due primarily to visual, hearing, or motor handicaps, to mental retardation, emotional disturbance, or to environmental disadvantage.

Basic to a theoretical philosophy is a working understanding of specific deficits. Educational management can be more effective with such theoretical understanding than through the blind application of material found in the "teacher's guide."

The theoretical philosophy of this section suggests two systems of language: *(1) an integrational or automatic-sequential level of language functioning*, which deals with the higher automatisms necessary for processes such as closure, short-term memory, and speed of perception, and *(2) a representational level of language functioning*, which deals with language found in comprehension, concept development, and abstraction. A knowledge of the distinction between these two systems is prerequisite to the teacher's *understanding* of the child's reading disabilities, and the planning of appropriate remediation.

The basis for this distinction rests on a doctoral study (Kass, 1962) of some psychological correlates of severe reading disability. That study was based on an adaptation (Kirk and McCarthy, 1961) of Osgood's theory of language (Osgood, 1957). The results indicated that children with severe reading disability have more deficits at the integrational or automatic-sequential level of language functioning than at the representational level.

The specific correlates of severe reading disabilities included impairment of:

1. Ability to use grammar (Grammatic Closure).
2. Ability to reproduce a series of symbols presented visually (Visual Sequencing).
3. Ability to predict a whole from a part (Visual Closure).
4. Ability to blend parts into whole (Sound Blending).
5. Ability to manually execute a visual prediction (Mazes).
6. Ability to reproduce a design from memory (Memory-for-Designs).
7. Ability to note likenesses and differences rapidly (Perceptual Speed).

These results indicate that learning to read involves more than the comprehension of the printed page and includes certain integrative functions which we associate with the skill of reading, or the identification of symbols. When basic deficits are diagnosed in a child with a severe reading problem, specialized remedial techniques can be applied.

The diagnostic test which revealed the deficits was the Illinois Test of Psycholinguistic Abilities (ITPA), plus some supplementary tests at the integrational level. A revision of the ITPA with subtests similar to these supplementary tests has since been published (Kirk, McCarthy, and Kirk, 1968). The ITPA model is a multidimensional one and has been described in a variety of sources. A summary of studies on the ITPA has been compiled by Bateman (1965). Briefly, this test was devised on the basis of a clinical model utilizing three dimensions: (1) the channels of communication, both receptive and expressive; (2) the psycholinguistic processes of decoding (obtaining meaning from sensory stimuli), association (internal relating of concepts and symbols), and encoding (expressing ideas); and (3) the levels of organization, which are named representational (semantic meaning) and integrational or automatic-sequential (structural meaning and memory).

As a very practical exercise in pretesting one's understanding of integrational language, the reader might consider several everyday activities which are performed automatically. The reader will find himself naming such activities as reading, writing, spelling, walking, talking, and playing a musical instrument. While context and personal meanings bias one's performance, the activities themselves are carried out in an overlearned habitual manner. Short-term memory, also part of integrational language (such as repeating digits), is prerequisite to overlearned habits or skills.

For success in reading, the child must first memorize the symbols of the language, and after overlearning these must remember the printed symbols in a secondary fashion as he comes to focus primary attention on the meaning of what he is reading. It was suggested earlier that children with reading disabilities frequently have difficulty at the integrational level of language functioning. By the time a child has reached school, certain habitual patterns of learning have already been incorporated by the central nervous system. The child with an integrational level deficit may have learned to compensate through the overuse of representational language. This is the child who may learn to read very well initially through the use of pictures and context clues, but who, to everyone's surprise, does not have word-attack skills when he reaches the second grade, and who does not seem to be able to master spelling. Many of these children seem to overlearn the initial sounds and then fall into the habit of guessing the rest of the word. Since they are not able to deal with all the graphemes representing the smallest units of sound within the word, it is easy to understand why they would not perceive the difference between such words as house and houses.

To aid the reader in understanding the difference between representational and integrational language levels, definitions of some words which could be classified under each level are presented. We recognize that all the words have multiple meanings but the definitions given relate to the particular level (adapted from English and English, 1958).

Some words and definitions at the representational level are the following:

Meanings. That which a symbolic act signifies.

Understanding. The process of apprehending or grasping a meaning.

Concepts. Any object of awareness together with its significance or meaning.

Reasoning. Problem solving by means of general principles.

Abstractions. The process of selecting or isolating a certain aspect from a concrete whole, as a process of evaluation or communication.

Comprehension. Knowledge or understanding of an object, situation, event, or verbal statement.

Some words and definitions at the integrational level are the following:

Perception. An event in a person controlled by the excitation of sensory receptors, yet also influenced by factors within the person.

Skill. Ability to perform complex motor acts with ease.

Memory. The general function of reviving past experience.

Body memory. Metaphorical expression for learned responses that take place automatically and without apparent conscious control or even awareness.

Reproductive memory. A memory that preserves both the form and content of the past without addition or distortion (but often with much omission).

Automatisms. An act performed without reflection or intent, often without realizing that it is taking place.

Habit. Tendency toward an act that has become, by repeated performance, relatively fixed, consistent, easy, almost automatic; or the enduring structural basis for such behavior.

Recall. The process whereby a past experience is elicited, specifically evoking or experiencing an image.

A study of "the mediation theories of learning," especially those of Osgood (1957) and Mowrer (1960b), provides further clarification of central language processes. The theories of learning which incorporate the concept of mediation help to explain what occurs *within* the reader as he identifies symbols. The words in reading are the "mediators" of inner as well as overt responses to the printed page. In reading, "the ability to call up a clear visual image (a mental picture) of a known word is closely related to the habits of scrutinizing word forms to remember details. The child who has carefully observed the details of the known word can usually develop the ability to call up a mental image of that word and to compare its form with that of a word that is before him in print" (Gray, 1960, p. 20). For example, reading the word *apple* may be recognized by combining phonemes and syllables which together form a pronounceable unit, later to be recalled and reproduced in a spelling test.

O. Hobart Mowrer's concept of "imagery" is particularly helpful (see his chapter, "Imagery, Memory, and Attention," 1960b). In this chapter, Mowrer defines an image as "conditioned sensation." Imagery includes two types of meaning according to Mowrer. One type of meaning he calls "cognitive," which refers to some object (or word) which an individual "sees" or otherwise "perceives" without the object (or word) being objectively present. This imagery involves memory and occurs at the integrational level of language functioning.

Mowrer's second type of meaning—"evaluative"—belongs under the representational level of language functioning. Evaluative meaning is emotionally based. Mowrer has suggested that emotions, particularly hope and fear, are the mediators of learning. In education, a great deal of emphasis has been placed on emotional meanings. There are reading materials for the reluctant reader called "high-interest, low-reading level" which appeal to the likes and dislikes of the student. The method described by Sylvia Ashton-Warner (1963) is one in which Maori children in New Zealand chose for their own first reading words those which had the most emotional meaning. The cognitive image of the letters in the word *apple* in the above paragraph is not the same as the evaluative meaning of an apple as something that is liked or disliked.

Osgood (1966, p. 212) describes how the integrative level may be modified:

> . . . sensory and motor integrative systems are assumed to be modifiable on the basis of experience—but modifiable according to sheer frequency and independent of motivation and reinforcement (in contrast to S-R type associations) . . . This is a behavioristic closure principle, and it is assumed to underlie the formation of tightly bound perceptual and motor units in language.
>
> . . . These integrative mechanisms provide the organism with an effective means for unitizing or "chunking" its decoding and encoding operations. They provide a mirror of "what ought to be" or what is predictable on the basis of frequent redundancies in past experiencing and past behaving. Of course, being merely predictive mechanisms, they will occasionally make errors—they will produce an illusory perception of familiar "sure" when the visually flashed stimulus was actually the unfamiliar "sere" and they will make for repeated typing of "ration" when "ratio" is intended, for example—but this is a small price to pay for predicting the future from the (related) past with overall efficiency.

Understanding the distinction between the integrational and representational levels of language functioning is not an easy task. The teacher who wishes to plan reading activities for the child who shows deficits at the integrational level will find some additional references helpful, such as Wiener (1954), Osgood and Miron (1963), and Osgood and Sebeok (1956, pp. 50-73).

EDUCATIONAL MANAGEMENT

From the above theoretical philosophy of language functioning, it is possible to derive procedures for educational management. Going beyond diagnostic test procedures and interpretations is necessary if the child with reading deficits is to overcome these and function normally, which we assume will be the outcome of remediation. Diagnostic procedures generally are well done, but unfortunately only up to the point of making an educational prescription. Then we may find the ambiguous statement, "Place this child in a remedial reading class if a vacancy can be found within the school system."

Organizing and carrying out remediation procedures according to the above theoretical philosophy requires the following three steps:

1. *Understanding the disability and making a decision regarding the specific language deficit.* Understanding of level disabilities comes from a synthesis and assimilation of theoretical foundations of language. One such theory has been presented in this section. For remediation purposes, a distinction must be made between representational and integrational language since the two levels require diametrically opposite techniques. Remedial techniques for deficits at the integrational, or automatic-sequential, level of

language functioning differ from the methods used for deficits at the representational. For example, a representational-level problem may be specifically related to listening comprehension and an integrational-level deficit may be specifically related to auditory memory. In the case of the comprehension difficulty, remedial exercises would focus on meaning and thought; however, in the case of the memory deficit, remediation would focus on an automatic process which has no meaning.

A decision regarding the level deficit can be made from the results of diagnostic testing. Once a decision has been reached about a level deficit, further analysis of the data will lead to hypotheses about specific deficits.

Table 1 analyzes a few diagnostic tests according to level functioning and specific abilities. Through an examination of the scores, the educator will be able to make decisions about which area requires remediation. This procedure of interpreting test results can be applied by the educator to other diagnostic tests.

Table 1. Representational and Integrational Subtests of Some Standard Diagnostic Tests

Tests	Level	Subtests for specific deficits
The Illinois Test of Psycholinguistic Abilities	Representational	Auditory Reception
		Visual Reception
		Auditory Association
		Visual Association
		Vocal Expression
		Motor Expression
	Integrational	Grammatic Closure
		Auditory Sequencing
		Sound Blending
		Visual Sequencing
Detroit Test of Learning Aptitude	Representational	Pictorial Absurdities
		Verbal Absurdities
		Pictorial Opposites
		Verbal Opposites
		Oral Commissions (understanding)
		Social Adjustments (A)
		Social Adjustments (B)
		Orientation
		Number Ability
		Oral Directions
		Likenesses and Differences
	Integrational	Motor Speed and Precision
		Auditory-Attention Span
		Oral Commissions (remembering)
		Visual-Attention Span
		Free Association

Table 1. *(Continued)*

Tests	Level	Subtests for specific deficits
		Memory-for-Designs Broken Pictures Likenesses and Differences
Gates Basic Reading Tests	Representational	Reading to Appreciate General Significance Reading to Understand Precise Direction Reading to Note Details Reading Vocabulary Level of Comprehension
Diagnostic Reading Examination for Special Difficulty in Reading	Integrational	Alphabet Repeat and Reading IOTA Word Test Letter Naming Recognition of Orientation Mirror Reading Number Reversals Word Discrimination Sounding

2. *Planning and carrying out remediation for specific deficits.* For each child, remediation begins with a specific technique, individually tailored. Since this section is concerned with deficits in the automatic process of reading, the principles used in remediation must be applicable to the integrational level of language functioning. At the integrational level especially, principles from the psychology of learning (Mowrer, 1960a) for unlearning habits often have to be applied. A common example of unlearning found in psychology textbooks is one which describes the typist who consistently types *hte* for *the* with the suggestion that this habit can be changed by typing *hte* several times consciously and purposely.

More specifically, the usual educational principles for deficits at the representational level are not appropriate at the integrational level. Principles applicable at the representation level include the following: (1) Begin with the simple and go to the complex, (2) find the child's level of achievement and proceed from there, and (3) capture the child's interest (Mowrer's evaluative meaning). However, deficits at the integrational level should be treated according to the following principles: (1) Begin with the complex, (2) find the child's expected level of achievement and begin there, and (3) use drill rather than high interest (Osgood's frequency of presentations.)

Reasons for beginning with the complex or the child's expected level of achievement can be found in Luria (1966). Different stages of development result in different remedial procedures. When a child reaches roughly 9 to 12 years of age, speech and language have developed to the point where more complex factors are related to learning. Therefore, working on simple tasks does not provide transfer of learning. For example, if a child of 10 can repeat only four digits in an auditory memory task, the remediation would begin not with 4 symbols but with a much longer series of 9 or 10.

Similarly, reasons for drill rather than high interest can be found in the writings of Osgood (1957) and Mowrer (1960b). Repetitive frequency causes pairing and chaining of responses and accuracy of response reflects adequate imagery of the cognitive type.

In metaphorical language, overcoming a specific deficit is like tipping a seesaw. The deficit is like the heavier weight which holds down one end of the seesaw. This weight must move toward the center in order for the other end to go down. The first movement is the most difficult because the incline is the greatest. Moving toward the center will lighten the effort of moving the weight. At a given point, the seesaw will tip. The weight will then automatically slide toward the lighter weight.

In applying this metaphor to remediation of specific deficits at the integrational level, the "bad" habit is the heavy weight and must be displaced so that a "good" habit can take its place. The first step in overcoming a bad habit is the most difficult. Some initial movement away from the bad habit is essential. This movement is a self-awareness in the child that something he is doing wrong can be done correctly. From then on, the goal of remediation is to remove the deficit by displacing the bad habit with the good habit. At the point of such displacement there is a "breakthrough," which means that the activity can now be performed automatically without error.

At the representational level, the point at which deficits are corrected takes place when semantic meaning occurs ("insight"). Remedial planning from the first step through the "breakthrough" or "insight" requires skilled, educational techniques, and it is this planning which separates the professional from the neophyte.

The choice of the specific deficit to be corrected is, in a sense, dependent upon the expertise of the examiner. However, if the diagnostic analysis is thorough, the lowest scores(s) will generally reflect the "bad habit" which is hampering the child's performance in reading. When all scores are depressed, educational management must be of a general nature.

For planning specific remedial techniques, the following rules are suggested:

1. Work on the lowest deficit(s) first. The child will read no better than his specific deficit(s) will allow him. Remediation, then, becomes urgent!

2. The remediation situation must utilize a specific technique different from the one the child usually encounters for "breakthrough" or "insight" to occur. Changes can be made in figure-background relationships (e.g., words can be written on newspaper as background); in setting (e.g., tutoring at home instead of at school); and in reinforcement procedures (e.g., accuracy might be rewarded rather than guessing).

3. The remediation must introduce changes into the child's sensory feedback system. Sensory masking procedures can be applied. For example, the child might be blindfolded while listening to a tape.

Some specific deficits are listed below with accompanying illustrative case material.

A Visual-Memory Deficit

Visual memory is the ability to hold in mind an image of one or more objects or symbols. On the ITPA, the Visual-Motor Sequencing Test is a measure of this ability. The most helpful reference for planning activities is Fernald (1943), whose method involves writing words from memory.

A modified version of this method was used with an 11-year-old boy, who was reading at the early second-grade level and whose lowest score was in visual memory. Kenneth was struggling along in a regular fourth-grade class. The tutoring situation was set up so that Kenneth would have to remember words under different circumstances than the ordinary learning situation. Instead of working on reading or writing, the tutor presented only spelling words to Kenneth. He was told that he could learn to be as good a speller as his classmates, but that he would have to remember words in his head instead of copying them from the book or board.

Since the child with a visual-memory deficit obviously does not know how to go about remembering words, the teacher must change the situation in such a way that the child will be forced to remember the word differently from his usual manner. For Kenneth, this was done by writing the word to be remembered on newspaper, which changed figure-background relationships. Tracing the words, as Grace Fernald (1943) suggests, changes the kinesthetic stimulation if the child has not been used to learning words in this way. However, Kenneth was in the habit of copying words from the board or book in an effort to remember them, and had been unsuccessful; therefore, the tracing method alone was not effective.

Most importantly, it was necessary to redirect the learning process so that visual memory would become part of the integrational language system. This was accomplished by having Kenneth count out loud while looking at the word to be remembered. This procedure is an auditory-feedback-masking mechanism. It is wise to work with only one or two words for the first several sessions so that the mind may acquire the idea of the technique of remembering words, rather than learning the words per se. The words should be long words to satisfy the principle of beginning with the complex. The mistakes which Kenneth made as he attempted to write the words from memory were also very important for remediation purposes. He was encouraged to check his word with the stimulus word and not to feel ashamed of discrepancies. By checking these discrepancies and gradually coming closer to the exact word, Kenneth learned to monitor his visual memory.

Having accomplished a "breakthrough" in visual memory, the tutoring sessions focused on remedial spelling. With the new habit, Kenneth could soon boast that he was at least as good a speller as his classmates.

Transfer to reading skills was made through the use of McGraw-Hill Programmed Reading Series. The important aspect in this tutoring was accuracy. Attention was called to each mistake for the purpose of self-correcting. Kenneth improved in reading two grade levels in a few months.

Other references which are helpful to the reader are Smith (1967) and O'Donnell and Towns (1963).

An Auditory-Memory Deficit

Auditory memory is the ability to recall letters, words, or numbers and sounds after hearing these. A common disability is in the area of sound blending. A 7-year-old boy at the end of the first grade was referred for tutoring because he could not identify letters of the alphabet. On the ITPA, Billy's lowest score was in auditory-vocal sequencing. Because the child's reaction to failure in reading class at school was negative, a different symbol system was introduced in the tutoring situation. The i.t.a. (Initial Teaching Alphabet) was used as a "secret code" between the tutor and the child. Following the successful learning of the first few sounds, the i.t.a. method introduces sound blending. In a matter of 3 weeks, Billy was pointing out "his symbols" in the newspaper spontaneously and reading simple i.t.a. books.

The "breakthrough" in auditory memory occurred through auditory training on a few sounds while varying the sensory feedback. For example, one procedure that was used was to have Billy listen to the sound and repeat it immediately, listen to it again, then walk around the room and repeat it. Sometimes Billy was asked to shut his eyes while listening to the sounds.

Other references which are helpful to the reader are Hegge et al. (1940) and Bloomfield and Barnhart (1960).

3. *Transferring specific remediation to the total learning environment.* There is no guarantee that overcoming one or two specific deficits will produce overall improvement in reading scores. What does happen is that broader-based education can be more effective when specific deficits are removed. After "breakthrough" or "insight" occurs, reading materials at the child's reading level may be incorporated into his program. A selection from a structured programmed reading set, a high-interest, low-reading-level set, or a basal reader set may be made for the purpose of helping the child "catch up" to his expected level of reading.

REFERENCES

Ashton-Warner, Sylvia. 1963. Teacher. New York, Simon and Schuster.

Bateman, Barbara. 1965. The Illinois Test of Psycholinguistic Abilities in Current Research, Summaries of Study. Urbana, Ill., Institute for Research on Exceptional Children.

Bloomfield, L., and C. Barnhart. 1960. Let's Read. Detroit, Wayne State University Press.

English, H. B., and A. C. English. 1958. A Comprehensive Dictionary of Psychological and Psychoanalytical Terms. New York, David McKay Co.

Fernald, Grace. 1943. Remedial Techniques in Basic School Subjects. New York, McGraw-Hill.

Gray, W. S. 1960. On Their Own in Reading. Chicago, Scott, Foresman and Co.

Harris, A. J. 1968. Diagnosis and remedial instruction in reading. *In* Robinson, H. M., ed., Innovation and Change in Reading Instruction. Yearb. Nat. Soc. Stud. Educ., 67(2):159-194. Chicago, University of Chicago Press.

Hegge, T., S. A. Kirk, and Winifred Kirk. 1940. Remedial Reading Drills. Ann Arbor, Mich., George Wahr Publishing Company.

Kass, Corrine. 1962. Some Psychological Correlates of Severe Reading Disability (Dyslexia). Unpublished Doctoral dissertation. Urbana, University of Illinois.

Kirk, S. A., and J. J. McCarthy. 1961. The Illinois Test of Psycholinguistic Abilities—and approach to differential diagnosis. Amer. J. Ment. Defic., 66:399-412.

———— J. J. McCarthy, and Winifred Kirk. 1968. The Illinois Test of Psycholinguistic Abilities, revised. Urbana, Ill., University of Illinois Press.

Luria, A. R. 1966. Human Brain and Psychological Processes. New York, Harper & Row.

Mowrer, O. H. 1960a. Learning Theory and Behavior. New York, John Wiley & Sons.

————1960b. Learning Theory and the Symbolic Processes. New York, John Wiley & Sons.

National Advisory Committee on Handicapped Children. 1968. First Annual Report, Special Education for Handicapped Children, January 1968. Washington, D. C., U. S. Department of Health, Education, and Welfare, Office of Education.

O'Donnell, Mabel, and W. Towns. 1963. Words to Read, Write and Spell. New York, Harper & Row.

Osgood, C. E. 1957. Contemporary Approaches to Cognition, a Behavioristic Analysis. Cambridge, Mass., Harvard University Press.

———— 1966. Contextual control in sentence understanding and creating. *In* Carterette, E. C., ed., Speech, Language, and Communication, pp. 201-230. Los Angeles, University of California Press.

———— and M. S. Miron. 1963. Approaches to the Study of Aphasia. Urbana, Ill., University of Illinois Press.

———— and T. A. Sebeok. 1965. Psycholinguistics, A Survey of Theory and Research Problems. Bloomington, Ind., Indiana University Press.

Smith, D. E. P., ed. 1967. Michigan Tracking Program. Ann Arbor Publishers.

Strang, R. 1964. Diagnostic Teaching of Reading. New York, McGraw-Hill.

Wiener, N. 1954. The Human Use of Human Beings, Cybernetics and Society. Garden City, N. Y., Doubleday and Co.

14: Educational management of writing deficits

Corrine E. Kass

In any language, writing is a complex process. First, it involves the reception and comprehension of auditory and visual symbols; next, the storage of these in the form of auditory and visual word images; and finally, the appropriate motor movements for the production of letters or words. It is one of the four language arts which Myklebust (1965) relates to the following language processes: (1) listening is an auditory-receptive process, (2) spoken language is an auditory-expressive process, (3) reading is a visual-receptive process, and (4) written language is a visual-expressive process.

In this section, writing deficits are defined as *specific integrational difficulties associated with writing as a skill or habit*. These deficits inhibit the development of a "smooth motor stereotype," which is described by Luria (1966) in the following paragraph:

> In the first stages of learning to write, the process of analysis of the sound-letter composition of a word is consecutive in character, and the child uses the method of articulating aloud the word to be pronounced. An investigation conducted in our laboratory has shown that the prevention of articulation at this stage increases by many times the number of mistakes made by the child during writing. As skill in the function of writing develops, this need, based on articulation, for a consecutive analysis of the phonetic composition of the word gradually becomes superfluous, the process is shortened, and in the adult person, highly skilled in writing, it may be converted into a smooth motor stereotype, dispensing with the phonetic analysis of the word; this is the structure found, for example, in a person's signature, in the writing of highly automatized words, and so on.

This section will include a *theoretical philosophy* about the types of writing deficit commonly found in children with learning disabilities[1] and three steps in the *educationa* *management* of such writing deficits.

For an analysis of research in handwriting, the reader is referred to Herrick (1963).

THEORETICAL PHILOSOPHY

In Chapter 13 a distinction was made between two theoretical levels of language: first, a *representational* level which deals with language found in comprehension, concep* development, and abstraction; and second, an *integrational* level which deals with the automatisms necessary for processes such as closure, memory, speed of perception. In this chapter the same theory of language will form the basis for educational management with the addition of a third language level—a *projection* level which deals with the automatic behavior resulting from imitation of a stimulus which is present.

Writing deficits can be classified into three types according to these levels: (1) those resulting from lack of ideas to be shared (representational level); (2) those resulting from sensory feedback distortion in visual, auditory, and kinesthetic channels (integrational level); and (3) those resulting from defective physical conditions necessary for the writing act (projection level).

Developmentally, the physical conditions of the projection level precede the sensory feedback of the integrational level and the "message" of the representational level. The physical conditions for writing include such factors as gross muscle control, fine muscle control, and environmental and spatial considerations. The motor involvement of the muscles is in tensing and relaxing the arms, wrists, feet, body, and fingers. Ease and speed of muscle efficiency comes from overlearning the motor act of writing. Environmental and spatial considerations include light, posture, writing tools, position of paper, and left-to-right movement. In a study of the practices in the teaching of handwriting in the United States, Herrick and Okada (1963) found that teachers paid more attention to the environmental and spatial factors of body and paper positions than to the physical conditions of the muscle control of feet, wrist, arm, and fingers.

In Chapter 13 words and definitions were given for better understanding of the difference between representational and integrational language levels. The following words and definitions, adapted from English and English (1958), help to explain the projection level:

---

[1] "Children with special learning disabilities exhibit a disorder in one or more of the basic psychological processes involved in understanding or in using spoken or written language. These may be manifested in disorders of listening, thinking, talking, reading, writing, spelling, or arithmetic. They include conditions which have been referred to as perceptual handicaps, brain injury, minimal brain dysfunction, dyslexia, developmental aphasia, etc. They do not include learning problems which are due primarily to visual, hearing, or motor handicaps, to mental retardation, emotional disturbance, or to environmental disadvantage" (National Advisory Committee on Handicapped Children, 1968).

Sensorimotor act—an act whose nature is primarily dependent upon the combined functioning of sense organs and motor mechanisms.

Copy—an imitation or reproduction of an object or act.

Imitation—action that copies the action of another more or less exactly.

At the integrational level, writing deficits are noted in sensory feedback, which is experienced mainly in three channels of communication: visual, auditory, and kinesthetic.

During the writing act, visual feedback comes from information from performance. A circular effect is set in motion when information from performance is compared with a visual standard. In spelling, for example, the visual image of a word precedes writing the word. The written word is then recognized as correct or incorrect through comparison with a standard (either in print or "in the mind"). When the child compares his own writing with a standard, better visual feedback occurs than when the teacher scores the paper. Unfortunately, the latter occurs all too regularly.

Auditory feedback occurs when an individual repeats the sounds or letters to himself. The letters must be thought in correct order to appropriately write words.

Kinesthetic feedback comes from the proprioceptive movement involved in forming a letter or word. The habitual motor patterns which are set up by this form of sensory feedback contribute to ease and speed of writing.

The final goal of writing is concentration on the message to be relayed rather than attention to the motor skills. The message involves the representational level of language functioning. For the act of writing, the child with deficits at the projection or integrational levels will *not* be able to compensate by a strength in representational ability. The message cannot be understood by the reader when the "marks" are not similar to the symbols he knows.

EDUCATIONAL MANAGEMENT

Organizing and carrying out remediation procedures according to the above theoretical philosophy require the following three steps.

1. *Understanding the disability and making a decision regarding the specific language deficit.* For remediation purposes, the educator must understand the differences among representational, integrational, and projection levels of language since different techniques for remediation must be applied at each level. Projection deficits may be corrected through copying and matching exercises; integrational deficits, through memory and imagery exercises; and representational deficits, through word-meaning activities.

Table 1 analyzes some test items by level of language functioning. Through an examination of the scores, an educator will be able to make decisions about remedial procedures. This method of analyzing items can be applied to other tests as well.

2. *Planning and carrying out remediation for specific deficits.* Projection-level deficits must be corrected first because early muscular habits in handwriting become cerebral automatisms. Should the child lack gross motor control, it is not reasonable to expect him to learn to write at the same time as his age peers. Training activities in gross motor

Table 1. Representational and Integrational and Projection Subtests of Some Standard Diagnostic Tests

Tests	Level	Subtests for Specific Deficits
Purdue Perceptual Survey Rating Scale	Projection	Entire Test
Marianne Frostig Developmental Test of Visual Perception, Third Edition	Projection	Eye-Motor Coordination Figure-Ground Discriminati Form Constancy Position in Space Spatial Relations
Picture Story Language Test	Representational Integrational	Productivity Scale Abstract-Concrete Scale Syntax Scale
Strauss, A. A., and Lehtinen, M. A. (Taken from Osgood and Miron, 1963, p. 196)	Projection	"Subject is asked to duplicate mosaic patterns with black and red marbles on board with holes allowing the insertion of marbles. 100 possible locations can be used."

control can be found in Kephart (1960) and Barsch (1965). Fine motor control at a readiness level can be trained through the use of Frostig Materials (Frostig, 1966).

It must be recognized that physical development varies and some children may not reach the readiness level for writing until age 8 or 9. For those children, remediation should not be started too early except for the gross motor level.

Tracing, copying, and matching are projection-level activities. For example, a child could be asked to copy the symbols F R E D without having to know the letters or word. At the integrational level, however, spelling the word *Fred* from memory is easier when the child remembers the letters, sounds, or word wholes.

Writing at the integrational level of language functioning requires visual, auditory, and kinesthetic imagery. The Orton (1937) method suggests a procedure for training kinesthetic feedback—the child copies from the blackboard while the paper on which he is writing is blocked from his view.

One of the best means for the correction of feedback deficits is to use spelling as the basis of remediation. There are a number of methods for teaching spelling, but the best sources for remedial procedures are Fernald (1943), Gillingham and Stillman (1960), and Hildreth (1947, 1955).

An example of a sensory feedback deficit was noted in a young man of 21 who referred himself to the writer because he could not continue his education and was about to lose his present job, which required written messages. An analysis of Ralph's symptoms and history revealed the following: (1) slight hearing loss, (2) known brain injury at age 13, (3) normal intelligence, and (4) spelling at the second-grade level.

No remediation was necessary at the projection level. Some hypotheses were made about sensory feedback deficits, and confirmed through informal testing. Both the auditory and visual channels were involved. Ralph appeared to write messages by phonetic guessing. The remediation involved learning correct spelling in individual sessions. Changes in the sensory feedback mechanisms were effected through the use of Remedial Reading Drills (Hegge et al., 1940). A modified Fernald technique was applied by requiring that Ralph write the words from memory as he slowly pronounced them. He then compared his written word with the printed word in the book.

As his spelling skill improved, Ralph was helped with his job reports for the purpose of transferring the skill of spelling to the representational act of writing.

3. *Transferring specific remediation to writing at the representational level.* Difficulties in writing ideas—as for example, in the Picture Story Language Test (Myklebust, 1965)—can be corrected through remediation at the representational level. Factors important in remediation include an increase in the number of ideas to be communicated and the manner in which descriptive and imaginative thoughts are written down.

For purposes of educational management, practice in verbal expression should be preliminary to improvement in written communication. Discussions should precede a written communication for effective utilization of the sensory feedback at the integrational level.

Mowrer (1963) suggests that it is possible to improve writing skills by setting aside a certain portion of the school day for written communication only. That is, the only language permissible to both teacher and pupils would be through note writing. This idea is readily applicable to the remedial situation.

Motivation cannot be ignored when correcting representational-level deficits. Mowrer (1963) writes: "When the *content* of a message is thought to be especially interesting, we know how feverishly human beings will work to crack the code in which it is being transmitted. Might not similar motivation be developed in school children in connection with their learning to read?" And to write, we might add.

REFERENCES

Barsch, R. H. 1965. A Movigenic Curriculum. Madison, Wis., Bureau for Handicapped Children.

English, H. B., and A. C. English. 1958. A Comprehensive Dictionary of Psychological and Psychoanalytical Terms. New York, David McKay Co.

Fernald, Grace. 1943. Remedial Techniques in Basic School Subjects. New York, McGraw-Hill.

Frostig, Marianne. 1966. The Developmental Program in Visual Perception. Chicago, Follett Publishing Co.

Gillingham, Anna, and Bessie Stillman. 1960. Remedial Training for Children with Specific Disability in Reading, Spelling and Penmanship. Cambridge, Mass., Educators Publishing Service.

Hegge, T., S. A. Kirk, and Winifred Kirk. 1940. Remedial Reading Drills. Ann Arbor, Mich., George Wahr Publishing Co.

Herrick, V. E., ed. 1963. New Horizons for Research in Handwriting. Madison, Wis., University of Wisconsin Press.

———— and Nora Okada. 1963. The present scene: practices in the teaching of handwriting in the United States—1960. In Herrick, V. E., ed., New Horizons for Research in Handwriting, pp. 17-32. Madison, Wis., University of Wisconsin Press.

Hildreth, Gertrude. 1947. Learning the Three R's, 2d. ed. Minneapolis, Minn., Educational Publishers.

————1955. Teaching Spelling. New York, Holt, Rinehart and Winston.

Kephart, N. 1960. Slow Learner in the Classroom. Columbus, Ohio, Charles E. Merrill Publishers.

Luria, A. R. 1966. Human Brain and Psychological Processes. New York, Harper & Row.

Mowrer, O. E. 1963. Learning theory and pedagogical practice. In Herrick, V. E., ed., New Horizons for Research in Handwriting, pp. 95-110. Madison, Wis., University of Wisconsin Press.

Myklebust, H. R. 1965. Development and Disorders of Written Language, Vol. I. New York, Grune & Stratton.

National Advisory Committee on Handicapped Children. 1968. First Annual Report, Special Education for Handicapped Children, January 1968. Washington, D. C., U. S. Department of Health, Education, and Welfare, Office of Education.

Orton, S. T. 1937. Reading, Writing and Speech Problems in Children. New York, W. W. Norton.

Osgood, C., and M. S. Miron. 1963. Approaches to the Study of Aphasia. Urbana, Ill., University of Illinois Press.

15: Medical management

Sylvia Onesti Richardson

Although children with language disabilities may have related or coincidental conditions which can be treated medically or surgically, there is no specific medical treatment for language disorders as such. We do not wish to embark on a therapeutic treatise to cover the gamut of possible pathological problems that one may encounter; the purpose of this chapter is to indicate the role of the physician in the care and management of the child with language disabilities.

The physician's primary responsibilities include the following: (1) prevention and early diagnosis of language disorders; (2) the detection of any disease process, physical handicap, or sensory impairment which might interfere with language development; (3) obtaining and coordinating all necessary studies and consultations; (4) parent counseling and continuing support; (5) careful attention to the child's physical health and to his emotional health and that of his parents; (6) attention to the child's special educational needs; and (7) periodic reevaluation.

As stated in an earlier chapter, the term language disorders is used here to include developmental dysphasia, dyslexia, and dysgraphia. These are closely related conditions, often found together in the same patient or in members of the same family, and in each the process of symbolization is impaired.

Children with developmental dysphasia are a heterogeneous group with the common symptom of failure to acquire meaningful spoken language by the age of 3 to 3½ years, and whose inability to speak cannot be explained on the basis of mental retardation, deafness, anatomic or peripheral neurologic involvement of the articulatory mechanism, psychosis, or environmental factors. A significant percentage of these youngsters may have a sensorineural hearing loss as well, for which management or "treatment" is in the province of the otologist, audiologist, and speech clinician.

A higher than random percentage of children with language disorders may have histories of difficulty at birth, encephalitis, meningitis, or other events known to cause damage to the brain. Many of these children will demonstrate minor or "soft" signs of possible neurologic damage, dysmaturity, or immaturity. Reports of this from various clinics range from 30 to 40 percent. Thus, although the language disability may be the child's major problem, there also may be evidence of other neurological dysfunction of varying type and severity.

Children with developmental dyslexia and/or dysgraphia often present no major problems to their parents or physician until they have started school. On the other hand, they may have a history of retarded speech development, and/or retention of immature articulation. If we summarize the current neurological and educational views regarding the "dyslexic" children in our schools, we may find (1) children with a familial or constitutional dyslexia ("pure" and uncomplicated by neurological and/or environmental handicap); (2) reading retardation along with other symbolic and behavioral problems, secondary to brain injury; (3) reading retardation, secondary to psychological, educational, and/or environmental causes. The latter would include anxiety, which can cripple a child, and unrealistic adult expectations in school or at home.

"Pure," or specific developmental dyslexia (Critchley, 1964), is less common than the lay literature might indicate. It is almost entirely confined to males and usually inherited dominantly in the male line. It persists into adulthood, and there is a peculiar and specific nature in the errors of reading and writing. The adjective "specific" refers to the circumscribed nature of the reading disability and reflects our ignorance as to its cause (Eisenberg, 1966).

Successful medical treatment, or any specific treatment for that matter, is dependent upon a definitive and accurate evaluation of exactly what it is that requires treatment. Diagnostic evaluation of these youngsters involves the concerted efforts of physicians, psychologists, speech clinicians, audiologists, educators, social workers, and others. The diagnostic process is not an end in itself, not simply a search for an accurate diagnostic label, but is a means to set in motion a continuing program of treatment, education, and habilitation.

Traditionally in medicine, therapeutic measures may be divided into the following categories: prevention, specific remedies, substitution products, drugs or procedures designed to correct abnormal functions, correction of dietary deficiencies, symptomatic remedies, reeducation of body and mind, surgical removal or repair, and, last but not least, rest and masterful inactivity to allow the biological processes a free hand to accomplish their end. Of these, the greatest contribution that medicine can make for children with language disorders is toward the prevention of prenatal, natal, and postnatal causes. Medication is largely nonspecific except for such conditions as errors of metabolism, endocrine disorders, or other physical imbalances or deficiencies. Early surgical intervention is indicated in such conditions as craniostenosis (premature closure of the cranial sutures), subdural hematoma, or intracranial tumor. Orthopedic, ophthalmological, dental, otolaryngological, or other services should correct defects whenever possible. Physiotherapy or occupational therapy may be indicated where the child demonstrates clumsiness, fine motor incoordination, or perceptual-motor difficulty that appears to be impeding normal language functions. Where the child or family's emotional health is impaired, psychotherapy may be a requisite for effective therapy. In some instances psychotherapy for the child and family is the primary therapy. The usual

Table 1. Some Medications for Hyperactivity and Short Attention Span

Generic name	Trade name
Anticonvulsants	
Diphenylhydation	Dilantin
Primidone	Mysoline
Mephenytoin	Mesantoin
Ethotoin	Peganone
Phensuximide	Milontin
Methsuximide	Celontin
Ethosuximide	Zaronthin
Acetazolamide	Diamox
Trimethadione	Tridione
Paramethadione	Paradione
Stimulants	
Dextroamphetamine	Dexedrine
Methylphenidate hydrochloride	Ritalin
Amphetamine	Benzedrine
Antihistamines	
Diphenhydramine hydrochloride	Benadryl
Tranquilizers	
Chlordiazepoxide hydrochloride	Librium
Thioridazine	Mellaril
Hydroxyzine	Vistaril
Meprobamate	Equanil
Meprobamate	Miltown

attention to good nutritional care, prevention and early treatment of infection is, of course, just as important for the child with a language disorder as for the normal child.

MEDICATION

When the child is unable to control his behavior and to integrate his experiences, this disintegrated behavior must be modified for language training to be successful. Psychotropic drugs may be useful in treating these children, but it must be pointed out that, in spite of the tremendous publicity about psychopharmacologic agents, drugs do not necessarily provide the solution for the control of hyperactive behavior.

Medications for hyperactivity and short attention span most commonly encountered in the literature include anticonvulsants, antihistamines, and the psychotropic drugs, tranquilizers and stimulants (Baldwin, 1967). Some of these are listed in Table 1.

Many difficulties are encountered in evaluating the effects of these drugs on behavior. For example, the tranquilizers have a sedative effect if given in large-enough dosage, and it may be difficult to distinguish between sedation and psychotropic effect. Theoretically, the tranquilizer relieves anxiety and agitation without impairing the thinking processes, but we have seen many children whose behavior is not affected until they become absolutely stuporous from large doses of medication. Such use of drugs may provide a chemical restraint, but this defeats the primary purpose of therapy, which is to assist the child to learn.

It is well known that the stimulants, amphetamine (Benzedrine) or dextro-amphetamine (Dexedrine), often have a paradoxical effect in calming a child and making his behavior better organized. Similarly, phenobarbital and other sedatives may have him "climbing the walls" with excessive hyperactivity. However, there are many exceptions to these generalizations. Unfortunately, we have no surefire prognostic device to tell us how a child will react to a specific drug.

Quite a few medications may be prescribed, singly or in combinations, but results are rarely consistent. Drug-evaluation studies yield a variety of contradictory results. Different practitioners will sing the praises of quite different drugs. One wonders if the success of a particular medication might not be directly proportional to the physician's faith in it. This could be called the "practitioner effect."

On the other hand, Eisenberg (1964) has described the "placebo effect" occasioned by the overoptimistic, overanxious mother who is so hopeful of a "cure" that she cannot be objective in her observations of the child. Almost anything seems to work for a while.

In order to evaluate the effectiveness of a given drug, one must rely on the judgment of those around the child. These judgments are often influenced by unpredictable environmental factors. For example, a teacher may feel that the child shows improved behavior in the classroom while the mother may report no change at home; at this time there may be undue stress in the home for various reasons, and this can influence parent judgment, as well as the child's behavior. Some parents resist the idea of using drugs or are afraid that the child will become addicted. As a result, they may "forget" to give the medication on a regular basis, thereby nullifying its effectiveness. Not infrequently different members of the family report different reactions in the child.

The use of drugs to alter behavior is, at present, a trial-and-error process, and repeated changes in medication may be necessary before a useful one is found. This requires close cooperation with parents and teachers. One can be fairly confident of results when reports of the child's behavior are similar from parents, teachers, therapists, or others. Many in clinical practice report favorable results when medication is used in a combined program with psychotherapy. Parent counseling is always a necessary and useful adjunct to chemotherapy.

The use of drugs in the treatment of behavior disorders which may accompany language disabilities is a relatively new field, still not accepted by many pediatricians, neurologists, or psychiatrists. Research is still needed in correlating various medications with behavior response, neurological findings, and electroencephalogram patterns. Studies are needed which will compare the response to chemotherapy, psychotherapy, and a combination of the two. Like aspirin, the psychotropic drugs may ameliorate symptoms, but neither effects a cure. However, when the psychotropic drugs are effective, they do permit easier training and education with a simultaneous increase in attention span. With thoughtful selection, careful regulation of dosage, and careful watchfulness for toxicity, they can add to the total plan of patient care.

PARENT COUNSELING

Since the pediatrician or the family physician is usually the first to see a child with a possible language disability, he initiates the diagnostic process and maintains contact with the family. The child will undergo a complete battery of laboratory examinations, he will be seen by various medical specialists, and he will undergo a full array of psychological tests, as well as thorough speech, language, and hearing evaluations. Throughout all of these sometimes prolonged procedures, it is important for the parents to have some guidance and, at the conclusion, correct interpretation of the findings. The importance of the latter cannot be overemphasized. One person with whom the parents have good rapport, and in whom they have confidence, should put together all the findings and recommendations in such a way that the parents can understand the nature and extent of the problem as well as the necessary steps in management. Hopefully, this person will be the child's physician.

The experienced physician's interpretation usually adds considerable weight to what has been said by others involved and is often the opinion most readily accepted by the parents. However, not every physician can be a successful interpreter, especially of the nonmedical results and recommendations. In such a case, the language clinician or the special educator should join the physician during some of the counseling sessions. In any case, the physician must be careful to communicate his findings, and also the way in which he has interpreted them to the parents, to the family physician, educators, psychologists, speech and hearing clinicians, and social workers involved.

The physician will arrange for periodic reevaluation and will provide continuing medical management of the child.

There must be close cooperation between the school and the physician, with recognition of where school responsibility and medical responsibilities begin, end, and overlap. There will be shifts in responsibility for parent counseling—but the physician, by virtue of his training, experience, and relationship with the family, is in a strategically favorable position to be of service in this regard.

PREVENTION

It is clear that optimum management of children with language disorders requires the concerted efforts of representatives from many disciplines. The physician has a direct responsibility to take a leading part in this team management. This will require persistent pediatric procedures for followthrough, along with acceptance of medical responsibility in the establishment of vigorous measures in prevention and early detection of language disabilities.

Pediatricians in every community should endeavor to participate in planning and executing more effective comprehensive maternal and child health programs to prevent the complications during pregnancy, delivery, and in the neonatal period that can cause damage to the infant central nervous system. We can no longer consider maternal and child health as simply another function of the government public health service. It is each community's problem and its solution requires the combined skills of each community's medical personnel, nurses, nutritionists, social workers, health educators, and others.

Speech and language clinicians should be included as consultants to maternal and child health programs to educate and assist parents to provide for their children home environments conducive to optimal language development. Such consultants should also be available to early childhood educators as well as to teachers in primary education.

Preschool programs should be available to all children. Facilities should be established in every community to provide comprehensive evaluation of each child before he enters kindergarten to determine his state of perceptual organization or "ripeness" (school readiness). Multiprofessional groups should be available to evaluate preschool children to determine each child's particular learning style, his assets and liabilities, and to transmit this information to the elementary school in useful forms (Richardson, 1968).

The preschool program can serve as enrichment for our underprivileged children. It can also enable the pediatrician to identify medical defects and to mobilize corrective or therapeutic measures.

Community emphasis should also be placed on improving programs in our elementary schools. Proper educational assessment, diagnostic teaching, and educational therapy or prescriptive teaching should be established and continued from preschool through the primary grades at least. In every case where a child demonstrates deviation or difficulty in learning, there should be an adjustment in the way he is taught.

Speech and language clinicians and other specialists can assist classroom teachers to utilize multisensorial techniques, to provide perceptual-motor training in the classroom, and especially to develop language-oriented programs. In every case, teachers should be encouraged to search continuously for methods of instruction that will fill a particular child's needs, rather than search for ways to make the child fit a particular method or curriculum.

If honestly administered, in principle and practice, a flexible ungraded primary from kindergarten through grade 3 might prevent or alleviate some of the language and learning disabilities that may be due to lags in maturation. If not the ungraded primary, a transition class could be provided, as suggested by de Hirsch et al. (1966).

SUMMARY

There is no specific medical treatment for language disorders as such. Medical management is dependent upon definitive diagnosis, which is a continuing process involving the concerted efforts of physicians, psychologists, speech clinicians, audiologists, teachers, social workers, and others in allied professions.

Where pathogenic processes or associated defects are found, these must be corrected whenever possible.

Medications can be useful to ameliorate symptoms of hyperactivity and short attention span, but have a limited role in the treatment of language and learning problems.

The physician's primary responsibilities are in prevention and early diagnosis of language disabilities, parent counseling, appropriate and timely referral to diagnostic centers, in careful attention to the child's special educational needs, his physical health, and to his emotional health and that of his parents. In order to fulfill these responsibilities for one child, he will need to work with others for all children in the community by directing his efforts toward better programs in maternal and child health, comprehensive preschool evaluation, and by working with educators to encourage improved and revised school programs.

REFERENCES

Baldwin, R. W. 1967. The treatment of behavioral disorders with medication. Selected Conference Papers: International Approach to Learning Disabilities of Children and Youth, pp. 111-118. Tulsa, The Association for Children with Learning Disabilities.

Benton, P. C., and Wanda McGavock. 1968. Medication in child psychiatry. Southern Med. J., April:347-353.

Bradley, C. 1937. Behavior of children receiving benzedrine. Amer. J. Psychiatr., 94:577.

———1950. Benzedrine and dexedrine in the treatment of children's behavior disorders. Pediatrics, 5:24.

Critchley, Macdonald. 1964. Developmental Dyslexia. Springfield, Ill., Charles C Thomas.

de Hirsch, K., et al. 1966. Predicting Reading Failure. New York, Harper & Row.

Denhoff, Eric. 1964. Drugs, behavior and the family. Drugs in Cerebral Palsy: Clinics in Developmental Medicine, No. 16: 62-71. London, The Spastics Society, in Association with William Heinemann Medical Books.

Eisenberg, Leon. 1964. Role of drugs in treating disturbed children. Children, 2(5):167-173.

———1966. The management of the hyperkinetic child. Develop. Med. Child Neurol., 8(5):593-598.

Kirman, Brian. 1961. Tranquilizers for hyperactive children. Cereb. Palsy Bull., 3(4):379-382.

McDermott, Mary. 1967. Medication—and the role of the occupational therapist. Selected Conference Papers: International Approach to Learning Disabilities of Children and Youth, pp. 104-107. Tulsa, The Association for Children with Learning Disabilities.

Paine, R. S. 1963. The contributions of neurology to the pathogenesis of hyperactivity in children. Clin. Proc. Child. Hosp. D. C., 14(9):235-247.

Richardson, S. O. 1968. Learning disorders and the preschool child. New Jersey Educ. Assoc. Rev., 41:6.

16: Social management

Empress Y. Zedler

A phenomenon in the history of child development as a scientific study is the keen interest and vigorous activity engendered in a particular problem area when the demands of society enforce a shift of focus. For example we are now witnessing a productive, exciting, and perhaps inevitably chaotic period in the history of man's concern with language disorders in otherwise normal children. The interest of the public in the problem is now intense, often rampant. Throughout our social structure there seems to have erupted a sudden awareness of the problem area and its deleterious effect upon the academic achievement of children.

As recently as 10 years ago, there was little public awareness of the nature, the etiology, or the incidence of language difficulties even as they were expected to occur in children with sensory or intellective impairment: the deaf, the blind, or the feeble-minded. But today parents and educators are demanding remedial procedures to alleviate, if not to eradicate, the scourge of language disabilities. And the individuals about which there seems to be most concern are children with basically adequate intellective, sensory, motor, and emotional equipment. These children have had the opportunity to learn by methods and under conditions which have been successful with others, but have nonetheless failed to acquire expected competence in one or more, and probably in all, of the aspects of language—understanding speech, speaking, reading, and writing—and their presenting complaint is overall academic deficiency.

The purpose of this chapter is to remind those who would identify and correct language disabilities in children that the primary goal of all education is social adequacy. The handicapped child can best be served by helping him gain social acceptance, by promoting his feeling of personal adequacy, and by encouraging him to develop his individual potentialities as fully as possible (Kaplan, 1959). Any procedures of management which do not achieve these goals are hurtful rather than beneficial. From the writer's 15 years of experience in working with language-disabled children and their parents comes awareness of the danger of creating more serious problems than those we seek to solve.

355

In teachers' and therapists' search for the best way to deal with deficient language function there is the danger of creating a category of pathology. We must face the possibility that too often we involve parents to the extent that they find the concept of a child with a disability rewarding. The satisfaction derived by parents from frenetic organizing, fund raising, and disseminating literature for lay persons is great indeed. One wonders if such children were returned to "normalcy" might not the parents find the children more difficult to accept than if they remained "disabled?"

In this chapter the proposition will be advanced that the development of characteristics conducive to social acceptance and to feelings of dignity and self-respect should be the primary concern of those who would help children with language disabilities.

GENERAL CONSIDERATIONS

The Abnormality of Normalcy

With the keen interest and vigorous activity now being shown in the problem of language difficulties the vast heterogeneity of the phenomena included under the rubric should not be overlooked. There is danger of constructing a homogeneous group of children defined by concepts of language disability, when academic failure or underachievement is actually the one common and dependable characteristic of the group.

When society recognizes a behavioral "disability" and sets about to prevent or ameliorate the symptoms, there must be an understanding of the continuum of individual differences within the trait or skill. Hirsch (1963) points out that individual differences are generated by properties of organisms which are fundamental to behavioral science. He warns against assuming uniformity of expression of any behavior under study. Workers in the area of language disabilities would do well to heed the warning regarding the "uniformity assumption," which is too often explicitly incorporated in the current outpouring of theories and models designed to formalize the study of language disabilities.

Implicit in the use of the term "normal" is reference to some region of a distribution arbitrarily designated as not extreme (Williams, 1956). And yet there is evidence that, through well-intentioned but misguided zeal for helping children, society may be creating horrendous labels and constructing arbitrary, nebulous classifications for qualitatively normal children whose language competencies are not high, but whose language incompetencies are not extreme. For example, in a publication widely distributed among lay persons, a new book (Ellingson, 1967) was reviewed:

> THE SHADOW CHILDREN is a new book ... about children—millions of children—with subtle learning disorders. "They are not blessed with the sunlight of normal perception; nor are they cursed with the total darkness of hopeless abnormality. They stand in the shadows between light and dark. They are educationally gray—the shadow children." The author writes about dyslexia, minimal brain dysfunction, testing, and teaching (ACLD Items of Interest, 1967).

What's in a name? Just as children tend to identify with their personal names, so do they identify with labels assigned to their educational groupings. To children there is no name more repugnant or injurious than "special." In the vernacular of public school children, it is synonymous with "stupid." By the same token "regular" means "I belong" and "Like us." Children react according to whether their companions approve or disapprove of the label. All labels associated with special education rate low in social approval (Dunn, 1968). No label is rated higher by a child's agemates, nor contributes more to his social acceptance, than a label which connotes ordinary, regular, to-be-expected normalcy.

The attaching of labels and the assigning of categories to children who are to receive language therapy evidences that educators assume relative uniformity between individuals for the behavior under study. The need for protest against such a counterfactual uniformity postulate is evident. The answer to this need may be found in studies of behavior which employ methods of both the behavioral and physiological sciences (Hirsch, 1963). We can probably best assist children to achieve social adequacy if we accept the concept that normal language behavior has no generality.

Understanding the Individual

The capacity for learning and using a language code is probably a biosocial intrinsic endowment of man (Chomsky, 1965) dependent upon several physiological systems which are variable, not uniform. There is little reason to expect that the many possible combinations and integrations of those systems that go to make up the members of a population will yield a homogeneously normal distribution of responses for behavioral measurement. "An organism richly endowed with the components of one subset of systems and poorly endowed with those of another is not expected to behave in the same manner as an organism with an entirely different balance of endowments" (Hirsch, 1963, p. 1438).

Individual differences are not accidental. They are generated by properties within the organism. If we would function as behavioral scientists in our dealings with children and their acquisition of language, our models and assumptions must be consistent with knowledge that is coming out of other sciences. The educator and the therapist must utilize in their work developments from fields which may previously have seemed remote from behavior. One such field is genetics.

The worker who would understand individuality should keep in mind that the behavior of any organism is determined by interaction of environment and the organism's complete genetic endowment. Whether genotypic differences are involved in language behavior is an empirical question to be settled separately for each population being studied. The matter of heredity and environment (nature and nurture), however, can no longer be settled by dogmatic attitudes and assumptions about uniformity. Through study of the distribution of genes in populations, and the mechanisms responsible for stability and for change in gene frequencies, genetics has provided the behavioral scientist with some understanding of the gene pools from which individuals come.

The most thorough and voluminous study about the heredity of children who are unable to learn to read normally (dyslexic) has been done by Hallgren (1950), reported by Zerbin-Rüdin (1967), and translated from the German by Vandenberg (1967). Hallgren studied 116 experimental subjects and 212 controls. His experimental group contained 79 children from the Stockholm Child Guidance Clinic, and 43 children from a Stockholm school which gave special attention to poor readers. On the basis of genetics Hallgren was able to divide his 116 experimental subjects into the following four groupings: (1) both parents were dyslexic (3 percent); (2) one parent was dyslexic (81 percent); (3) at least one case of dyslexia was found among siblings, uncles, aunts, or grandparents (6 percent); and (4) isolated cases (10 percent). In the predominant majority, 81 percent, there was at least one parent with the same disability. Furthermore, it was pointed out that this represented a minimum value, "since adults have largely compensated for their original difficulties and often have forgotten or repressed them." For example, the mother of one of Hallgren's experimental subjects denied in good faith that she had ever had difficulty with reading, while ensuing testing brought out clearly that she did.

Almost all studies find more males than females affected by language disabilities. Among Hallgren's experimental subjects, the boys outnumbered the girls by 76 percent (89 boys, 27 girls). Furthermore, the difference between the number of males and females, while less, was still significant when the affected parents of group 2 and the siblings of group 3 were put together; 47 percent were males and 37 percent were females. However, complete or partial sex linkage was rejected by Hallgren on the basis of thorough calculations. He explained the excess of boys by (1) the higher manifestation and stronger expressivity in males, and (2) the one-sided selection of dyslexics, especially in clinics but also in schools. In other words, Hallgren implied that the inability to learn to read is more socially stigmatizing to boys than to girls.

The findings of Hallgren, as well as other researchers (Zerbin-Rüdin, 1967), point clearly to the transmission of specific dyslexia by an autosomal, dominant gene with almost complete manifestation. Genetic recessiveness has only rarely been proposed (Stephenson, 1907; Tkacev, 1948).

When reading behavior is investigated a continuum of gradations is found from superior to alexia. For this reason some investigators assume polygenetic inheritance as in the case of intelligence.

Zerbin-Rüdin (1967) contends that the latest findings do not support the theory that congenital word blindness is a symptom of brain damage. According to the German studies "social conditions such as separation of parents, poverty, too early a start in school, being a single child, number of other children, and so forth, apparently are of no importance for the etiology of specific dyslexia, nor are physical illness, neurological or sensory defects."

The scientist in genetics reminds us that man with his 23 chromosome pairs produces gametes with any of 23 alternative genomes. This makes exceedingly small the chances that even siblings, other than identical twins, will be genetically identical. According to Hirsch (1963) the probability that the second offspring born to the same parents will have exactly the same genotype as the first offspring is less than 1 chance in over 70

trillion. And the probability that two unrelated individuals will have the
endowment is operatively zero. Therefore, before we begin to intervene witl
experiences for children with language difficulties, we must remembe
organisms are intrinsically variable before they undergo differentiating exp
example, some will learn better by visual or auditory cues, others by predominantly
kinesthetic cues. As our methods of observation become more reliable, the more evident
it will be that the children we seek to study are the products of their gene pools but that
each differs from the other. The concept of a normal individual has no generality.

The Dilemma of Labeling

Before theories of management can be implemented it seems important to ask how
society can help those language-disabled children who could benefit from identification
and corrective education without injuring with indefensible labels that sizable group of
children within the normal distribution who must function at a relatively low linguistic
level. A model is needed which will generate a theoretical "two-group approach" to the
distribution of facility in language. Such a model has been propounded by Zigler (1967)
for the distribution of intelligence, as an approach for understanding and working with
mental retardates. He suggests that some order could be brought to the area of mental
retardation if a distinction were maintained between pathologically defective persons and
those representing the lower, but nonetheless integral, part of the distribution of
intelligence that we would expect from the normal manifestation of the genetic pool in
our population. Such a model could and, this writer proposes, should be applied to the
language function. The two-group approach would recognize that group of children who
fail to acquire language, and would treat them as pathologically impaired. However, in
addition to this group which forms a minority of all children classified as language-
disabled, there would be recognized that much larger group of children who have
acquired language but whose language acquisition is below levels attained by their age
peers in their speech community. This second and larger group would not be labeled
defective, but would be treated as just as much an integral part of the normal distribution
as those who are superior in language abilities, or as the more numerous group of children
who are considered to be average in language skills. Such a two-group approach would
help to dispel the fallacious formulation that all children who are low in language facility
compose a homogeneous class of subnormals qualitatively different from persons having
higher language abilities.
   Children with no primary sensory, motor, intellectual, or emotional deficits who by
the age of four have not learned the phonological, semantic, and syntactic components of
a language well enough to understand and speak that language certainly comprise a
population who are pathologically defective in the acquisition of language. Such children
should be identified and treated as language-disabled children. It is warranted to suppose
that they would derive more benefit than harm from such diagnosis and labeling.
Furthermore, those children who meet the same criteria of adequate sensory, motor,
intellectual, and emotional equipment and who have attended school for 2 years but who

by the age of 8 have not learned to read and write should also be identified and clinically taught as language-disabled pupils.

It has been the experience of the writer that the nonreading and nonwriting 8-year-olds in school are likely to be the same children who at the age of 4 could not communicate with others in their speech community (Zedler, 1968b). Since reading and writing are in essence particular systems for recording speech, it is logical to expect pathology of language function to cut across all modalities. Schuell et al. (1964) found that aphasia in adults resulted in generalized reduction of available language and was not modality centered. Research done at Southwest Texas State University with school children who had neurologically based learning disorders revealed that those who had been unable to learn to read and write were also disabled in understanding speech and in speaking (Zedler, 1968b). There are strong implications that children who are pathologically defective in acquisition of written language could be identified and treated in preschool years on the basis of their failure to acquire spoken language. If treatment were effective such children could be spared the social trauma of identification and labeling as language-disabled school children. If identified and treated before entering school it is possible that children with language disabilities might be absorbed into the socially acceptable group who are "below average but normal" on the language continuum. It is reasonable to believe that, even after effective treatment, children who were pathologically defective in language acquisition will not be highly proficient in language skills. However, being classified among "the normal" can do much to alleviate the social ineffectiveness of children with inadequate language.

The Epidemic of Language Disabilities

The medical profession has long been aware that certain otherwise normal children fail to acquire the language faculty. Educators and psychologists, however, have been slow to manifest similar awareness. At the turn of the century a physician, Dr. Pringle Morgan, a general practitioner in Seaford, England, reported that his experience in preparatory schools had brought to his attention an intelligent 14-year-old-boy who was incapable of learning to read (Critchley, 1961). Important studies followed and were reported by ophthalmologists and neurologists. These early studies, however, had no impact upon educators. Critchley (1961), in attempting to explain the failure of these studies to influence educational policy, states that the reporting neurologists did not put forth their views clearly or forcefully enough. In 1961 (Critchley, 1961) he deplored that scientific attitudes toward reading disabilities had "oscillated like a pendulum over the past 60 years." Although Orton (1937) had called attention to the correlation between neurological organization and the reading, writing, and speech problems of children, the concept had had little influence upon the educational management of children.

Theoretical efforts in the remedial education of children who could not read, write, or spell were hampered by a variety of conceptual ambiguities. Soon after publication of Orton's (1937) concept that the learning of language is dependent upon integrity of the central nervous system, opinions of a different sort generated the proposition that failure to learn language skills was a sociological problem and the product of environmental factors. Language difficulties not attributable to sensory loss were envisaged on a continuum between neurosis and mental deficiency. Educators with little but ambiguity to guide them were understandably either confused or opinionated in their thinking, and fortuitious in their management of pupils with learning disabilities.

Although a coming together of medicine and pedagogy in the joint study of children with language disabilities has been a slow process, it has come to fulfillment in the present decade. Interdisciplinary communication has been realized in national conferences, in a vast body of professional literature, in joint research projects, and on the local level in diagnostic and evaluative centers. Any person now closely associated with public and private schools which provide for the special education of children with language or learning disabilities is impressed with the increasing number of such children being "discovered." In some localities the diagnosis is so widely diffused and rapidly spreading that it has reached proportions of an epidemic.

It seems warranted to apply some of the principles of epidemiology to language disabilities which are now recognized as afflicting so many school children. According to Gruenberg (1954) epidemiology is not only a study of the distribution of prevalence rates of a disease or disorder in a human community but it also seeks to understand the forces that make those prevalence rates higher in one population than in another. Behavior can be contagious in a group and the contagion is most likely when "the size, structure and atmosphere of the group favor the behavior" (Gruenberg, 1954). We would do well to ask why language disabilities have become so prevalent among school children in the present decade. What has changed in the past 20 years? Neither the nature of children nor the English language has changed. Dunn (1968) suggests that the epidemic is generated within the school by educators who refer problem children out of regular classes, thus reducing the need for dealing with individual differences. The school acts as a case-finding agent, and what the school designates as a disability might not be detected by the rest of the community. The possibility must be seriously considered that the present high prevalence rate of children's behavioral abnormalities, such as hyperactivity, short attention span, perceptual disorders, motor incoordination, and specific difficulty in learning what their teachers think they should learn, may be a functional disequilibrium between the child and his environment.

It is clear, for example, that in a society increasingly dependent upon literacy, a handicap in reading is a major disorder and worthy of special attention in the school's curriculum. In present-day society, which emphasizes individual striving and upward economic mobility, any child is stigmatized who is unable to progress in school at the same rate as others. One of the consequences of a society's more complex industrialization is the demand for people with specific technical skills. This requires universal compulsory education with more complex curricula, the consequence of which is the identification of numbers of pupils who cannot fit into the new environment nor respond adequately to the new demands for learning.

It would seem that the vast heterogeneity of the phenomena included within the rubric of language difficulties should be carefully considered before a scholastically underachieving child is assigned an additional stigma of "language-disabled." There has been a widespread tendency to place children who have acquired language but who are low in language facility into self-contained "special" groups for educational purposes. Research has not supported the hypothesis that such grouping is beneficial to the children. In fact, there is strong evidence that it may be more harmful than helpful (Zedler, 1967).

The decision as to whether a child is to be categorized as language-impaired and eligible for a special education class is often based as much upon his general level of social adjustment as upon his facility in language. Identification of the language-impaired child is similar to that of the mentally retarded about which Maher (1963, p. 238) stated:

> What constitutes mentally retarded behavior depends to a large extent upon the society which happens to be making the judgment. An individual who does not create a problem for others in his social environment and who manages to become self-supporting is usually not defined as mentally retarded no matter what his test IQ may be.

As with mental retardation, language disability is largely a socially defined phenomenon. The person who is adept in making satisfactory social relationships is not likely to be judged disabled even though his scholastic achievement may be such that he will require extensive, individual, supportive teaching to meet minimal requirements for scholastic promotion with the slowest of learners in a regular general classroom. With social adequacy he may escape the stigma of "subnormalcy."

As with mental retardation (Zigler, 1964), the prevalence of language disabilities fluctuates widely across age categories and according to locality. This may well be explained on the basis of the children's success in meeting social demands. For example, the low prevalence of language difficulties reported by parents and preschool teachers for children under 5 years of age may reflect lack of social demands made on young children. The age range of most subjects reported in research related to language disabilities is from 9 to 15 years, with the mean age at 10 years. This is the age at which more social demands are made upon children in school, in the home, and in the community at large. This is the age at which society's demands for success in school are the greatest. If there were some way of helping children at this age to meet society's demands at a minimal level of adequacy, the prevalence rate of school children detected and labeled as disabled in verbal behavior might be substantially reduced. To the extent that adequacy in verbal behavior is a social concept, there will be fluctuating thresholds of society's tolerance. With appropriate management only those children with the most profound impairment in communication need be classified as other than normal. Few children with high social competence are referred for diagnosis and evaluation of their language abilities. Perhaps a child's social incompetence would be more easily investigated and treated than his language disabilities.

Although the concern about language facility in children has reached all but epidemic proportions, still no thoroughly satisfactory instrument has been developed for assessing language development in children. Stark (1966) concluded, from his use of the Illinois Test of Psycholinguistic Abilities (McCarthy and Kirk, 1961) with aphasic children, that the performances of these children were highly individual, and that no typical pattern emerged. He concluded that, in spite of theories to the contrary, "we do not know how stimuli are received, processed, and stored in the central nervous system." The how's and why's of individual differences are enormously complex in the normal as well as in language-impaired children and adults. Certainly the language process is complicated and highly individual in each learner. One who has worked extensively with developmental aphasia in children or with adult aphasics would agree with Schuell et al. (1964) that aphasic persons "make the same kinds of errors as nonaphasics make under conditions of fatigue or inattention, but with far greater frequency."

It would seem, therefore, that we who would attack the problem of management and corrective education of children with language difficulties should weigh the notion that the nature of the disability is a system working below the efficiency level set by the social environment. With this concept as a premise we may direct our energies (1) to altering society's attitudes toward individual differences in language abilities of children, and (2) toward teaching children how to compensate for language deficits through social competence.

A Concept of Socialization

If we are to help in the social management of children with language deficits, an understanding of the socialization process in general is necessary. The traditional concept of socialization is to define it in terms of the acquisition of social values and conformity to certain norms; these cultural norms are passed from one generation to the next (Blatz, 1944; Dager, 1964). As Zigler and Harter (1968) point out, however, such a point of view leaves little room for a consideration of individual differences in the socialization process. The child with a language disability should be viewed as an essentially normal person whose ultimate socialization pattern is influenced by his difficulty in learning to understand speech, speak, read, and write, but whose socialization process is mediated and/or influenced by precisely the same variables as influence the socialization of individuals who are more proficient in language.

By understanding the experiences, the motivation, and the personality of the child, and also the relationship of these factors to his language disabilities, insight will be gained as to his socialization. A frenzy of effort is being expended to improve language modalities of children, often at the expense of certain motivational and personality factors which are highly relevant to social adjustment. On the other hand, certain classroom teachers, parents, and clinicians are achieving outstanding success in the unspectacular social management of children who are low in language facility. As pointed out by Penrose (1963, p. 282), the most important work "is not highly technical but requires unlimited patience, good will, and common sense." While the child may not become highly competent in language skills, his personal adjustment to social life may become tremendously rewarding to him and to his family.

Socialization prepares a person to take part as fully and usefully as possible in human affairs. Any procedure which emphasizes improvement of language function at the cost of social adjustment is harmful. There is little demonstrable value in the concept of social competence since it is so value-laden and differs so much among social groups. Perhaps the best operational definition of social competence is related to whether or not the person can manage to function within the regular group of his age peers. Such functioning will depend upon his ability (1) to participate independently within his group, and (2) to abide by the group's values, that is, to behave within the limits set by the authority figures of the group.

To acquire social competence the child must be loved and in turn learn how to love; he must be accepted as a needed member of the group; and he must have the opportunity to do things for himself and receive approval for his efforts even though he may have fallen far short of success. If these needs can be met, any child, with or without language disabilities, can become an "optimistic, hopeful individual, one who can contribute something to the world at large and to those nearest to him" (English and Pearson, 1955, p. 6).

The needs which, if met, preserve and develop a child's psychological and social well-being are (1) affection, with which he bestows and derives interpersonal satisfaction; (2) acceptance, which is synonymous with group status; and (3) approval which results in feelings of personal worth, and leads to self-development (Kaplan, 1959). How then can society provide the three A's—affection, acceptance, and approval—for the child with language disabilities?

SPECIFIC CONSIDERATIONS

Affection, or Interpersonal Satisfactions

All children seek love and affection from those who are important to them. Parents are the source of the love which makes their children feel warm and wanted, secure and strong. Yet the parents of children who cannot communicate adequately in the language code often have difficulty transmitting love. Parents of children with language disabilities need to be counseled in how to make their children aware that they are beloved.

It is important for parents, as well as those who counsel them, to understand the four attitudinal stages through which parents go when they realize that their child may have any type of disability. These stages are disbelief, guilt, martyrdom, and, hopefully, objectivity; the first three are not conducive to communication of affection from parent to child. The four attitudes occur in sequence. They are common to all parents and are not influenced by social class or intellectual status. No one of the four sequential attitudes can be slighted. Nor can a parent be informed, shamed, or counseled out of one stage into another. Each stage must run its course until the next emerges. It is helpful only to have some supportive person standing by who can react with empathy as parents struggle through each attitude. Group therapy is especially helpful for parents with similarly disabled children, for, from other parents, they may gain insight into their own feelings. A group leader who can mirror parents' feelings can do much to hasten progression through the impotent stages of disbelief, guilt, and martyrdom, and into the objective stage where parents can enjoy their children.

Disbelief is parents' first reaction to a child's disability. Parenthood is an egoistic experience. Whether the pregnancy was planned or accidental, wanted or resented, the inevitable expectancy is for a child who will incorporate all that is desirable and nothing that is undesirable from each of his procreators. As surely as a gambler watches the roulette wheel with anticipation, just so prospective parents expect a winner from their contribution to the child's genotype drawn in the lotteries of the mating ritual and meoisis. This child will be better than either of themselves. This child will have all that they did not have. What does it matter if neither parent went to college, or if one or both dropped out of high school because the going was rough? The great American dream is a high school diploma for all, and college for everybody who is anybody.

Parents tend to forget about one or the other's having failed one or more grade levels in school. If questioned or reminded of it a parent recalls that he did not fail, but was "kept back" for one or more years because of illness, change of residence, or any of many good rationalizations. Grandparents may recall that one of the child's parents was a late talker, but that was because there were older children to do the talking for him, or some other equally plausible but unscientific explanation. So it is unbelievable that this child, who is the product of themselves, is disabled in the acquisition of oral and/or written language. Thus precious time is dissipated in the parents' stage of disbelief.

Time which could be spent in productive therapy is wasted waiting for speech or reading and writing to emerge. And professionals unwittingly encourage the futile waiting by endorsing without evidence such vague concepts as "immaturity" and "readiness," thus implying, if not advising, "wait-and-see" tactics. It is in this stage of disbelief that parents all too often impoverish themselves seeking panaceas and cults—anything to assure them that there is no basic trouble, or that, if there is trouble, it can be easily and quickly remedied if they but pay and persist.

Why do scientists not counter with valid information about the onset and remediation of language disabilities, since the sooner sound corrective measures are begun the better is the prognosis for improvement? The truth is that the scientific community has produced no simple formulas for the remediation and management of language disabilities. Available knowledge from controlled studies indicates that there are no easy to follow, well-defined techniques. Procedures are complicated and arduous, calling for the combined efforts of many workers in various professional disciplines. Consensus and limited data do not provide sufficient bases for the promulgation of corrective procedures. Controlled, unbiased research promises the only valid basis for the correction of language disabilities. And research so far has emphasized only the difficulties and complexities of the problem rather than the solutions. In the urgency for positive action, therefore, the public, and in some instances professionals are too often responsive to methods based upon dogma set forth by their promulgators, remedies which make up in the heat of their proponents' enthusiasm what is lacked in grasp of the complex issues they seek to solve (Zedler, 1967). And parents, in the stage of disbelief, provide a ready market for the nostrums.

When disbelief gives way to credence, parents enter the second attitudinal phase—the stage of guilt. "What did I do or not do that caused my child to be less than normal?" This uncomfortable feeling of having done wrong, and the disability's being the parent's punishment, seems to afflict mothers more frequently than fathers. Perhaps this is because the child's prenatal and perinatal experiences are inseparable from the mother.

Fathers, however, are not immune to feelings of guilt. Deeds of omission and of commission are recalled and ruminated. In this period all those responsible for the care of the mother during pregnancy and delivery are subject to incrimination. These feelings of irrational blame are incited further by untenable terms such as "brain injury" which are often applied, without supportable evidence, to children with language disabilities (Denhoff and Robinault, 1960).

As long as there are feelings of blame there will be irrational attempts at restitution for the damage done. Each parent tortured by a sense of badness, of having "injured" the child, must take some action to be rid of the sense of guilt. Such action often takes the form of aggression toward the other parent, the partner equally responsible for the procreation of the "injured" one. "What did I do to injure my child? I chose the wrong parent for him!" If the stage of parental guilt does not ultimately result in separation or divorce of the parents it invariably leads to disharmony, bickering, and belligerence—a poor climate for the affection which is any child's first and most basic psychosocial need.

And following guilt—martyrdom. "We believe; we now know that our child is disabled. We shall not, however, torture ourselves with blame and guilt. Instead we shall repress all hostile aggressive feelings toward each other and, of course, toward this unfortunate child. Instead we shall do everything in our power to compensate for the misfortune which has befallen our child."

Thus the child and his disability become a cause for which parents renounce all else, and devote themselves to its perpetuity. It is in the stage of martyrdom that previously bewildered, buffeted parents often seek and find autonomy in activites devoted to fund-raising, organizing, and publicizing in behalf of their child's disability. While zealous devotion may compensate parents for their feelings of guilt, it is questionable that their children benefit from it.

It is from the stage of martyrdom that parents may be helped to progress into an attitude of objectivity—of viewing their child, who is low in language ability, as a part of the normal population, as a fine and likeable person who is probably no more disabled than they themselves are or once were. By seeing themselves in their child parents may become aware of the child as he is: less endowed with language ability, but endowed nonetheless with many fine and desirable qualities. Parents may be guided into knowing their child as an interesting, likeable person who can be enjoyed. In being enjoyed the child becomes aware that he is loved. In being loved he can return love. In loving he learns to live a rich and rewarding life.

Therapy for the child's language deficits should be provided by professionals outside of the home. The parents should not be involved with therapeutic and teaching procedures. Parents' direct attempts to teach their own children to talk, read, write, and/or compute are seldom satisfactory, and, if effective, are too costly in emotional flareups. According to Ginott (1967) direct help from parents may only convey to the child that on his own he is helpless. Homework assigned by the school or the clinic should be strictly the responsibility of the child and his teachers. Parents should not supervise or check the homework unless the child asks them to do so. For a parent to criticize or correct a child for his poor speech, reading, writing, or school marks is tantamount to conditional love. A child interprets such criticism and correction as the withholding of parental love until certain standards are achieved. This is certain to engender hostility and feelings of insecurity.

Are parents, then, incapable of extending help to their child with language and/or learning disabilities? Actually the parents are the first and basic source of help, but their assistance must be extended indirectly and skillfully. To ignore or to deny that the child has a problem is to reject the child. To tell him that he is a poor speaker who cannot be understood, or a nonreader who will not be able to progress in school until he learns to read, is to convince him that he is stupid, a feeling that he probably harbors about himself anyway. He is likely to give up his efforts to learn, feeling that if he does not try he can avoid failure. To praise the child for an improvement in language skill is often a signal for him to cease his efforts to learn, to disprove the parents' praise, since he is well aware that his achievement is far below that of those he would like to emulate. Parents should not teach; they should not ignore; they should not criticize; they should not praise.

What then *should* parents do to assist their language-impaired child? Perhaps the most desirable thing to do is to mirror the child's feelings about himself (Ginott, 1967). In such mirroring they can prepare the child for the clinical teaching or therapy which the parents themselves cannot do but which they can seek for their language-disabled child. This mirroring should be done without fault-finding and without compliments; but with unemotional understanding and objective reflection of the child's feelings, such as

I know it makes you feel bad when people don't understand what you say.

No wonder you refused to play, when the rules are so hard for you to understand.

It must be embarrassing to be laughed at because you cannot read like the others.

I'll bet you wanted to tear this report card up. You worried so about bringing it home.

If you'd like to have some help we will find a special teacher who can teach you all by yourself before or after school. It may be hard work for you, like our work is for us, but if it helps you will not mind doing it. Let us know if you want the special help.

The child knows he is loved by parents who clearly understand his feelings, and who refrain from upbraiding him for his shortcomings. Furthermore, these loving parents have provided him with an opportunity for self-initiating an improvement program. The child can now make the first move toward assuming responsibility for his own learning. Without rejection or criticism he has been treated as an individual, who may now choose an acceptable solution for his problems. Parents who are capable of such behavior have progressed into the desirable stage of objectivity where mutual affection and respect are possible between parents and child, and where the child may profit from clinical teaching.

Some children may resist proffered clinical help, in which case parents should not become insistent, but should adopt a lenient attitude of noninterference, always leaving the door open for the child to try the help of a clinical teacher. After remedial procedures have been tried for a reasonable length of time, the child should be the judge as to whether the supplementary individual work has resulted in improvement. The burden of proof as to the effectiveness of therapy should be entirely upon the school, the clinician, and the child. The home can then remain a place of warm security and affection—a place where the child may always go for recharging of inner strength to face life's unavoidable failures.

It should be clearly understood that parental attitudes of leniency and laissez-faire toward the child's behavior apply only to those activities for which the school and the clinical teachers are responsible. Parents have an obligation to set and enforce limits, not upon the child's thoughts, feelings, or speech, but upon any act which may result in harm to self, harm to others, or violation of property rights. In the setting and enforcing of appropriate limits parents should convey authority while preserving their own and the child's dignity and self-esteem. This requires skill, insight, and self-control; but this is part of the difficult role of parenthood. If played competently and consistently parents will have no time to be concerned with home tutoring and the affairs of the school.

All children need a clear understanding of acceptable and unacceptable behavior. They feel secure only when they know the limits within which they may operate, and beyond which the parents who love them will not permit them to go. Parents of all children usually can profit from counseling as to what to limit and how to set and enforce limits, but for parents of language-handicapped children such counseling is imperative. In their eagerness to help the child compensate for language deficits, parents try to discipline for good manners, in the hope that through politeness their child may gain peer friendships and the approval of society in general. Parents of a child who is delayed in the development of speech often mistakenly insist that he try to say "I'm sorry," "please," "thank you," and "good-bye" before he can produce a simple structured utterance to influence his environment for practical needs. Nothing could be more frustrating or meaningless to the child. Children learn politeness and good manners from the desire to imitate parents who are themselves polite. Matters of courtesy should be in the realm of parental behavior not discipline. Parental discipline is the process whereby the child learns right from wrong, and eventually, with maturity, is able to impose self-restraints upon himself.

The following is a dependable sequence for parents to follow in conveying affection through discipline.

1. Restrict only that behavior which meets one or more of the following criteria: (a) hurts self, (b) hurts others, or (c) violates property, including those things which are forbidden by law, ethics, or social acceptability. Such acts should be unequivocally forbidden. Behavior which does not fall into one or more of these three zones, however, should be sanctioned or, at least, tolerated. When parents are instructed to keep a record of the number of times they start to limit their children but refrain from doing so because the behavior does not meet any one of the three criteria, and can therefore be tolerated if not sanctioned, they begin to realize how much of their relationship with their child is

taken up in unnecessary criticism and nagging. With this realization comes the first step toward a relationship in which parents can enjoy their children.

2. Parents should present a united front in the setting of limits. It is fortunate for children that parents come in pairs, for much of the child's personality development will depend upon his awareness that he has two parents, each of whom fulfills different needs for him, but both of whom are equally involved in loving and protecting him.

First, the child will become attached emotionally to the parent of the opposite sex, and feel resentment and jealousy toward the other parent. In the acting out of this love triangle, however, the preschool child discovers that happiness comes from identifying with the parent of the same sex. With this discovery the child moves into the next important stage of his psychosocial development—the period of identification when the little boy becomes aware of his maleness, that he is like Daddy, and the little girl of her femaleness, that she is like Mother. With awareness and appreciation of his or her own sex, the ground is laid for the important peer status that must emerge by the time the child starts school: "I am a boy and I like all boys; we boys must stick together," and vice versa for girls.

Unfortunately for the boy with language disorders, his father seldom interrelates enough with his son for the crucial identification to take place. Because the boy cannot communicate adequately his father often shys away, leaving the field entirely to the mother, as though the child were physically ill and in need of nursing. Thus both father and son miss out on much joy and satisfaction. Often the only self-pride which a language-disabled boy can claim is in his masculinity. After all he is a *boy*, and that is *something*! Mothers cannot provide this pride for their sons; it comes only from identification with the father or a father figure.

Parents who are in the stage of guilt tend to incriminate one another by "passing the buck" one to the other for setting limits. This leaves the child with feelings of ambivalence, and with no criterion for making decisions. Out of the child's presence, both parents should agree upon or come to a compromise as to what is to be limited. Then the limit may be set by either parent who firmly states, "We have decided that . . . " or "We cannot permit . . . ." This gives the child a secure feeling that both parents love him and will protect him from wrongdoing.

3. The child must clearly understand the limit. This presents a momentous problem to children with language disorders. Their poor retention and recall of auditory stimuli and their misunderstanding of much that they hear make it inordinately difficult for them to honor limits which are set verbally. Consequently they soon get the undeserved reputation of misbehavers and "nonminders." As time progresses, they find it rewarding to live up to this reputation, for with it comes at least some recognition. "Do you understand?" "Didn't we tell you . . . ?" "Can't you remember?" "Don't forget!" and "I'll tell you one more time!" are futile expressions of parental frustration. It is important that all who work with language-impaired children set limits in a manner (a) to ensure that the child comprehends what is expected of him, and (b) to provide some reinforcement for recall. The following procedures are usually effective in setting limits:

(a) Speak briefly, in simple syntax.

(b) Give only one instruction at a time.

(c) Blandly ask the child to repeat what has been said to him before attempting to respond. This "reauditorization" (Johnson and Myklebust, 1967) of instructions serves several useful purposes. It lets the authority figure know whether or not the child has understood what has been said. It also provides the child with reinforcements from sensory feedback which may serve him well in organizing and recalling.

(d) If possible give the child some visual reinforcement, such as a picture or a diagram to carry with him as a reminder. Language-impaired as well as presumed-to-be-normal persons profit from visual stimulation, not so much because they are more visile than audile, but because the visual stimulus is permanent and can be referred to indefinitely, while the auditory stimulus is fleeting.

4. Give the child some leeway within the boundaries of the limit. By recognizing the urges which prompt children to defy limits, by giving them the privilege without punishment of freely expressing their resentment of limits, and by pointing out acceptable alternatives without bribing or withdrawing the limits, children may be led to voluntary acceptance of the need to discipline themselves. This is the first step toward developing inner standards for self-regulation.

5. Expect the child to honor the limit. If it is a fair limit, if both parents have presented a united front, if the child understands what is expected of him, and if he has not been handled with high-handed arbitrariness, most children will honor the limit; all children should be extended the courtesy of expecting them to do so. Many parents convey doubt and suspicion in their very tone of voice, as though in spite of everything, the child, being the ornery person that he is, will surely not conform. This leaves the child no choice but to live up to his parents' expectations.

Even though the parents have exerted all patience, common sense, and goodwill in the setting of limits, there will be times when the child will transgress a clearly stated and understood restriction. Many parents in the stage of martyrdom make no attempt to enforce the limit, but accept the child's transgression as a part of his disability. Nothing could be more unjust to the child. The parents should not relinquish the role of the loving but steadfast authority figures who set limits and who intend to enforce them. When enforcing limits all discussion, argumentation, explanation, and verbal defending of position by parents are out of order. The parent now moves in to enforce firmly, unemotionally, and physically if necessary. The young child who will not leave the playground can be led or carried away. The older child who has not returned from his bicycle ride can be hunted by his parents, or by a policeman called by the parents, and escorted home.

When parents consistently enforce appropriate limits which they have set it conveys to the child the parents' deep and abiding affection. It is as though the parents have said, "We know that you may not always be strong enough to limit yourself, but we are here to keep you from going too far. You have nothing to fear, for we love you and will keep you safe from wrongdoing." Although the child with language disabilities may not understand such spoken words, the setting and enforcing of limits can convey the message nonverbally, and the child may grow into a self-regulating individual. It requires self-discipline for the language-impaired child to be able to accept and profit from the rigorous clinical teaching which he must have, in addition to his regular classroom participation, if he is to be socially competent.

Acceptance, the Need for Group Status

Growing out of the child's need for love and affection is his need to belong first to his parents and family, and later to a gang and his peer-age group in school. Only if his needs to belong are met can he finally become a contributing member of that larger social group—a community. As noted by Kaplan (1959):

> Status in a group gives a child assurance that he is an acceptable being. He gains personal strength from being wanted by others, from identifying with others, and from being a part of something larger than himself. Without the companionship of other people he becomes lonely, loses self-confidence, and begins to question his own adequacy.

And it is precisely these feelings of loneliness, inadequacy, and lack of self-confidence that become incorporated in the personality structure of most school-aged children with language disabilities, and that prevent their developing emotional security.

With alacrity to provide special classes for academically underachieving children with language disorders, schools unintentionally, but nonetheless certainly, deny satisfactory group status to these children.[1] By the creation of special classes in which all members are low in language abilities, the school limits each member's choice of friends and close companions, for children choose their associates from among their classmates. Nor can the socially stigmatizing practice of homogeneous grouping of disabled pupils be justified by providing certain periods during the day when members of the "special class" are permitted to participate with members of the "regular class." Such procedures but call attention to the "special" child's alienage, and preclude his forming close friendships with those children who could exert the most beneficial and corrective influence upon him. All parents with perspective would concur with Ginott (1967, p. 88) that "a child needs opportunities to associate with personalities different from, and complementary to, his own." Just as a withdrawn child needs the frequent company of outgoing friends, so the child who is low in language abilities needs close daily association with age peers who are facile in language. Furthermore, such friendships can be mutually beneficial. For example, children who are normal or precocious in language skills, and who rely heavily on imagination, fantasy, and excitement, can benefit greatly from close association and friendship with children below normal in language facility, who almost invariably are prosaic, unimaginative, and matter-of-fact.

[1] The writer is well aware that this opinion may run counter to that of the majority of the special education community. Being the chairman of a department of special education in a state university, and having investigated this matter in depth, however, she feels constrained to speak out on this policy.

Table 1. Description of Experimental and Control Subjects at Beginning of Study

Experimental subjects: Each subject in regular public school class receiving individual instruction after school		Control subjects: Each subject in a special education class for pupils with minimal neuro- logical impairment	
N = 48 (36 males, 12 females)		N = 50 (39 males, 11 females)	
Mean C.A.[a]	9.61 yr	Mean C.A.[a]	9.92 yr
Mean ed. age	8.00 yr	Mean ed. age	8.14 yr
Mean ed. grade	2.90	Mean ed. grade	3.04

Mean scholastic achievement
   test average
	24.57	Mean scholastic achievement
		   test average
			26.50

Mean IQ WISC full scale	93.72	Mean IQ WISC full scale	92.84
Mean learning rate	0.83	Mean learning rate	0.82

[a]Chronological age.

This writer can find no study in the literature which supports the advantage derived from isolating a learner or group of learners from the mainstream of normal environment. There are numerous studies negating advantage to be gained from isolation or self-contained grouping (Bruner et al., 1967; Goldstein, et al. 1965; Meyerowitz, 1967; Zedler, 1968a). More than a decade ago, Brosin (1957) showed that brain function in normal adult college students is affected by social interaction. When the students were isolated in cubicles away from normal social interaction, with physical stimulation kept at a low level, their intellect deteriorated as well as their problem-solving abilities and their powers of concentration.

Educators who would assign language-disabled pupils to classes composed of children with similar disabilities, in special rooms—many of which are equipped with isolation cubicles presumed to improve powers of concentration—would do well to search the literature for controlled research studies supporting such practices. In so far as this writer has found, the studies reporting favorably on the use of isolation, reduced stimulatory techniques, and homogeneous grouping (Strauss and Lehtinen 1947; Cruickshank et al., 1961) did not measure gain made by the experimental subjects against that made by control subjects with the same disabilities who remained in the socially stimulating mainstream of regular education and received supportive but not isolative treatment.

A 2-year study was conducted at Southwest Texas State University (Zedler, 1968a) to test the relative efficacy of teaching scholastically underachieving, language-disabled children with medically diagnosed neurological impairment (1) in regular, heterogeneously grouped classes, supplemented by clinical teaching after school, or (2) in homogeneously grouped special education classes. A description of the experimental and control populations at the beginning of the study is shown in Table 1.

The stated purpose (Texas Education Agency, 1965) of the special education classes from which the control subjects were selected was twofold and as follows:

(1) to provide appropriate school placement for children who give evidence of being unable to adjust to or profit from a regular school program, and

(2) to provide an instructional program in an educational setting that will meet the needs of such children by assisting them to function educationally and emotionally in such a way that they will be prepared to return to the regular school program.

To those who proposed the controlled study, two implications within the stated purpose of the special, homogeneously grouped classes seemed vulnerable to challenge. First was the implication that such children could not profit from a regular school program, and therefore, for their own welfare, needed to be removed from the regular class of their peers. Second was the implication that the curricula offered in the special education classes prepared the children to return to the regular school program.

This study (Zedler, 1968a) proposed to test the first implication by investigating whether or not such children could make more academic and intellective progress by remaining in the regular classroom and receiving supplementary teaching after school, than by being removed from the regular classroom and assigned to special education classes. Results of the investigation, shown in Fig. 1, strongly supported the hypothesis

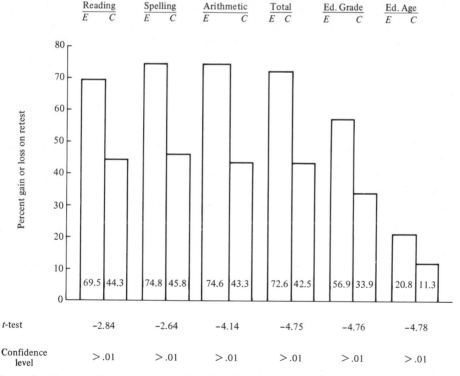

Figure 1. Comparative gain on academic achievement test for experimental (*E*) and control (*C*) groups.

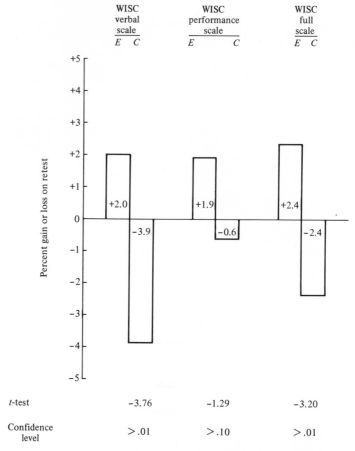

	WISC verbal scale		WISC performance scale		WISC full scale	
	E	C	E	C	E	C

Figure 2. Comparative gain on intelligence scale (Wechsler, 1949) for experimental (*E*) and control (*C*) groups.

that the experimental subjects, who were not removed from the intellectually stimulating and highly varied social interaction of the regular classroom, made significantly greater improvement in academic achievement than the control subjects, who were in special classes. Furthermore, as shown in Fig. 2, the experimental subjects gained while the control subjects deteriorated in intellective functioning. Results of this study would seem to support Orton's (1937) observation that children with language disabilities who do not learn concepts of their environment deteriorate mentally because of deprivation of information. The information which such children need to prevent intellective deterioration seems to be available in regular rather than special classes.

The second implication, that self-contained special education classes would prepare children to return to the regular school program, was tested by ancillary data accumulated 6 months after termination of the 2-year study. Data are shown in Table 2. After 2½ years in the special education program, only 16 percent of the control group of pupils had been returned to regular classrooms. This percentage is much too low to support the

Table 2. School Placement of Experimental and Control Subjects at the Beginning, and 6 Months after Termination, of the Study

	Experimental (%)		Control (%)	
	1964	1967	1964	1967
Special education unit (MBI)	0	10	100	82
Regular classroom	100	88	0	16
Lost	0	2	0	2
Total	100	100	100	100

second stated purpose of the special classes: to prepare children to return to the regular program.

There are strong and unsavory implications that, under the guise of attempting to "meet the needs" of scholastically underachieving, language-disabled pupils by removing them from interaction with normal peers in regular classrooms, the school may be (1) avoiding an appraisal of the internal structure of its regular curriculum and teaching procedures, and (2) creating a category of deficiency which must perpetuate itself by a search for, and a clinging to, customers. Once a special education unit has been established in a school system a minimum number of handicapped pupils must be maintained, according to formula (Texas Education Agency, 1965), for the school to receive the state funds provided by statute for such classes.[2] It is shocking but true that in some school systems under the unit formula problem pupils may be referred out of regular classes in response to edicts from administrative quarters to refer additional pupils for special education because numbers are needed to maintain state support for the unit. Fortunately new legislation is moving to change this procedure (Texas Education Agency, 1970).

In the Southwest Texas study (Zedler, 1968a), there were intangible factors which could not be measured for statistical significance which favored regular classroom enrollment, even though it had to be supplemented by clinical teaching after school. Unbiased, trained social workers interviewed the parents and children in the experimental and control groups of the study. Parents and children were questioned as to whether or no they considered their respective educational programs for the 2 years of the study as beneficial (helpful) and socially rewarding (fun), or unsuccessful (not helpful) and stigmatizing (bad). Table 3 shows in percentages the results of these interviews. The group status provided by being a participating member of a regular rather than a "special" school class was so rewarding and ego-strengthening for most of the children and their parents in the experimental group that it offset the extra time which had to be spent after school in study with the clinical teacher.

[2] Under Senate Bill 230 (Texas Education Agency, 1970) by September 1976 the formula for financing special education programs in Texas will be based on the local school districts' total average daily attendance for the preceding year, rather than upon the numbers of handicapped pupils identified by type of disability (T.E.A. 1970, p. 29).

Table 3. Parents' (*P*) and Children's (*Ch*) Opinions of Educational Programs

	Experimental (%)		Control (%)	
	P	Ch	P	Ch
Positive	86	84	64	34
Negative	4	10	34	30
Ambivalent	10	6	2	36
Total	100	100	100	100

The evidence is strong that if schools are to help children develop the social livin; skills which are necessary to succeed in society, all children with normal intelligence mus be accepted and wanted within their normal age group. Referral to a "special class" i tantamount to being unwanted and rejected by the group to which the child needs t belong. When a child reaches school age his greatest psychosocial need is to be accepter by the gang as "normal." Members of special education classes are not gang members; o the contrary, they are likely to be objects of the gang's derision. As Dunn (1968) point out, we cannot ignore the evidence that removing a child "from regular grades for specia education probably contributes significantly to his feelings of inferiority and problems o acceptance."

Skillful classroom teachers were integrating children with language disabilities int normal, regular classrooms long before the public or school administrators were aware o special education. Clinical teachers and language therapists are successfully using pro cedures with language-disabled children which might be equally beneficial and at least no detrimental to pupils with adequate language skills. There is need for a meeting of minds as well as methods, between regular classroom teachers and clinicians to stem the epidemic of referrals of children out of the mainstream of education into group-statu; oblivion.

Approval, the Need for Self-Development

One of the strongest fundamental forces which motivates man's behavior is the need to be independent and self-sufficient. But equally strong is his need for the people he holds dear to approve of his efforts to establish his own adequacy. This need is most difficult to fulfill for the child with a language disability, because man's social adequacy is so closely tied to his ability to influence his environment through use of the language code.

Kaplan (1959, p. 231) maintains that "at each stage of life, as the growing organism gains awareness of his potentialities and capacities, there arises a compelling urge to test and use these powers." Those who study the developing child observe the sense of personal worth he derives from doing things for himself. He initiates activities to test his newly discovered power to direct himself and at the same time to influence and maneuver his environment. In no form of behavior is this more evident than in recently acquired speech of the young child. The baby who commands "Go! No! Mine! Gimme! I do!" effuses feelings of personal power. And when his listening subjects obey his orders with approval the baby commander is on his way toward developing his own adequacy. He seems to go through a stage of verbal megalomania in which he takes issue with all around him, declaring his unshakable feeling that his word is supreme—"no!" to every *yes*, and "mine" to all property. When authority figures must intervene to enforce appropriate limits upon his *no*'s and *mine*'s no defeated general in a field of battle is more crest-fallen and desolate than the child, until he rallies his verbal powers and discovers that within certain limits he is again master of his environment.

Most children move rapidly to expand their linguistic competence by learning to derive meaning from utterances of others, and to express their own intended meanings. Menyuk (1968) theorizes that as the child acquires the grammar of his language he detects and recognizes abstract features in the language he hears, and stores them in memory as linguistic data for future use. With maturity he rejects, adds to, refines, and elaborates his linguistic data until, by the age of 2, he is relatively competent, and by 4 years he has acquired expertise as a speaker-listener.

We are concerned, however, with the children who, as speaker-listeners, are so markedly deviant in basic capacities underlying the acquisition of language that they are unable to experience the feeling of power and self-worth which comes from manipulating others through speech. Some of them, those who are lowest on the distributional curve of language abilities, may be so lacking in linguistic competence that they will not try to interact verbally, but satisfy their needs for self-development by asocial behavior, as though they had no need for their fellow men.

A much larger group of children, although they are below the norm in language ability, have, as Tikofsky (1968) points out, the competence to generate language but are lacking at the performance level. These are the children who try to communicate verbally, but whose performance is ineffective. Because of their poor performance they do not receive the social approval which is necessary if their self-initiated and self-directed behavior is to result in feelings of personal worth and adequacy. These are the sad, defeated children who have tried and failed, in whom the desire to talk is present but inhibited as protection against further failure and social disapproval.

If the child's language deficits could be discovered and appraised, and corrective measures initiated before the age of 3, many failures in self-development might be circumvented. Whether the child's deficit is at the competence or performance level, it is the responsibility of professionals in speech and language pathology to meet the language-disabled child's need for approval of self-initiated attempts to communicate. Only the highly competent pathologist and clinician can be expected to assume this responsibility. As Menyuk (1968) and Tikofsky (1968) assert, those who seek to modify linguistic behavior must actively incorporate in therapy the descriptions and theories developed by linguists, psychologists, and physcholinguists. The clinician must understand not only the structure of the language on the phonologic, semantic, and syntactic levels, but also the developmental course of a child's acquisition of language.

Many practicing speech therapists attack the awesome task of treating children who have not acquired speech, or who are delayed in the development of speech, without being able to evaluate the child's total linguistic system to ascertain the extent of his competence or the level of his performance. Many failures in therapy with such children must be attributed to professional ineptness. Speech pathologists should take a complete look at the child's linguistic environment to determine where, how, and if he deviates from his norm. It has been well demonstrated that a child who is acquiring language understands and produces utterances at his level of competence, and that syntax influences the child's ability to recall what has been said to him.

Those who would assist a child in the acquisition of language frequently sabotage the process by withholding approval of the child's futile but independent attempts to use the linguistic code. Such ineptness on the part of well-meaning but misguided adults may be observed in their dealings with language-disabled children at all levels and in all modalities of language. Parents and less than competent therapists often concern themselves with trying to correct vocabulary and phoneme production, instead of rewarding with approval any attempt which the child makes to communicate. Teachers of reading erroneously expound that unless the child learns to read rapidly, silently, and accurately the doors of knowledge will never open to him, instead of providing the poor or nonreader with someone who will read aloud to him so that he will not be deprived of information to be gained from reading. Teachers of written spelling usually award grademarks on an all-or-nothing basis of exact spellings rather than on a continuum, such as

1. No credit if no attempt has been made to write the word.
2. Minimal credit if the word has been attempted but irrelevantly spelled.
3. More than minimal credit if the spelling is partially correct.
4. Still more credit if the word is "phonetically" spelled.
5. Maximal credit for correct spelling.

Teachers of written composition too often stifle ideas, which might find their way into words, by penalizing the writer for errors in the mechanics of spelling and grammar, and withholding approval for expression of thoughts.

A highly promising technique has evolved at Southwest Texas State University for initiating the development of speech in young children who hear but who have shown no signs of acquiring language, and for stimulating further development of the language process in those who are slow in acquiring functional speech. The therapeutic procedure is termed "imitation therapy." It is based upon the premise that if the child has the potentiality for learning language it can be developed (1) if he becomes aware of his independent, self-sufficient power, (2) if he has opportunities to test his many capacities for manipulating others, and (3) if he is aware that the adults in his environment are noting his manipulations approvingly.

In imitation therapy there are four distinct stages each of which may last a few days or several weeks. Although these stages develop in sequence, the clinician may return to an earlier stage in therapy any time the child evidences anxiety or insecurity. In the first stage the clinician is the only imitator, and is at the complete command of the child so long as the activity is not injurious to person or property. In the second stage the clinician is the major imitator, and the child is a part-time imitator for brief periods. In the third stage the clinician is again the only imitator, but is at the child's command only for behavior involving phonation or movements of the face and speech organs. In the fourth stage the clinician and the child reciprocate imitations of any behavior involving voice, face, or mouth.

The results of experimentation with this procedure indicate that only after the child has progressed through the following sequence of experiencing approval is he ready to participate in direct language therapy. He must experience approval (1) for being the leader in self-initiated—at first relatively unlimited but later limited—activities, and (2) for being the follower—first in gross activities and later in activities involving phonation but not speech. While the child is in imitation therapy he becomes aware of his potentialities and capacities for influencing others appropriately. He has the opportunity to give vent to his compelling urge to test those powers. While he is testing he is supported by approval and encouragement from those who are being manipulated.

A brief description of the four sequential stages in imitation therapy as it was developed at Southwest Texas State University is offered here as a guide for professional speech and language pathologists who would experiment further with the process. All therapy takes place in a small clinical room with one mirrored wall, two chairs, a table, and several pairs of matched toys or easily manipulated objects.

In the first stage of therapy the clinician imitates everything that the child does, as long as it does not damage property or harm the child or the clinician. No sound is made unless the child makes it, in which case the clinician makes the same sound in the same manner as the child has made it. The clinician makes no move except in imitation of a move the child has made. No activity of the child escapes the alert clinician, who immediately "follows the leader." When the child touches or manipulates one of the paired toys or objects, the clinician imitates the activity with its mate. Often the child will commandeer both of a pair of toys, thus making his first probing test of power. In which case the clinician retrieves one of the pair with no show of authority but with precise imitation of the child's movements, sounds, and facial expression. It has been surprising to the experimenters that the child does not react negatively but seems to delight in this reciprocal, grabbing exchange of paired objects. Observers seem to accelerate rather than deter the child's progress in this first stage of therapy. Occasionally the child welcomes participation of observers as imitators, and will encourage others to involve themselves as followers of his command. He soon abandons leadership of the group, however, and devotes himself to manipulating only the clinician.

A sign that progress is being made in this stage of therapy occurs when the child changes an activity and watches to see that the clinician makes the same change. The mirrored wall assists both the imitator and the imitated in keeping check on each other. It is a sign of additional progress when the child uses the mirror to watch himself and the obedient clinician.

When the child becomes fully aware of his potency as a commander it is not unusual for him to become exultant, unwilling to release the imitator for a moment of rest or to terminate the session. He moves frantically from one activity into another. He eagerly devises new and more complicated activities for his exhausted but still approving imitator. The child is permitted several sessions of such megalomanic sprees before he is enticed into the second period of therapy, where cautious limitations are imposed upon his command.

In the second stage of therapy the clinician sits in front of the mirror and motions for the child to sit in a chair which also faces the mirror. If the child complies he is rewarded by the clinician's imitation of any activity the child performs while seated. If the child does not comply by sitting the clinician initiates some other simple activity such as hand clapping, head patting, or nose touching, clearly demonstrating that it is the child who is to be the imitator of this act. If the child complies by imitating any activity, the clinician again becomes the follower and the child is permitted to assume the command. Excessive indulgence to the point of frenzy is not permitted in this stage, however. When the child-commander begins to "carouse," the clinician sits in front of the mirror and refuses to be manipulated.

The mirror is extremely important in all stages of imitation therapy as a source of visual feedback for matching performances. One of the implications from this procedure has been the value of parallel viewing in a mirror rather than reciprocal viewing across a table. Parallel viewing seems to reinforce the self-monitoring or feedback process by which behavior is scanned, compared, and corrected to match or approximate a standard pattern (Van Riper and Irwin, 1958). The goal of this second period in the sequence of therapy is to impose minimal self-control upon the child's self-initiated activities by encouraging him to explore the imitating process briefly as a follower.

In the third stage of imitation therapy the child is again permitted to take full command as the leader, but only in behavior involving phonation, or activity of the head, face, or speech organs. The clinician sits in front of the mirror during this period, faithfully imitating all the child's posturings and expressions of head, face, and mouth, and accurately reproducing any sound the child makes with his mouth or throat (with the exception of negative emotional sounds such as weeping and screaming). The clinician blandly ignores all other activities of the child.

In this third stage the child is encouraged to come into close physical contact with the mirror—to blow on it, and to touch the precipitation with his tongue. Often the first voluntary manipulative phonations made by the child are produced against the mirror. This suggests that the child may receive rewarding reinforced auditory and tactile feedback from the cold, wet, resounding glass.

When the child is aware that the clinician is again the imitator and he the initiator he usually shows great versatility with face and voice. It is not unusual in this stage for the child to touch the clinician's face and mouth, often exploring her teeth, lips, and tongue with his own fingers. The clinician accepts these oral explorations without touching the child's mouth. Often following his exploration of the clinician's mouth, the child will explore his own mouth manually in front of the mirror. If this occurs, the clinician imitates by exploring her own mouth, with face close to the child's in front of the mirror. This usually leads to the making of "funny faces" with accompanying oral sounds. The clinician is careful to consistently associate a specific sound with a particular facial posture.

The goal of the third stage of imitation therapy is to limit the range of the child's self-initiated, manipulative activities to acts closely related to speech, thus focusing attention upon the mouth and voice as potent organs for exerting approved influence over others.

In the fourth and last stage of the imitation therapy process, the clinician initiates facial expressions and oral sounds, taking care to avoid all phonemes or phonations with which the child may have had unpleasant experiences associated with "trying to get him to talk." The child is given an opportunity to imitate the clinician, but no pressure is placed upon him to do so. If the child makes no attempt to imitate the oral sounds, the clinician explores simpler, more primitive activities such as sticking out the tongue, an act in which the child usually delights. Growling, hostile, animal-like sounds are often effective for encouraging imitation by the child. The imitating child will usually repeat the sound, adopting it as though he had originated it and the clinician were the imitator. In this way the child is enticed into imitating nonsense, oral sounds produced by the clinician. As soon as possible the clinician associates each sound with a particular toy or activity, to establish the sound as a signal. This introduces the child to a code. If the imitation therapy has been successful the child is now ready to initiate communicative sounds.

Care must be taken at each stage of therapy to maintain the child's confidence in his own capacity for effective, self-directed, independent action which meets the approval of adults in his environment. Without criticism or correction the language-disabled child thus gains the stamina and inner strength which he must have if he is to undergo the critical corrective rigors of direct clinical teaching, which will be necessary if he is to take his place as an effective, productive member of society. He may always be lower in all language abilities than the majority of his age peers, but he can still be a participating member of his "normal" social group.

GLANCES INTO THE SOCIAL DEVELOPMENT OF ONE LANGUAGE-DISABLED CHILD

The opinions expressed in this chapter were formed by the writer during 15 years of general association with and observation of language-disabled children in a university clinic, and during 7 years of close daily association in a longitudinal study of one child. This child was a boy who had acquired no functional language until he was 5 years old. By the age of 12 years he was still unable to read, write, or compute. The following vignettes, taken from the extensive records kept on The Boy (Davis, 1962), are recounted here as illustrations from the vast evidence which formed a basis for the writer's ideas regarding social management of language-disabled children.[3]

At the age of 5 in a kindergarten his speech was relatively unintelligible jargon. During his sixth and seventh years, both of which were spent in the first grade of a public school, his oral language developed deviantly, with numerous errors in phonology, semantics, and syntax. There is no evidence that the orthodox phoneme-and-vocabulary-centered articulation therapy which he received during those 2 years in the first grade of a public school took into account The Boy's total linguistic system, his competence in generating grammar, or the degree to which his verbal performance deviated from the norm. That he was unable to learn to read or write with age peers was not considered to

[3]Information recounted here is factual except that precautions have been taken to guard the child's identity. He is now achieving average success in his second year in the technical institute of a junior college.

be a responsibility of major concern to the speech therapist. After 4 years of traditional speech therapy, he produced all phonemes correctly in most words, but his cluttered speech was often unintelligible. He omitted unstressed syllables in utterances. That he did not understand much of what was said to him went undetected, since tests of his auditory acuity were negative.

After repeating the first grade he was able to read only four words—*stop* and *go*, which he had learned from traffic signals, his own first name but not his last, and the word *the*. He explained in later years that he had learned to read *the* in dire extremity to be sure that his book was not upside down. "It's 'barrassing for somebody to walk up and say 'Ha, your book's upside down!' How did I know, 'cause I didn't often find *stop* or *go* and I never did find . . . (his first name); but look how often you find *the* and see how crazy it looks upside down!"

When he was 8 years old he was medically diagnosed as having "motor and sensory aphasia." At a loss to know whether or how to deal with him, the school placed him in a special education class for mentally retarded pupils where he remained for 5 years. At the close of these 7 unproductive years in school he could read only the same four words, and he could do no spontaneous writing.

When he was 12 years old, at the suggestion of his physician and with the consent of his parents, he volunteered to serve as an experimental subject for those of us who were trying to formulate methods whereby language-disabled children with normal intelligence could be taught with normal age peers in the framework of regular classrooms. His participation in this pilot study required that he spend from 3 to 5 hours each day after school in individual work with a clinical teacher. This was a risk we took in the face of admonitions from psychologists that The Boy "could not profit from the average classroom . . . " and should have "all pressure removed" as far as school work was concerned. At the end of 18 months in this highly "pressurized" program he had made up 6 legitimate grade levels and was achieving with the slow learners in a regular sixth grade. From then until his graduation from high school he was able to maintain a C average. He never complained about having to pay the price of long after-school hours with a clinical teacher in return for that most desirable of all labels—"Normalcy."

It is better to read The Boy's story in his own words. The following essay was composed by him to fulfill an English assignment in the eighth grade to write his "autobiography, including early life, family, early school days, junior high school days, interests, hobbies, plans for future life, and ideals, with a special paragraph devoted to a self analysis as to 'the type of person you think you are.' " He accomplished the assignment—as he did all others when permitted to do them as homework—by first recording it orally, then writing it from the recording paying no attention to inevitable misspellings, and finally correcting all misspelled words. The assignment required about 9 hours of work. The product was as follows:

I'M DIFFERENT[4]

Of course everyone is different from every one else. But most people are enough alike for their families to know what to expect of them. But my

---

[4] His chronicle of family history has been omitted to respect privacy.

family had some surprises in store for them when I came along. Until July, 1960 the surprises had not been happy ones. By that time my family no longer expected me to be able to do what other children my age could do. But something wonderful began to happen to me when I was twelve and a half years old, and it is still happening. The surprises about me are now happy ones. I'm beginning to get used to the idea that I can do what other fellows can do, but I don't think my family is over the shock yet.

I couldn't talk until I was five years old. I didn't learn to read until I was twelve. But I have gone to church all my life. I said prayers in my heart when I couldn't say them with my tongue. My prayers were always that some day I could learn to read. My prayer has been answered.

My early school days were sad surprises for my parents. I couldn't learn in the first grade, even though I tried it for two years. I could learn anything that didn't include words. Although I could hear I couldn't understand what people said. It was like they were talking into a microphone but the wires were dead. My teachers thought I wasn't paying attention. I tried but it didn't do any good.

I pretended to read. If my book didn't have any pictures in it I sometimes held it upside down. I had the same primer for four years. Finally my teachers gave up and I was sent to a room for mentally retarded pupils. I stayed there five long years.

My friends were children in regular classrooms. I tried to keep them from knowing I couldn't read. I had only one friend who knew my secret. He was _____ and he is still my friend. My other dear friend was a white-tail deer that I raised from a fawn. She is still my friend. She brought her twin fawns up to the ranch house to show me.

Neither my parents nor I could believe I was stupid. In July 1960 my doctor sent me to the speech clinic at the college in San Marcos.

By studying five hours a day with a language therapist I have been able to pass the sixth and seventh grades in San Marcos. I live in the home of one of the college professors. I visit my family in _____ on holidays. I miss them, but it is worth it. I am not stupid! I can learn! At last I've been able to give my parents a good surprise! Now their second son is not much different from other eighth grade boys.

I have joined the Teen Club. I found out I like to dance.

All the subjects in eighth grade are hard for me, because I still read and write very slowly. My favorite subject is any one in which I have improved.

So many wonderful things have happened to me in the last three years that I haven't been able to catch up with my new self. On the day I learned to read a sentence I felt reborn. That makes the new me about three years old.

Three-year-olds are not supposed to know what type they are. I only know that I am thankful to God for answering my prayers.

I have no plans for traveling except to see my family in _____ . The place I would most like to go is to High School.

My hobbies are nature study and swimming. I learned to talk to animals when I couldn't understand words. Nature's language needs no words. When my wild white-tail deer let me pet her fawns I knew my hobby was a success.

My plans for the future are indefinite. My parents will share the ranch with me. I do not know yet if I can be a good rancher. I hope I can be as good a citizen as my father.

My parents are my ideals. I was different from any child they had known before. They might have given up trying to teach me, but they didn't. They taught me right from wrong. They taught me the love of God not only in church but in nature. They taught me to laugh and enjoy life.

None would dispute that The Boy's phenomenal acquisition of language and scholastic achievement were possible only because his basic needs for affection, acceptance, and approval had been met throughout his exceptional life. Furthermore, he had good insight as to how these needs had been met. He never failed to reveal this awareness in the many compositions which he wrote during his years in junior and senior high school. All his writings pertained to himself and his experiences. Subjects which he could not relate to himself were difficult for him, and he avoided them.

The following is his poignant story of his pet fawn:

WHITE TAIL

The boy was eight years old. He was sitting on the corral fence watching his father and the ranch hands work the sheep.

Ewes, bucks, and lambs were milling around in the pen. They were bleating from fear, as the men separated the bucks from the flock.

The boy jumped down to help. He wasn't any help but he thought he was. He liked it here because he thought he was doing something. There were times when he knew he was a failure because he could not read. Reading was not important on the ranch.

The boy saw brown and white spots among the sheep. Four slender legs darted under the sheep. The neck was long. Two pointed ears topped a little face shaped like a heart. It was a baby fawn. It had been caught in the roundup of sheep. One of the men grabbed the fawn and gave it to the boy. It was his very own, and he held it tight.

The boy took the fawn to the house. He found a coke bottle and filled it with milk. He fixed a nipple out of a finger of a glove. So the boy tended the fawn. The little white tail waved from side to side. He called the fawn White Tail.

They played chase through the long summer days. The peaches ripened. They were White Tail's favorite food. She ate them from the boy's hand. The boy learned to make sounds like the deer.

The boy left for a far off town to learn to read. The deer disappeared into the rolling hills of the ranch.

The boy returned on vacation. The peaches were ripe. The boy made the sound of the deer loud and clear. Down from the hills came a doe. Behind her were twin fawns. Two tiny white tails waved like flags as they ran behind White Tail.

In the interest of trying to change society's attitudes toward children with individual differences, The Boy at 13 years of age, was asked to try to recall and relate his feelings and his attempts to compensate, before he learned to read and write. The following are taken verbatim from his oral recounting[5] :

I don't like to 'member them, but I will if telling about them will help some other child who may be sitting in a mentally 'tarded room maneuvering to keep other people from knowing.

For seven years I tried to maneuver around the fact that I couldn't read, so that people wouldn't find out. Everybody else my age could read. I didn't want to be an outcast—somebody different. I tried to keep away from people that wanted me to read. I mean away from having to read things like signs, billboards, names of picture shows—just little things you see everyday.

I went to this boy's house once. He sensed I couldn't read. He said, "Read what's on the back of this soapbox." I made up silly lines, making fun of soap. I went home as soon as I could.

I'd lie if I had to. I was selling tickets once. I went to this lady's house, knocked on her door, and told her it was a raffle. She asked me to read the information on the ticket. I said, "I've been to the eye-doctor and he dilated my eyes and I can't read." She bought the ticket.

I remember when I was seven years old and in the regular first grade for the second year. The teacher wrote the Easter story on the board. It was in four units. We were 'posed to copy it. I wrote a whole page—two days—steady

[5] As he told them his anecdotes were recorded on tape, or taken in shorthand and transcribed for filing.

writing. I got down in the first unit I didn't know what I wrote but people could read it! "Where's the rest of it?" they'd say. I'd say, "I lost it." I was proud. They could read it. But I didn't know what I wrote.

His despair over being placed in a special class pervaded his recollections.

In a mentally 'tarded room you plant seeds. Weave. Play baseball with a soft ball. Make footscrapers out of bottle tops. Scrape out the cork. Nail 'em top side down on a board. Sell 'em and buy some more 'terial to weave baskets. No hope. Same 10 o'clock milk and drinks. Same book about TIP.

Mentally 'tarded rooms are OK if you can't learn. They don't work in those rooms. If you think maybe you COULD learn, but your're in school in a room that doesn't work, you feel bad—bored.

I wish something could be done to get children that can learn out of those rooms and teach them. Anybody who can learn shouldn't be in a special room. They don't even get to walk home with normal children. They get out of school at 2:30. The regular rooms get out at 3:30. When anybody asked me why I was out early, I said my teacher got sick.

Fear and self-doubt occasionally threatened but did not overwhelm him.

I couldn't make change. Sometimes I got the notion I was cheated. But I didn't say anything. I couldn't prove it.

Moods came over me. I began to think I'd have to leave home. I thought I'd never learn and wouldn't be any good in this world. So I planned to be a hobo. A hobo is a man who keeps moving from place to place. He never stays anywhere long enough for people to find out he can't read.

Before I was 12 I always thought I'd just live at home with my parents. But after I was 12 I knew they wouldn't want a grown man living in the house with them. On the night after my twelfth birthday I thought a lot about when to start being a hobo. But I never could decide to leave, 'cause I love my family.

The integrity of The Boy's personality was reflected in his belief in himself and in his hope for something better.

Was I hopeless. No. From day to day I went on, always praying to be normal. Please, God, help me to be normal like _____ (his friend).

I was hoping that I could go to a normal school and bring home books and lots of homework and lead a normal life. That's all anybody should want. I would just pray to God that I would learn to read and write and be a normal boy.

Fantasy often provided escape from his educational dilemma.

I was lucky enough to be a child who could stand pressure. But in the mentally 'tarded room there was no pressure. I'd pretend I was writing. I'd fill pages with little squiggles. That's the way other people's writing looked to me. I'd 'magine the numbers they gave me to write were complicated problems like 140, or 400 billion, or in algebra like my brother and sister had to do. In daily life I'd see problems in stores and garages, like what is the cost of a drive shaft or tires. I'd 'magine I was figuring those.

My sister had spiral notebooks tucked away to save. And every page was filled with writing and problems. I found those notebooks and I kept them hid in my room because they looked good. I'd pull them out when nobody was in there. And I'd look at them, and 'magine I wrote all of that. I couldn't really write. But I kept in my mind "I wrote these sitting at a desk in school. I wrote these." In my mind I was writing them. This was a good feeling. I liked the feeling so much that when it was the night before we was to move into our new house I was afraid the notebooks would be left behind, so I got out of bed and got the notebooks. I was in my pajamas. I went out to the car and hid the notebooks behind the seat. In our new house I put the notebooks in the closet in my room. And I'd pull them out and look at them. I still got the good feeling. It was the kind of feeling you have when you see a painting. You don't wish you made it. You know you couldn't. You just look at it because it looks pretty. My sister's high school notebooks were like pictures to me.

But the day came when The Boy kept notebooks of his own—high school notebooks. But he tells his school story much better than anyone can tell it for him. He told it in a theme assigned in tenth-grade English. He entitled the composition *Dreams* and wrote as follows:

DREAMS

The idea of moving was not a good one when I heard it. But the future could not be worse than the past.

I remember the first day I enrolled in school. The first few months it was pleasant. But things got worse. My grades were failing. It was no fun.

After school it was a different story. I was carefree and loved it. The battle of brains was over for the day. I could walk by the river, talk to my friends, and do anything that came into my mind.

Thinking about the future was a nightmare. What could a boy do that couldn't read or write? I asked myself how could I learn to read and write? I couldn't answer that question. I didn't know if anyone could.

The question was answered one day. But it meant moving away, away from my hometown, away from my friends and the places that I loved, to a town that I hadn't even heard of, to a place where I had no friends.

But all of that was changed when I enrolled in San Marcos. I learned to read and write at the college clinic. I skipped the first five grades and entered the sixth grade because I was already 12 years old. I worked long hours trying to catch up.

I had no time for homesickness until school was out in the afternoons. Then when I saw the rest of the people going home I wished that I could go with them. But I had work to do. One of my dreams had come true. I had learned to read and write. I was dreaming another dream, a dream of going to high school. I dreamed of being a member of a high school class, and included in things high school people do.

Two years later this great dream came true. My picture was in the annual among the freshmen of San Marcos High School. I was going with my Ag. class on a summer trip.

I was one year older than others in the freshman class. Some people teased me about this. But that was a small price to pay for a dream that had come true.

As we were returning from the summer Ag. trip the sponsor said he had a surprise for me. We were going back through my hometown. How proud I was! The boy who had left home a failure was returning as a success.

Before I had a chance to enjoy my new found pride it was time for my Ag. class to leave for San Marcos. I had had just enough time to say hello to my family. I had seen none of my old friends. I could stay at home for the rest of the summer. How I wanted to!

Summer school was beginning the next day. Another dream had been haunting me. If I went to summer school for two summers I might make up the year I was behind. I had just enough time to kiss my mother goodbye. That's the way with dreams that come true. One always leads to another.

There came a day when he was no longer permitted to record orally, then to transcribe into writing, and finally to correct his misspellings. The English assignment was to write, during class period, a short essay on one of three topics which the teacher wrote on the board—Pride, Courage, Honesty. The Boy wrote as follows:

Courage

Courage is not the absence of fear it's controll of fear. You can't put your finger on courage. Its a feeling that you have within you. Courage comes out in many forms. Its courage that helps you go on when you are trying to diagram a hard sentence in English. Its courage that makes you try to brake a record in track when the ods are agians you. Courage is also present in the battle field when a man gos after a wonded solger. So courage is every were but so is fear and there is a constint battel between them. At times fear wins the battel but thank God that courage wins the majority of them.

To the courageous boy and his parents this chapter is gratefully dedicated.

REFERENCES

ACLD Items of Interest. 1967. Newsbriefs on the child with learning disabilities. Tulsa, Association for Children with Learning Disabilities, November 16, 1967.

Blatz, W. 1944. Understanding the Young Child. New York, Morrow.

Brosin, H. W. 1957. The primary processes and psychoses. Behav. Sci., 2:62-67.

Bruner, J. S., R. R. Oliver, and P. M. Greenfield, 1967. Studies in Cognitive Growth. New York, John Wiley & Sons.

Chomsky, N. 1965. Aspects of the Theory of Syntax. Cambridge, Mass., The MIT Press.

Critchley, M. 1961. Inborn reading disorders of central origin. Trans. Ophthal. Soc. U.K., 81:459-480.

Cruickshank, W. M., F. A. Bentsen, F. H. Retzburg, and M. T. Tannhauser. 1961. A Teaching Method for Brain-Injured and Hyperactive Children. Syracuse, N. Y., Syracuse University Press.

Dager, E. Z. 1964. Socialization and personality development in the child. *In* Christenson, H. T., ed., Handbook of Marriage and the Family. Skokie, Ill., Rand McNally.

Davis, E. L. 1962. Teaching language skills to a neurologically deficient child with adequate intellect. Master's thesis, San Marcos, Texas, Southwest Texas State College.

Denhoff, E., and I. P. Robinault. 1960. Cerebral Palsy and Related Disorders; A Developmental Approach to Dysfunction. New York, McGraw-Hill.

Dunn, L. M. 1968. Special Education for the mildly retarded—is much of it justified? Except. Child., 35:5-22.

Ellingson, Careth. 1967. The Shadow Children. Chicago, Topaz Books.

English, S. O., and G. H. J. Pearson. 1955. Emotional Problems of Living. New York, W. W. Norton.

Ginott, H. G. 1967. Between Parent and Child. New York, Macmillan.

Goldstein, H., J. W. Moss, and L. J. Jordan, eds. 1965. The Efficacy of Special Education Training on the Development of Mentally Retarded Children. Urbana, Ill., University of Illinois Institute for Research on Exceptional Children.

Gruenberg, E. M. 1954. Epidemiology of mental disease. Sci. Amer., 190(18):38-42.

Hallgren, B. 1950. Specific dyslexia: A clinical and genetic study. Acta Psychiat. Scand. Suppl., 65:1-287.

Hirsch, Jerry. 1963. Behavior genetics and individuality understood. Science, 142:1436-1442.

Johnson, D. J., and H. R. Myklebust. 1967. Learning Disabilities. New York, Grune & Stratton.

Kaplan, L. 1959. Mental Health and Human Relations in Education. New York, Harper & Row.

Maher, B. A. 1963. Intelligence and brain damage. In Ellis, N. R., ed., Handbook of Mental Deficiency. New York, McGraw-Hill.

McCarthy, J. J., and S. A. Kirk. 1961. The Illinois Test of Psycholinguistic Abilities. Urbana, Ill., University of Illinois Press.

Menyuk, P. 1968. Theories of language acquisition and practices in therapy. ASHA, 10:200-201.

Meyerowitz, J. H. 1967. Peer groups and special classes. Ment. Retard. 5:23-26.

Orton, S. T. 1937. Reading, Writing, and Speech Problems in Children. New York, W. W. Norton.

Penrose, L. S. 1963. The Biology of Mental Defect. London, Sidgwick & Jackson.

Schuell, H., J. J. Jenkins, and E. Jimenez-Pabón. 1964. Aphasia in Adults. New York, Harper & Row.

Stark, Joel. 1966. Performance of aphasic children on the ITPA. Except. Child., 33:153-158.

Stephenson, S. 1907. Six cases of congenital word-blindness affecting three generations of one family. Ophthalmoscope, 5:482.

Strauss, A. A., and L. E. Lehtinen, 1947. Psychopathology and Education of the Brain-Injured Child. New York, Grune & Stratton.

Texas Education Agency. 1965. State Plan for Special Education. Austin, Texas Educational Assoc.

Texas Education Agency. 1970. State Plan for Special Education. Austin, Texas Education Agency.

Tikofsky, R. S. 1968. Discussion of Menyuk's paper. ASHA, 10:201-202.

Tkacev, R. 1948. [Cited by Solms, H., Beitrag zur kongenitalen Worblingheit. Mschr. Psychiat. Neurol., 115:1.]

Vandenberg, S. G. 1967. (Dept. of Pediatrics, University of Louisville Medical School, Louisville Twin Study, Louisville, Ky.) (Unpublished paper.)

Van Riper, C., and J. V. Irwin. 1958. Voice and Articulation. Englewood Cliffs, N. J., Prentice-Hall.

Wechsler, D. 1949. Wechsler Intelligence Scale for Children. New York, The Psychological Corp.

Williams, R. J. 1956. Biochemical Individuality. New York, John Wiley & Sons.

Zedler, E. Y. 1967. Conference charge. *In* Final Report, Research Conference on Dyslexia and Related Disorders in Schools of U. S. San Marcos, Texas, Southwest Texas State College.

―――1968b. Screening underachieving pupils for risk of neurological impairment. *In* Hellmuth, J., ed., Learning Disorders, Vol. 3. Seattle, Special Child Publications.

―――1970a. Educational programming for pupils with neurologically based language disorders. J. Learning Dis., 3:618-628.

Zerbin-Rüdin, E. 1967. Congenital word-blindness. *In* Becker, P. E., ed., Homangenetik, Vol. 2. Stuttgart, Georg Thieme Verlag.

Zigler, E. 1964. Mental retardation: current issues and approaches. *In* Hoffman, M. L., and L. W. Hoffman, eds., Review of Child Development Research. New York, Russell Sage Foundation.

―――1967. Familial mental retardation: a continuing dilemma. Science, 155:292-298.

―――and S. Harter. 1968. Socialization of the mentally retarded. *In* Goslin, D. A., and D. C., Glass, eds., Handbook of Socialization Theory and Research. Skokie, Ill., Rand McNally.

Index